Recent Advances in

Orthopaedics 4

Recent Advances in

Orthopaedics 4

Gregg R Klein MD
Vice-Chairman
Department of Orthopaedic Surgery
Hackensack University Medical Center
Associate Professor
Department of Orthopaedic Surgery
Hackensack Meridian School of Medicine
Rothman Orthopaedic Institute
Montvale, NJ, USA

P Maxwell Courtney MD
Assistant Professor
Department of Orthopaedic Surgery
Rothman Institute
Thomas Jefferson University
Woodbury, NJ, USA

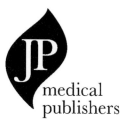

JP
medical
publishers

London • New Delhi

© 2022 Jaypee Brothers Medical Publishers

Published by Jaypee Brothers Medical Publishers,
4838/24 Ansari Road, New Delhi, India

Tel: +91 (011) 43574357   Fax: +91 (011)43574390

Email: info@jpmedpub.com, jaypee@jaypeebrothers.com
Web: www.jpmedpub.com, www.jaypeebrothers.com

JPM is the imprint of Jaypee Brothers Medical Publishers.

The rights of Gregg R Klein and P Maxwell Courtney to be identified as the editors of this work have been asserted by them in accordance with the Copyright, Designs and Patents Act 1988.

ISBN: 978-1-78779-174-9

British Library Cataloguing in Publication Data
A catalogue record for this book is available from the British Library

Library of Congress Cataloging in Publication Data
A catalog record for this book is available from the Library of Congress

Development Editor: Nikita Chauhan
Editorial Assistant: Keshav Kumar
Cover Design: Seema Dogra

Preface

Recent Advances in Orthopaedics 4 is intended to serve as a practical source for "Orthopaedic surgeons", students, residents and fellows. It is a detailed overview of the newest information in the field of "Orthopaedics", arranged by sub-specialty.

We have sought to provide the reader with an informed perspective on the most pertinent "hot topics" in our field, written by renowned thought leaders. This edition is focussed on "What is new in…". Topics cover the majority of sub-specialties in "Orthopaedic Surgery" including: spine, hip preservation, hip and knee arthroplasty, sports medicine, shoulder and elbow, foot and ankle, hand and wrist, oncology, trauma, and a section about COVID-19. We are excited to have contributions from internationally renowned surgeons in Europe, Asia, and South America. This lends to a truly international perspective to this work and informs the readers of similarities and differences from different parts of the world.

It is our sincerest hope that *Recent Advances in Orthopaedics 4* will serve as a compendium of the newest advances in adult reconstruction. We hope that you will find this to be a unique, practical source for the latest information as you care for your patients.

Gregg R Klein
P Maxwell Courtney
May, 2022

Contents

Acknowledgements

We would like to express our sincere appreciation to the talented contributors to *Recent Advances in Orthopaedics 4*, without whom this wonderful work would not have been possible.

Chapter 1

What is new in spine surgery?

Zachary T Grace, John D Koerner

TRENDS IN SURGICAL TREATMENT

With advances in techniques and technology as well as an ageing population, the rate of spine surgery continues to increase, particularly for lumbar spine pathology. In an analysis of the National Inpatient Sample (NIS) in the United States (US) from 2004 to 2015, Martin et al found the number of elective lumbar fusion cases to increase by 62.3% (122,769 cases in 2004 to 199,140 in 2015), with the highest increase in patients >65 years of age [1]. The largest increases in fusion in the US for this time period were seen for the indications of spondylolisthesis and scoliosis [1], but the accuracy of diagnosis codes in the NIS given for lumbar fusion procedures is questionable [2]. Another study using the same database found an increasing number of lumbar fusion procedures among octogenarians from 2004 to 2013, but the length of hospital stay decreased (from 6 to 4.5 days) with increases in hospital charges [3]. There are also fewer isolated decompressions being done. The percentage of patients with lumbar spinal stenosis undergoing decompression alone decreased from 47.5 to 34.6% from 2010 to 2014 in the NIS database, with increases in both simple fusions (35.3–47.2%) and complex fusions (>3 vertebrae or 360°) (5.7 to 7.1%) [4]. These findings of an increasing number of fusions in an older population are consistent around the world. A database analysis from Japan between 2004 and 2015 found a 1.9 times increase in the total number of spine surgeries, with patients in their 70s being the most popular age group [5].

These findings of fewer decompressions and more fusions are not limited to the elderly. For patients with continuous 12-month insurance coverage aged 40–64 years between 2010 and 2014, the proportion of patients with lumbar stenosis undergoing decompression alone decreased linearly. The rates of complex arthrodesis also increased significantly each year, along with increased complications and higher costs [6]. There are also significant regional differences in the rates of arthrodesis, being more commonly performed in the South (48%), the Midwest (42%), versus the Northeast (36%) and the West (31%) [7].

The rate of cervical spine surgery has actually decreased slightly over the course of 2001–2013 (75.34 to 72.20 per 100,000 adults) [8] (**Figure 1.1**). However, the total number of fusion procedures still increased when looking at cervical spondylotic myelopathy (CSM)

Zachary T Grace BS, Hackensack Meridian School of Medicine, Nutley, New Jersey, US
Email: zachary.grace@hmhn.org

John D Koerner MD, Rothman Orthopaedic Institute, Paramus, New Jersey, US
Email: john.koerner@rothmanortho.com

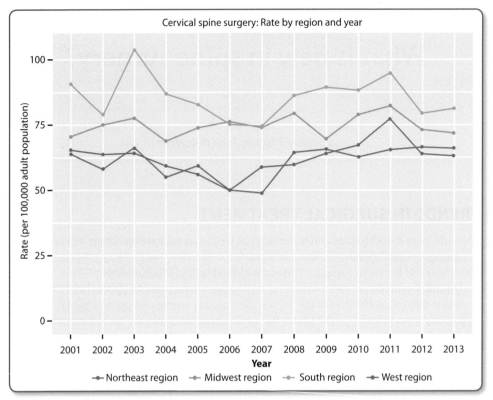

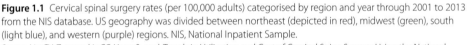

Figure 1.1 Cervical spinal surgery rates (per 100,000 adults) categorised by region and year through 2001 to 2013 from the NIS database. US geography was divided between northeast (depicted in red), midwest (green), south (light blue), and western (purple) regions. NIS, National Inpatient Sample.
Source: Liu CY, Zygourakis CC, Yoon S, et al. Trends in Utilization and Cost of Cervical Spine Surgery Using the National Inpatient Sample Database, 2001 to 2013. Spine (Phila Pa 1976) 2017; 42:E906–E913.

(3,879–8,181 from 2003 to 2013), with slight increase in the average age (58.2–60.6 years), and significant increases in hospital charges [\$49,445 to \$92,040 ($p < 0.001$)] [9]. Trends in surgical treatment for single-level cervical radiculopathy have changed recently. Based on data from the National Surgical Quality Improvement Program (NSQIP) database from 2010 to 2016, there was an increase in the percentage of cervical disc replacement (7.7–16.1%), with a decrease in posterior cervical foraminotomy (20.3–10.6%), and relatively stable rate of anterior cervical discectomy and fusion (ACDF) procedures (72.0–73.3%) [10].

ROBOTICS

Robot-assisted spine surgery has become increasingly popular over the past several years. Pedicle screw placement by free hand or fluoroscopic guidance is relatively safe, but still has a risk of misplacement which can lead to neurologic or vascular injury, dural tear, or inadequate fixation. The accuracy of free hand versus robot-assisted pedicle screw placement has been evaluated by many studies and numerous robotic platforms. A meta-analysis of ten articles demonstrated significantly greater accuracy with the robot-assisted group compared to free hand with fluoroscopic guidance (odds ratio 95%, "perfect accuracy" confidence interval 1.38–2.07, $p < 0.01$; odds ratio 95% "clinically acceptable" confidence interval: 1.17–2.08, $p < 0.01$) [11]. This analysis only included studies with postoperative computed tomography (CT), and had two separate accuracy measurements: perfect accuracy (completely within the pedicle) and clinical acceptance (<3 mm of screw outside the pedicle without complication). In addition to the potential benefit of accuracy within the pedicle, there may be a decreased rate of proximal facet violation when using robotic assistance. In a randomised control trial of minimally invasive posterior lumbar interbody fusion (MIS-PLIF) comparing the Mazor robot with freehand technique, there were no proximal joint violations when using the robot (74 screws), but 13/82 (15.9%) in the freehand technique [12].

The ROSA robot (Medtech) uses an intraoperative O-arm (Medtronic Inc.) to produce a 3D reconstruction. The Globus Medical Excelsius GPS (Globus Medical, Audobon, PA) system uses similar techniques requiring a pre-operative CT, but uses a rigid arm without the need for k-wire placement, and provides real-time feedback (**Figure 1.2**). One study evaluating the first 54 cases performed using this system demonstrated a 98.3% accuracy with minimal offset from the pre-operative plan and no complications [13]. These platforms are gaining popularity but cost may be a limiting factor to widespread use.

SPINAL CORD INJURY TRIALS

There have been two recent clinical trials for acute spinal cord injury (SCI), evaluating the Rho inhibitor VX-210 and Riluzole. The enzyme Rho is activated after SCI during the secondary inflammatory phase. This enzyme can inhibit axonal regeneration and, therefore, an investigational agent VX-210 which inhibits Rho was the focus of a clinical trial of SCI [14]. The initial phase 1/2a safety trial included 48 patients with acute SCI with an American Spinal Injury Association Impairment Scale (AIS) grade A undergoing surgery where a single dose of VX-210 was applied to the dura mater [15]. Initial results were promising with improvement in motor strength in patients with cervical SCI. The phase 2b/3 Spinal Cord Injury Rho Inhibition Investigation (SPRING) trial then investigated the safety and efficacy of VX-210 treatment [14] (**Figure 1.3**). Unfortunately, the interim analysis failed to demonstrate efficacy and the trial was terminated.

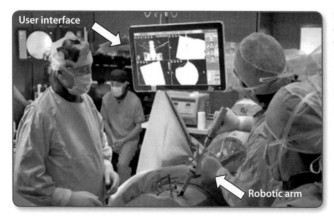

Figure 1.2 Intraoperative utilisation of the Globus Medical Excelsius GPS (Globus Medical, Audobon PA) system. Arrows depicting robotic arm assistance with 4-panel interactive user interface for real-time feedback. With permission from Benech CA, et al. (2019)

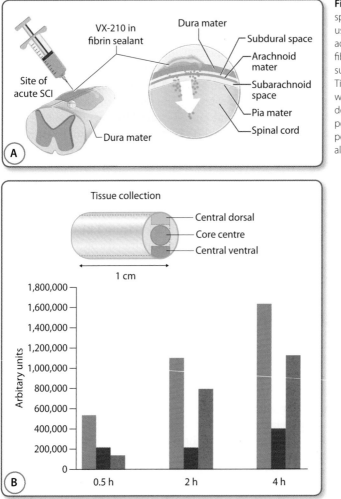

Figure 1.3 Depiction of acute spinal cord injury (SCI) treatment using VX-210. (A) Topical administration of VX-210 in a fibrin sealant to the extradural surface of the spinal cord. (B) Time-sensitive gradient levels were measured to assess 1-mg dose of VX-210 penetration in a post-mortem pig model. With permission from Fehlings MG, et al. (2018)

Riluzole, a sodium channel-blocking agent, demonstrated safety and possible efficacy for treatment of acute SCI in a phase I trial, and the subsequent phase IIB/III double-blinded randomised controlled trial [Riluzole in Acute Spinal Cord Injury Study (RISCIS)] is ongoing [16]. Currently, no results are available.

Numerous trials evaluating stem cell treatment for chronic SCI have been completed with significant variability in results [17]. One acute-phase trial used allogenic umbilical cord-derived mesenchymal stem cells (MSCs) within 24 hours of injury and found recovery of two patients from American Spinal Cord Injury Association (ASIA) A to ASIA C [18]. However, there is significant variability in the types of cells, methods, and timing of implantation to make any definitive conclusions at this time.

The use of steroids for acute SCI is still controversial, and popularity today has decreased. However, a systematic review on the use of methylprednisolone sodium succinate for the treatment of acute SCI led to the creation of three suggested guidelines: (1) do not offer steroids to adult SCI patients presenting after 8 hours; (2) offer patients presenting within 8 hours of acute SCI steroids as a treatment for 24 hours; and (3) do not offer a 48 hour infusion of steroids [19]. It is important to note that these are "suggestions" only, and are not strong recommendations.

SPINAL CORD INJURY: PRECLINICAL

There are numerous preclinical studies evaluating methods of treatment for acute SCI. Electrical stimulation has been evaluated in animal models as a treatment for SCI. In a rat SCI model, epidural electrical stimulation stimulated the Wnt signalling pathway and increased brain-derived neurotrophic factor (BDNF) and fatty-acid amide hydrolase (FAAH), which may help in recovery after SCI [20] (**Figures 1.4** and **1.5**). Electro-acupuncture also demonstrated benefits in reducing oxidative stress in a rat SCI model [21]. Other preclinical studies have evaluated the role of tumour necrosis factor-α-induced protein 8 (TNFAIP8) in SCI [22], selective agonists of the P2Y purinergic receptor [23], and proanthocyanidins (PACS) to inhibit ferroptosis in SCI and promote recovery [24], as well as ascorbic acid to promote axonal sprouting in SCI [25].

Mesenchymal stem cells have been studied for the treatment of neurodegenerative diseases [26]. The ideal timing of therapeutic treatment for SCI is still unknown. A rat study attempted to measure the chondroitin sulphate (CS) and dermatan sulphate (DS)

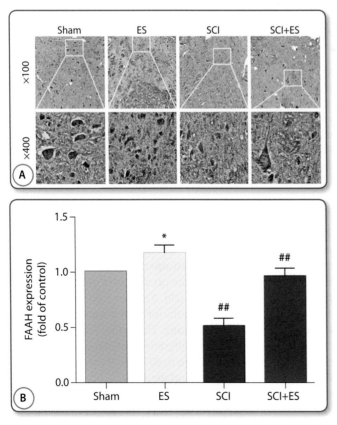

Figure 1.4 Electrical stimulation (ES) use on fatty-acid amide hydrolase (FAAH) expression in a rat model after spinal cord injury (SCI). (A) Immunohistochemical stain of FAAH among different groups. (B) FAAH expression levels among different groups.

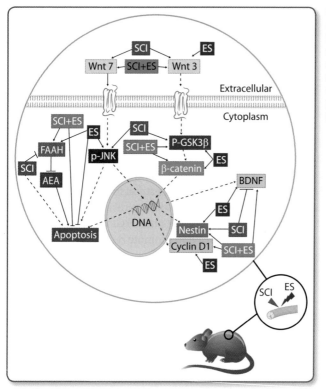

Figure 1.5 Summarisation of molecular and gene pathways involved and the effects of spinal cord injury (SCI) and electrical stimulation (ES). With permission from Ghorbani M, et al (2020) (FAAH, fatty-acid amid hydrolase; BDNF, brain-derived neurotrophic factor).

levels at different time periods in order to identify the ideal timing for intervention, and found higher levels of DS compared to CS starting at 2 weeks after SCI, which suggests that week 2 after SCI may be ideal [27]. Adipose-derived mesenchymal stem cell (ADSC) transplantation for SCI has been studied in several animal models. In a mouse SCI model, ADSCs were injected into the lesion site immediately after injury and were found to survive at least 28 days. Several pathways were studied resulting in decreases in proinflammatory cytokines and increased neuron survival [28].

PREDICTIVE ANALYTICS

Predictive modelling and machine-based learning have been applied to the field of spinal surgery to predict outcomes post-operatively. One such framework called "SpineCloud" used perioperative imaging along with post-operative functional and pain outcomes to try to predict outcomes. By incorporating the preoperative demographics, there was significant improvement in prediction ability [29]. Another study attempted to predict outcomes, surgical parameters, and reoperations for patients undergoing decompression for lumbar stenosis using machine learning. The authors were able to predict patients achieving minimal clinical important difference (MCID) from 51 to 85% in various outcome measures, predict rate of reoperation in 63–69% of cases, predict with 78% accuracy cases that were prolonged surgery, and predict 77% of patients that required an extended hospital stay [30]. Machine learning can also be used to aid in medical decision making using electronic medical records [31]. These are promising technologies that may help physicians and patients to better understand peri-operative risks and post-operative outcomes.

DISC REPLACEMENT

Motion preservation techniques continue to gain momentum, but the number of fusion procedures still greatly outnumbers non-fusion procedures. Based on data from the NIS database from 2006 to 2013, approximately 132,000 ACDFs are performed each year versus only 1,600 cervical disc arthroplasties (CDAs), but the number of CDAs performed over that time period increased by 190% versus 5.7% for ACDF [32].

Longer follow-up studies are becoming available as well and have shown good results and durability. 10-year outcomes of the single-level Prestige LP cervical disc remained stable compared to the 7-year data, with patient satisfaction above 90% [33]. Additional benefits may be seen with disc replacement with multilevel procedures. The two-level Prestige LP cervical disc at 10 years also demonstrated a higher rate of overall success compared to ACDF (80.4% vs. 62.2%), as well as fewer secondary surgeries at adjacent levels (9.0% vs. 17.9%) [34]. Similarly, in the 7-year follow-up study for the Mobi-C Cervical Disc, the overall success analysis demonstrated clinical superiority of two-level disc replacement versus ACDF, and non-inferiority of single level [35] (**Figure 1.6**).

A meta-analysis of eleven randomised controlled trials of CDA versus ACDF with at least 4-year follow-up showed no difference in neurological improvement, but significantly greater improvement in Neck Disability Index (NDI) and Short Form 36 Health Survey physical component [36]. The authors also found a lower rate of secondary surgical procedures in the CDA group, but similar rates of adjacent segment degeneration. Another meta-analysis started to find differences of adjacent-level operation at 5 years favouring CDA for single level pathology, which was also evident at 7 years (4.3% vs. 10.8%) [37]. Similar findings were seen with two-level CDA at 7 years for adjacent-level operation (5.1% vs. 10.0%) (**Figure 1.7**).

A 10-year follow-up study of the Bryan CDA found significantly higher incidence of adjacent level ossification disease (ALOD) after ACDF compared to CDA (68.2% vs. 11.1%, $p = 0.0003$) but there were no significant differences in NDI, VAS-arm, or neck pain in high- versus low-grade ALOD. This suggests that ALOD is only a radiographic finding which does

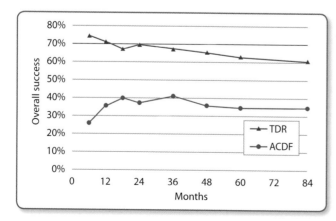

Figure 1.6 Overall treatment success of Mobi-C© cervical disc in two-level disc replacement versus anterior cervical discectomy and fusion (ACDF) surgery among 330 patients. TDR, total disc replacement. With permission from Radcliff K, et al (2017).

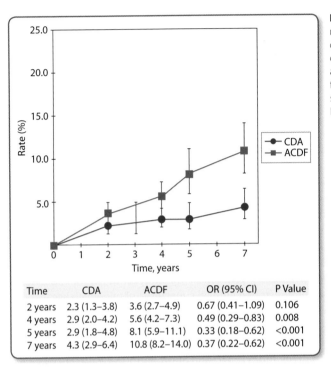

Figure 1.7 Data from nine randomised trials comparing rates of adjacent-level reoperation for cervical disc arthroplasty (CDA) with anterior cervical discectomy and fusion (ACDF) in one-level cervical spondylosis. With permission from Badhiwala JH, et al (2020).

Time	CDA	ACDF	OR (95% CI)	P Value
2 years	2.3 (1.3–3.8)	3.6 (2.7–4.9)	0.67 (0.41–1.09)	0.106
4 years	2.9 (2.0–4.2)	5.6 (4.2–7.3)	0.49 (0.29–0.83)	0.008
5 years	2.9 (1.8–4.8)	8.1 (5.9–11.1)	0.33 (0.18–0.62)	<0.001
7 years	4.3 (2.9–6.4)	10.8 (8.2–14.0)	0.37 (0.22–0.62)	<0.001

not affect outcomes [38]. Heterotopic ossification was also assessed at 10 years following Prestige LP cervical disc at the index levels. The authors found a 39% incidence of severe (grade 3 or 4) HO at 10 years, but no differences were found in outcomes compared to those with less severe or no HO (grades 0–2) [39].

BIOLOGICS FOR SPINAL FUSION

Biologics to enhance fusion rates continue to be developed. Platelet-rich plasma (PRP) is one augment that has been used extensively to enhance fusion rates; however, there is conflicting evidence on its efficacy. A recent meta-analysis of 11 studies and 741 patients actually found a higher fusion rate in patients treated without PRP, with no significant changes in VAS scores or estimated blood loss [40]. However, another meta-analysis of 14 studies found a higher fusion rate in the studies that used a high-platelet concentration compared to those that used a low concentrate [41]. One prospective randomised study of 50 patients found a significantly higher fusion rate (94% vs. 74%, $p = 0.002$) in patients undergoing one- or two-level posterolateral fusion (PLF) for lumbar spondylosis, as well as a greater fusion mass and faster time to fusion in those treated with PRP versus not [42]. Another meta-analysis of seven studies with patients undergoing posterior lumbar interbody fusion found no difference in fusion rate with PRP, but a shorter time to union (1.62 months) as well as lower back pain in those treated with PRP [43]. Another meta-analysis of 12 studies found no difference in fusion rate or pain levels with treatment of PRP [44]. There may be variability in the platelet concentration or technique that can explain the contradicting results from many of these studies.

Recombinant human bone morphogenetic protein-2 (rhBMP-2) continues to be a popular augment for spinal fusion procedures, but there is still concern for potential complications. A retrospective cohort study of 191 patients undergoing transforaminal lumbar interbody fusion (TLIF) showed high fusion rates with or without the use of rhBMP-2 (92.7% vs. 92.3%), with a slightly higher rate of seroma and radiculitis in the rhBMP-2 group [45]. The optimal dosage of rhBMP-2 is still unknown for posterior lumbar procedures. In a systematic review and meta-analysis of 22 articles and 2,729 patients undergoing PLIF or TLIF, the fusion and complication rates were not different between different dosages of rhBMP-2, and the minimally effective dose was found to be as low as 1.28 mg/level [46].

Allogeneic cellular bone grafts have also become more popular with varying degrees of clinical efficacy. One retrospective study from 150 consecutive patients undergoing posterolateral lumbar fusion found a successful fusion rate of 98.7% based on radiographs with Vivigen allograft (Lifenet Health) [47]. Osteocel (Nuvasive, San Diego, CA), Trinity Evolution (Orthofix, Lewisville, TX), and Bio4 (Stryker, Kalamazoo, MI) are allograft tissue products that contain live stem cells and have shown success in several studies [48]. However, the cost associated with these products can be substantial, and further evidence is needed before widespread acceptance.

DISC DEGENERATION TREATMENT

Intervertebral disc (IVD) degeneration continues to be a widely studied topic with numerous approaches. IVD degeneration is known to be at least partially due to an increase in cytokines and matrix metalloproteases, which is mediated by the nuclear factor kappa B (NF-kB) pathway. In a study of discarded human lumbar discs and rat discs, the NF-kB inhibitor NEMOE-binding domain peptide was found to reduce interleukin-1β (IL-1β) and matrix metalloprotease levels, increase cell viability, and downregulate IL-6 [49]. This may represent a potential target to prevent and treat disc degeneration.

Mesenchymal stem cells have also been evaluated for the treatment of IVD degeneration, but it is still unclear as what the exact mechanism. One study demonstrated a paracrine effect of MSCs, and not ECM remodelling in a disc degeneration model [50]. Growth factors have also been studied as a potential treatment to prevent or reverse degeneration of discs. The growth differentiation factor (GDF) family has been shown to promote disc regeneration by upregulating healthy cell marker genes in degenerated discs and by MSC induction to nucleus pulposus cells [51].

Autologous PRP has also been studied for chronic discogenic back pain. In one laboratory study, human bone marrow-derived mesenchymal stem cells (hMSCs) with leucocyte-poor PRP, enhanced hMSC proliferation, and hyaluronic acid production compared to leucocyte-rich PRP [52] (**Figures 1.8** and **1.9**).

SPINE REGISTRIES

The American Spine Registry and the North American Spine Society (NASS) Registry have both been established to improve patient outcomes. The American Spine Registry is a collaboration of the American Association of Neurological Surgeons (AANS) and the American Academy of Orthopaedic Surgeons (AAOS), and will incorporate the Quality Outcomes Database Spine Registry. The key distinction between the two registries is that

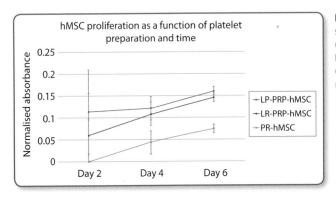

Figure 1.8 Human mesenchymal stem cell (hMSC) proliferation using normalised absorbance of PrestoBlue 570-nm across 6 days. (LP, leucocyte poor; LR, leucocyte rich; PRP, platelet-rich plasma).

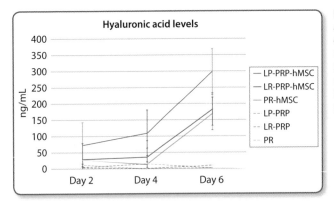

Figure 1.9 Hyaluronic acid levels among platelet preparation across 6 days. With permission from Dregalla RC, et al (2020). (LP, leucocyte poor; LR, leucocyte rich, PRP, platelet-rich plasma; hMSC, human mesenchymal stem cell, PR, platelet rich).

the American Spine Registry is procedural based and the NASS Registry is diagnosis based. Both registries will allow providers to compare their results to others within the registry.

NORTH AMERICAN SPINE SOCIETY GUIDELINES

The NASS publishes evidenced-based clinical guidelines on topics that are important to clinicians and can be found on their website (https://www.spine.org/Research-Clinical-Care/Quality-Improvement/Clinical-Guidelines). Previous guidelines have included antithrombotic therapies in spine surgery, diagnosis, and treatment of cervical radiculopathy from degenerative disorders, diagnosis, and treatment of degenerative lumbar spine stenosis, diagnosis, and treatment of lumbar disc herniation with radiculopathy, diagnosis, and treatment of degenerative spondylolisthesis, diagnosis, and treatment of adult isthmic spondylolisthesis. The most recent guideline is on the diagnosis and treatment of low back pain. The guidelines address several questions regarding low back pain including the diagnosis, imaging, medical and psychological treatment, physical medicine and rehabilitation, interventional treatment, surgical treatment, and cost utility. Several additional topics are under development including the diagnosis and treatment of neoplastic vertebral fractures in adults, diagnosis and treatment of osteoporotic vertebral compression fractures in adults, and a revision to the anti-thrombotic therapies in spine surgery.

REFERENCES

1. Martin BI, Mirza SK, Spina N, et al. Trends in lumbar fusion procedure rates and associated hospital costs for degenerative spinal diseases in the United States, 2004 to 2015. Spine (Phila Pa 1976) 2019; 44:369–376.
2. Gologorsky Y, Knightly JJ, Chi JH, et al. The nationwide inpatient sample database does not accurately reflect surgical indications for fusion. J Neurosurg Spine 2014; 21:984–993.
3. Kha ST, Ilyas H, Tanenbaum JE, et al. Trends in lumbar fusion surgery among octogenarians: a nationwide inpatient sample study from 2004 to 2013. Glob Spine J 2018; 8:593–599.
4. Al Jammal OM, Delavar A, Maguire KR, et al. National trends in the surgical management of lumbar spinal stenosis in adult spinal deformity patients. Spine (Phila Pa 1976) 2019; 44:E1369–E1378.
5. Kobayashi K, Ando K, Nishida Y, et al. Epidemiological trends in spine surgery over 10 years in a multicenter database. Eur Spine J 2018; 27:1698–1703.
6. Raad M, Donaldson CJ, El Dafrawy MH, et al. Trends in isolated lumbar spinal stenosis surgery among working US adults aged 40-64 years, 2010-2014. J Neurosurg Spine 2018; 29:169–175.
7. Raad M, Reidler JS, El Dafrawy MH, et al. US regional variations in rates, outcomes, and costs of spinal arthrodesis for lumbar spinal stenosis in working adults aged 40–65 years. J Neurosurg Spine 2019; 30:83–90.
8. Liu CY, Zygourakis CC, Yoon S, et al. Trends in utilization and cost of cervical spine surgery using the national inpatient sample database, 2001 to 2013. Spine (Phila Pa 1976) 2017; 42:E906–E913.
9. Vonck CE, Tanenbaum JE, Smith GA, et al. National trends in demographics and outcomes following cervical fusion for cervical spondylotic myelopathy. Glob Spine J 2018; 8:244–253.
10. Mok JK, Sheha ED, Samuel AM, et al. Evaluation of current trends in treatment of single-level cervical radiculopathy. Clin Spine Surg 2019; 32:E241–E245.
11. Fan Y, Du JP, Liu JJ, et al. Accuracy of pedicle screw placement comparing robot-Assisted technology and the free-hand with fluoroscopy-guided method in spine surgery. Medicine (United States) 2018; 97:e10970.
12. Kim HJ, Jung WI, Chang BS, et al. A prospective, randomized, controlled trial of robot-assisted vs freehand pedicle screw fixation in spine surgery. Int J Med Robot Comput Assist Surg 2017; 97:e10970.
13. Benech CA, Perez R, Benech F, et al. Navigated robotic assistance results in improved screw accuracy and positive clinical outcomes: an evaluation of the first 54 cases. J Robot Surg 2019; 14:431–437.
14. Fehlings MG, Kim KD, Aarabi B, et al. Rho inhibitor VX-210 in Acute Traumatic Subaxial Cervical Spinal Cord Injury: Design of the SPinal Cord Injury Rho INhibition InvestiGation (SPRING) Clinical Trial. J Neurotrauma 2018; 35:1049–1056.
15. Fehlings MG, Theodore N, Harrop J, et al. A phase I/IIa clinical trial of a recombinant Rho protein antagonist in acute spinal cord injury. J Neurotrauma 2011; 28:787–796.
16. Fehlings MG, Nakashima H, Nagoshi N, et al. Rationale, design and critical end points for the Riluzole in Acute Spinal Cord Injury Study (RISCIS): A randomized, double-blinded, placebo-controlled parallel multi-center trial. Spinal Cord 2016; 54:8–15.
17. Yamazaki K, Kawabori M, Seki T, et al. Clinical trials of stem cell treatment for spinal cord injury. Int J Mol Sci 2020; 21:3994.
18. Xiao Z, Tang F, Zhao Y, et al. Significant Improvement of Acute Complete Spinal Cord Injury Patients Diagnosed by a Combined Criteria Implanted with NeuroRegen Scaffolds and Mesenchymal Stem Cells. Cell Transplant 2018; 27:907–915.
19. Fehlings MG, Wilson JR, Tetreault LA, et al. A Clinical Practice Guideline for the Management of Patients With Acute Spinal Cord Injury: Recommendations on the Use of Methylprednisolone Sodium Succinate. Glob Spine J 2017; 7:203S–211S.
20. Ghorbani M, Shahabi P, Karimi P, et al. Impacts of epidural electrical stimulation on Wnt signaling, FAAH, and BDNF following thoracic spinal cord injury in rat. J Cell Physiol 2020; 235:9795–9805.
21. Cheng M, Wu X, Wang F, et al. Electro-Acupuncture Inhibits p66Shc-Mediated Oxidative Stress to Facilitate Functional Recovery After Spinal Cord Injury. J Mol Neurosci 2020; 70:2031–2040.
22. Xue W, Tan W, Dong L, et al. TNFAIP8 influences the motor function in mice after spinal cord injury (SCI) through mediating inflammation dependent on AKT. Biochem Biophys Res Commun 2020; 528:234–241.
23. Zhao Z, Hu X, Wu Z, et al. A Selective P2Y Purinergic Receptor Agonist 2-MesADP Enhances Locomotor Recovery after Acute Spinal Cord Injury. Eur Neurol 2020; 83:195–212.
24. Zhou H, Yin C, Zhang Z, et al. Proanthocyanidin promotes functional recovery of spinal cord injury via inhibiting ferroptosis. J Chem Neuroanat 2020; 107:101807.

25. Hong JY, Davaa G, Yoo H, et al. Ascorbic acid promotes functional restoration after spinal cord injury partly by epigenetic modulation. Cells 2020; 9:1310.

26. Reyhani S, Abbaspanah B, Mousavi SH. Umbilical cord-derived mesenchymal stem cells in neurodegenerative disorders: from literature to clinical practice. Regen Med 2020; 15:1561–1578.

27. Rezaei S, Bakhtiyari S, Assadollahi K, et al. Evaluating chondroitin sulfate and dermatan sulfate expression in glial scar to determine appropriate intervention time in rats. Basic Clin Neurosci 2020; 11:31–40.

28. Zhou Z, Tian X, Mo B, et al. Adipose mesenchymal stem cell transplantation alleviates spinal cord injury-induced neuroinflammation partly by suppressing the Jagged1/Notch pathway. Stem Cell Res Ther 2020; 11:212.

29. De Silva T, Vedula SS, Perdomo-Pantoja A, et al. SpineCloud: image analytics for predictive modeling of spine surgery outcomes. J Med Imaging 2020; 7:031502.

30. Siccoli A, de Wispelaere MP, Schröder ML, et al. Machine learning-based preoperative predictive analytics for lumbar spinal stenosis. Neurosurg Focus 2019; 46:E5.

31. Schwartz JT, Gao M, Geng EA, et al. Applications of machine learning using electronic medical records in spine surgery. Neurospine 2019; 16:643–653.

32. Saifi C, Fein AW, Cazzulino A, et al. Trends in resource utilization and rate of cervical disc arthroplasty and anterior cervical discectomy and fusion throughout the United States from 2006 to 2013. Spine J 2018; 18:1022–1029.

33. Gornet MF, Burkus JK, Shaffrey ME, et al. Cervical disc arthroplasty: 10-year outcomes of the Prestige LP cervical disc at a single level. J Neurosurg Spine 2019; 31:317–325.

34. Gornet MF, Lanman TH, Kenneth Burkus J, et al. Two-level cervical disc arthroplasty versus anterior cervical discectomy and fusion: 10-year outcomes of a prospective, randomized investigational device exemption clinical trial. J Neurosurg Spine 2019; Online ahead of print.

35. Radcliff K, Davis RJ, Hisey MS, et al. Long-term evaluation of cervical disc arthroplasty with the Mobi-C© cervical disc: A randomized, prospective, multicenter clinical trial with seven-year follow-up. Int J Spine Surg 2017; 11:31.

36. Byvaltsev VA, Stepanov IA, Riew DK. Mid-term to long-term outcomes after total cervical disk arthroplasty compared with anterior diskectomy and fusion. Clin Spine Surg 2020; 33:192–200.

37. Badhiwala JH, Platt A, Witiw CD, et al. Cervical disc arthroplasty versus anterior cervical discectomy and fusion: a meta-analysis of rates of adjacent-level surgery to 7-year follow-up. J Spine Surg 2020; 6:217–232.

38. Boody BS, Lee EN, Sasso WR, et al. Functional outcomes associated with adjacent-level ossification disease 10 years after cervical disc arthroplasty or ACDF. Clin Spine Surg 2020; 33:E420–E425.

39. Gornet MF, Lanman TH, Burkus JK, et al. Occurrence and clinical implications of heterotopic ossification after cervical disc arthroplasty with the Prestige LP Cervical Disc at 2 contiguous levels. J Neurosurg Spine 2020; Online ahead of print.

40. Yolcu YU, Wahood W, Eissa AT, et al. The impact of platelet-rich plasma on postoperative outcomes after spinal fusion: a systematic review and meta-analysis. J Neurosurg Spine 2020; Online ahead of print.

41. Manini DR, Shega FD, Guo C, et al. Role of platelet-rich plasma in spinal fusion surgery: systematic review and meta-analysis. Adv Orthop 2020; 2020:8361798.

42. Kubota G, Kamoda H, Orita S, et al. Platelet-rich plasma enhances bone union in posterolateral lumbar fusion: A prospective randomized controlled trial. Spine J 2019; 19:e34–e40.

43. Pairuchvej S, Muljadi JA, Arirachakaran A, et al. Efficacy of platelet-rich plasma in posterior lumbar interbody fusion: systematic review and meta-analysis. Eur J Orthop Surg Traumatol 2020; 30:583–593.

44. Ji-jun H, Hui-hui S, Qing L, et al. Efficacy of using platelet-rich plasma in spinal fusion surgery—a preferred reporting items for systematic reviews and meta-analyses–compliant meta-analysis. World Neurosurg 2020; 30:583–593.

45. Khan TR, Pearce KR, McAnany SJ, et al. Comparison of transforaminal lumbar interbody fusion outcomes in patients receiving rhBMP-2 versus autograft. Spine J 2018; 18:439–446.

46. Lytle EJ, Lawless MH, Paik G, et al. The minimally effective dose of bone morphogenetic protein in posterior lumbar interbody fusion: a systematic review and meta-analysis. Spine J. 2020; 20:1286–1304.

47. Hall JF, McLean JB, Jones SM, et al. Multilevel instrumented posterolateral lumbar spine fusion with an allogeneic cellular bone graft. J Orthop Surg Res 2019; 14:372.

48. Shah VP, Hsu WK. Stem cells and spinal fusion. Neurosurg Clin N Am 2020; 31:65–72.

49. Glaeser JD, Salehi K, Kanim LEA, et al. NF-κB inhibitor, NEMO-binding domain peptide attenuates intervertebral disc degeneration. Spine J 2020; 20:1480–1491.

50. Teixeira GQ, Pereira CL, Ferreira JR, et al. Immomodulation of human mesenchymal stem/stromal cells in intervertebral disc degeneration insights from a proinflammatory/degenerative ex vivo model. Spine (Phila Pa 1976) 2018; 43:E673–E682.
51. Hodgkinson T, Shen B, Diwan A, et al. Therapeutic potential of growth differentiation factors in the treatment of degenerative disc diseases. JOR Spine 2019; 2:e1045.
52. Dregalla RC, Uribe Y, Bodor M. Human mesenchymal stem cells respond differentially to platelet preparations and synthesize hyaluronic acid in nucleus pulposus extracellular matrix. Spine J 2020; 20:1850–1860.

Chapter 2

Hip preservation: An evidence-based update

Robert L Parisien, Joshua S Hornstein

INTRODUCTION

Over the course of the last two decades, there has been a rapidly expanding understanding of the spectrum of hip pathomorphology and the surgical treatment thereof. In addition to open surgical options, advances in arthroscopic skill and techniques have expanded the surgeon population attempting to understand and manage these disorders. In this review, we provide an update on recent evidence and clinical implications of hip preservation surgery for the management of young adult hip pathomorphology including hip dysplasia, intra-articular and extra-articular hip impingement, as well as the sequelae of paediatric hip disease.

DYSPLASIA

Dysplasia of the hip joint typically manifests as decreased anterior and lateral coverage of the femoral head. Radiographic parameters consistent with dysplasia include a lateral centre edge angle (LCEA) <20°, anterior centre edge angle (ACEA) <20°, sharp angle >45°, and Tönnis angle >10° [1]. Since its introduction >20 years ago, the Bernese periacetabular osteotomy (PAO) has been adopted as the preferred contemporary surgical treatment in adults with symptomatic hip dysplasia and without signs of osteoarthritis (OA). The surgical goals of PAO include pain relief and improved function and quality of life while preventing or delaying secondary development of OA. As such, we have seen a nearly four-fold increase in the number of operations completed in the adult population since 2005. Advantages of this osteotomy include maintenance of the blood supply to the articular fragment and an intact posterior column providing construct stability, thus allowing early patient mobilisation. Furthermore, the PAO technique enables acetabular reorientation such that both anterior and lateral coverage can be achieved. By normalising acetabular coverage, the PAO technique may decrease femoroacetabular chondral and labral contact stress, which may delay the onset of hip OA [2]. In evaluation of return to play (RTP) in 46 patients with a mean age of 26 years

Robert L Parisien MD, Orthopaedic Surgery and Sports Medicine, Icahn School of Medicine at Mount Sinai, New York City, New York, USA
Email: Robert.Parisien@MountSinai.org

Joshua S Hornstein MD, Orthopaedic Surgery and Sports medicine, Rothman Institute, Bordentown Township, NJ, USA
Email: Joshua.Hornstein@RothmanOrtho.com

following PAO, Heyworth et al reported RTP in 80% of patients at a median of 9 months with 73% successfully returning to the same level of competition [3]. Abraham et al [4] and Knight et al [5] emphasise the need for longer follow-up using biomechanical analysis to better understand the role of PAO in preventing OA. Troelson et al [6] reported hip joint survival rates of 81.6% at 9.2 years. Negative predictive factors included age >45 years, preoperative LCEA < 0°, post-operative LCEA <30°, or >40°, pre- or post-operative joint space <3 mm, pre-operative Tönnis OA grade ≥II, and pre-operative os acetabuli. Steppacher et al [7] reported the long-term results of 68 hips followed for a minimum of 19 years. At 20 years, there was a one-grade difference in Tönnis OA grade with a 60.5% hip survival rate and consistently good patient-reported outcomes (PROs). Factors predictive of poor surgical outcomes include age >30 years, patients with preoperative Merle d'Aubgné and Postel scores of 14 or less and those with preoperative Tönnis OA grade of 2 or more. As a complement to radiographic Tönnis grading, Cunningham et al [8] found the delayed gadolinium-enhanced magnetic resonance image of cartilage (dGEMRIC) index to be the most important predictor of failure of PAO surgery. Their follow-up study identified anterior dome cartilage as the most important factor contributing to survivorship. In evaluation of 75 hips treated with PAO, Lerch et al [9] identified that 33% reported good clinical results, no progression of OA, and no conversion to total hip arthroplasty (THA) at 30-year follow-up. Negative prognostic indicators included age at surgery > 40 years, pre-operative impingement signs or limited range of motion (specifically IR < 20), Tönnis grade > I, postoperative acetabular retroversion, and low preoperative PROs.

Addressing intra-articular pathology at the time of PAO

Periacetabular osteotomy is performed to restore the normal acetabular coverage of the femoral head. The reorientation of the acetabulum, however, may create iatrogenic femoroacetabular impingement (FAI) [10]. Additionally, pre-existing chondrolabral lesions can cause symptoms that mitigate the clinical success of PAO. As such, arthrotomy and arthroscopy prior to performance of a PAO may be utilised to address intra-articular chondrolabral lesions. Redmond et al [11] performed a recent systematic review of eight articles (775 patients) and reported a substantial presence of chondrolabral injuries at the time of PAO with arthroscopy able to more accurately identify such lesions as compared to arthrotomy. Furthermore, Ginnetti et al [12] reported on a retrospective series of 151 patients who underwent PAO and hip arthrotomy and compared the outcome to 39 patients who underwent PAO alone. A decreased head–neck offset was identified and corrected with femoral osteochondroplasty in 85% of patients but the effect on survivorship and symptomatology was not well understood. Literature on this topic continues to present controversy with differing outcomes among studies. Kain et al [13] performed an interesting analysis in which they sought to determine the effectiveness of PAO follow failed hip arthroscopy for labral pathology in dysplastic patients. The authors identified no difference in PROs in those patients undergoing a PAO following prior failed hip arthroscopy as compared to those undergoing primary PAO without previous arthroscopy. Therefore, PAO may be a reasonable treatment option for hip joint preservation following failed arthroscopic labral debridement. Thus, in 2020, there remain differing approaches for the management of intra-articular pathology at the time of PAO.

Periacetabular osteotomy for acetabular retroversion

Patients with significant acetabular retroversion often have anterior overcoverage and deficient posterior wall coverage evident via the radiographic cross-over sign. The PAO allows reorientation of the acetabular surface relative to the femoral head relieving abnormal anterior impingement and restoring normal posterior coverage. Siebenrock et al [14] reported on a series of 29 hips (22 patients) that underwent an anteversion-producing PAO. At a minimum follow-up of 2 years, 26 of 29 hips experienced good or excellent results. Peters et al [15] reported the results of reverse PAO for acetabular retroversion in 30 patients and found significantly improved clinical outcomes (based on Harris hip scores) and 28 of 30 hips experienced good or excellent outcomes.

Borderline dysplasia and the role of arthroscopy

In the setting of borderline hip dysplasia (BHD) (LCEA, 20–25°), the labrum may hypertrophy in response to increased load and subsequently assume a more important role as a weight-bearing surface in addition to providing a greater contribution to joint stability. Decreasing acetabular coverage leads to greater joint reaction forces imparted on the labrum, raising the risk for developing labral tears, degeneration, and detachment. Additionally, the reduced acetabular articular surface results in increased contact pressure, which may result in articular cartilage degeneration.

An early series by Byrd et al [16] of 48 hips having undergone hip arthroscopy for either symptomatic dysplasia or BHD identified an improvement in the modified Harris hip score (mHHS) with no difference noted in outcomes between dysplastic and borderline dysplastic hips. An additional evaluation by Hwang et al [17] analysed the utility of arthroscopy in patients with symptomatic BHD. A total of 162 patients having undergone arthroscopy for labral pathology were included. The authors found no difference in lateral labral thickness between the dysplastic group as compared to non-dysplastic controls. At a mean follow-up of 87 months, patients reported increased clinical outcome scores without demonstration of increased rates of OA, thus supporting hip arthroscopy for BHD. Similarly, a recent study by Beck et al [18] evaluated clinical outcomes of patients who underwent hip arthroscopy for BHD. Compared to matched-controls with adequate acetabular coverage, patients with BHD demonstrated no significant difference in clinical success at 5-year follow-up. With regards to revision arthroscopy, a recent analysis compared revision hip arthroscopy in patients with BHD with both primary arthroscopy in patients with BHD and revision hip arthroscopy in patients without BHD [19]. The authors reported that BHD patients having undergone revision arthroscopy demonstrated clinical improvement but were less likely to achieve PASS metrics for several PROs as compared to the BHD primary and non-BHD revision group. Furthermore, Cvetanovich et al [20] reported on arthroscopic treatment of FAI hips with BHD and compared them to a matched group of non-dysplastic hips with FAI. The authors reported no difference at minimum 2-year follow-up in hip outcome score activities of daily living (HOS-ADL), percentage of patients demonstrating clinical improvement, and those requiring subsequent surgery. While PAO remains the optimal treatment for acetabular dysplasia, debate remains in the literature regarding the appropriate intervention for BHD with concomitant intra-articular pathology. In a recent study comparing dysplastic hips managed via PAO alone or arthroscopy with subsequent PAO, a statistically significant difference in mHHS, HOS, and international hip outcome tool (iHOT) scores was realised at 1 year [21]. Fujii et al [22] further reported on 121 hips having undergone a combined PAO and arthroscopy at the index procedure. Arthroscopic findings of exposed subchondral bone and full-thickness labral tears and pre- and post-operative joint incongruity were strongly correlated to OA progression with unsatisfactory clinical scores at a mean follow-up of 9.9 years.

FEMOROACETABULAR IMPINGEMENT

Femoroacetabular impingement can be found in a number of patterns: Cam, Pincer, and mixed Cam–Pincer type FAI. Other unusual sources of intra-articular impingement may also be found (psoas tendon or ligamentum teres), and more recently emphasis has also been placed on identification and treatment of extra-articular sources of symptomatic impingement.

Intra-articular femoroacetabular impingement

Classic FAI is an osseous pathomorphologic variant predisposing the joint to potentially symptomatic intra-articular pathology, specifically labral tears and chondral lesions that lead to early hip arthritis and need for THA [23]. In Cam-type FAI, impingement most commonly occurs with hip flexion and internal rotation when an aspherical portion of the femoral head enters the acetabulum causing increased shear forces to the acetabular chondrolabral margin (**Figures 2.1** and **2.2**) [24] The impingement often occurs at the anterolateral acetabulum and frequently spares the capsular margin of labrum until late in the disease process. Cam-type FAI has been shown to produce a characteristic chondral injury, hyaline cartilage delamination, at the area of impingement, which can adversely affect surgical treatment outcome and complicate surgical decision making.

Pincer-type FAI is an acetabular-based pathomorphology where the acetabular rim and labrum impact the femoral neck or head-neck junction (**Figure 2.3**). This impingement mechanism may lead to labral attenuation, gradual ossification, and over time, the potential for posterior joint damage (contrecoup injury pattern) due to shear forces as the hip levers at the anterior neck–rim contact [24]. Pincer-type FAI can arise from acetabular retroversion, focal or global acetabular overcoverage. Pincer-type FAI is often radiographically characterised by findings consistent with acetabular retroversion (crossover sign, a posterior wall sign, and an ischial spine sign) and acetabular overcoverage (LCEA >40°, negative

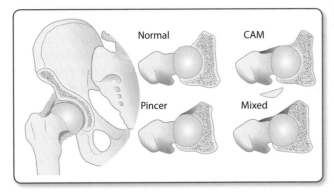

Figure 2.1 Bony morphology of femoroacetabular impingement.

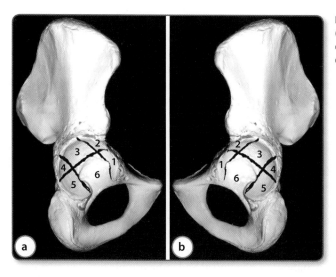

Figure 2.2 The right (a) and left (b) hemipelvis with an en face view of the acetabulum divided into 6 distinct zones.

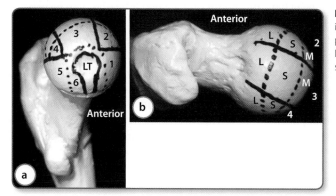

Figure 2.3 Proximal femur divided into 6 distinct zones around the projection of the acetabular fossa. LT, ligamentum teres; M, medial; S, superior; L, lateral.

acetabular index, and acetabular protrusio). While coxa profunda (defined as medial acetabular fossa in contact or projecting medial to the ilioischial line) was often considered diagnostic of Pincer-type FAI, several recent studies show that it is both a common and non-specific finding [25,26].

Often hips have components of both Cam- and Pincer-type FAI, which has been termed Mixed-type FAI. The pincer component combined with the Cam lesion can lead to earlier impingement with intra-articular shear forces consistent with Cam FAI. This can lead to an array of chondrolabral injuries including labral tears, labral detachments, and acetabular delamination [23,24]. Typically, femoral articular cartilage is preserved until very late in the disease process.

Open treatment of FAI

The understanding of FAI evolved from treatment of dysplasia and a growing understanding of young hip pathology, including Perthes and slipped capital femoral epiphysis (SCFE) (retroversion, FAI). This understanding highlights the need for a surgical intervention to address not only intra-articular lesions, but also correct the underlying deformity which was leading to pathologic impingement. Open surgical dislocation and osteochondroplasty (SDO) was initially proposed by Ganz et al [27], SDO revolutionised treatment and understanding of FAI, and has proved a workhorse for the treatment of FAI and its more dramatic causes including SCFE and Perthes. With the advent of minimally invasive techniques, SDO has fallen out of favour as the primary approach to FAI except in very select clinical scenarios.

Non-surgical treatment options for FAI

Not every patient diagnosed with FAI needs or desires surgical intervention. A number of authors have recommended and been successful with nonoperative treatment modalities such as rehabilitation and selective hip joint intra-articular injection. Tangtiphaiboontana and colleagues found 48% of adolescents with hip pain had prolonged symptom improvement after intra-articular corticosteroid injection of the hip. Interestingly, over 90% of patients without bony deformity had improvement and did not require surgery [28]. Kraeutler et al found in a group of patients with clinical and radiographic proof of intra-articular hip pathology underwent in-clinic hip injection with 98% of patients obtaining at least a 70% improvement in pain level [29]. This group showed that injections can be very valuable for both diagnosis and therapeutic reasons.

Physical therapy has been shown to be a valuable adjunct in the treatment of FAI. Hoit et al performed a systematic review of 124 patients from five studies on the efficacy of physical therapy in the treatment of FAI. They concluded that a supervised program focussing on active and core strengthening versus a passive program would be the best model for the non-operative treatment of FAI [30]. On a related note, Malloy found significant unilateral muscle atrophy on the CT scans of patients with unilateral symptomatic FAI. The authors concluded that the muscle atrophy could be addressed prior to or potentially in place of surgery to address the patients' muscular imbalances and deficiencies [31,32].

Labral refixation versus debridement

Larsen et al [33] noted good to excellent results in 68% of the focal debridement group and 92% of the refixation group at a mean 3.5-year follow-up. Despite reports to the contrary, the labrum does not appear to regenerate after excision and hips after excision have inferior results compared to hips that underwent labral repair or reconstruction.

Current trends in the treatment of FAI with labral tears has strongly favoured labral repair over debridement. In fact, some authors have begun to recommend labral reconstruction over repair as a primary treatment [34]. This recommendation has not been without controversy and debate [35].

Labral reconstruction

Labral reconstruction using allograft or autograft tissue, iliotibial band [36,37], allograft tendon/tissue, indirect head of rectus tendon [38,39], and even capsular advancement to the rim have all been described with varying degrees of clinical follow-up and success. From both a biomechanical and clinical perspective, best results at re-creating normal mechanics and preserving hip function and longevity are permitted by retaining as much labrum as possible and reconstructing the deficient labrum. Some authors have recommended either segmental [40] or circumferential reconstruction [41]. An attempt at gaining a general consensus on reconstruction technique, graft type, and outcomes have been attempted by a number of authors [42,43]. Circumferential intact labral tissue seems to give the best outcomes, however, this question needs to be clearly answered by future studies.

Chondral lesion patterns

Chondral lesions of the hip were historically graded using the Outerbridge Classification System borrowed from sports medicine for the grading of knee chondromalacia from 0-IV: 0 is normal cartilage, grade I is softening, grade II is superficial fraying, III is partial thickness loss, and grade IV is areas of full loss down to bone. Beck et al [24] proposed a now well-accepted grading scale for acetabular articular cartilage involvement: Beck score – 1, normal cartilage – 2, softening or malacia – 3, debonding or carpet lesions – 4, cleavage/flap lesions with free edge – 5, and full-thickness defect. The location of involvement is described using a clock face description with 3 O'clock always being anterior regardless of right or left hip. Lesions are described as from X to X O'clock and distance from the rim that the lesion extends. Additionally, Beck et al [24] classified labral involvement: Beck score – 1, normal labrum; – 2, degeneration, thinning or frayed labrum – 3, full-thickness tearing of labrum – 4 labral detachment – 5, labral ossification. These were used with the clock face to describe location and extent of labral lesions. An acetabular zone classification has been championed by Illizaliturri et al to improve the description and communication of these types of lesions. Based on location, the outcome of different treatment modalities can be evaluated as well [44].

With regards to predictive models of those patients at greatest risk of intra-articular chondral damage, Utsunomiya et al [45] evaluated patient-specific data of 2,396 hips having undergone arthroscopy. They found that chondral damage (Outerbridge III and IV) was more commonly present on the acetabulum as compared to the femoral head with older age identified as an independent risk factor. Male sex, increased body mass index (BMI), and increased alpha angle were found to be significantly associated with increased risk of chondral damage to the acetabulum. Decreased CEA and increased Tönnis angle were predictive of chondral damage to the femoral head. An additional multicentre cohort analysis of 802 patients attempted to determine the effect of hip morphology on acetabular chondral wear [46]. The authors reported significantly increased acetabular chondral debonding in patients with Cam (93%) and mixed (97%) impingement as compared to those with Pincer (75%) type pathology. Furthermore, superolateral chondral defects were more commonly identified in patients with Cam (90%) and mixed (91%) morphology as compared to Pincer (60%) impingement.

CHONDRAL TREATMENT OPTIONS

Debridement and microfracture

Unstable cartilage cannot heal autonomously and so careful cartilage probing and examination is required to locate these lesions. The goal of debridement of chondral lesions is to eliminate unstable cartilage that will progress to loose bodies or instability of adjacent cartilage while preserving stable cartilage. Using larger shavers and shavers of various angles avoids gouging the cartilage or clogging the shaver tip.

The goal of microfracture in the treatment of cartilage lesions of the hip is to perforate the cortical bone at the base of the lesion to permit undifferentiated mesenchymal stem cells (MSCs) and growth factors to fill the defect with fibrocartilage, a reparative cartilage of inferior biomechanical quality to hyaline cartilage. Ideally, the lesion should be focal and contained so that the bleeding bone can form a chondrogenic clot and not larger than 4 cm^2 [47]. Additionally, there is some evidence that drilling causes less distortion and damage to the subchondral plate than microfracture with an awl. Specially developed arthroscopic drill bits and guides are now available to drill perpendicular to the bone.

One of the earliest studies on microfracture for acetabular high-grade cartilage lesions was published by Philippon et al [48], which demonstrated good filling of lesions by fibrocartilage but without clinical results. 11 out of 12 studies showed good results after microfracture of chondral lesions in 267 patients undergoing arthroscopy for FAI in a systematic review by MacDonald et al [49]. All publications used focal high-grade lesions as the indication for microfracture and limited weight-bearing after surgery for some period, usually 4–8 weeks. A study by Levinson and colleagues [50] showed the chondral flap associated with chondrolabral disruption had reasonable chondrocyte viability but the extracellular matrix was disorganised. The authors questioned the clinical efficacy of replacing these chondral flaps with fibrin glue sealant. Finally, O'Connor et al performed a systematic review on the outcomes of chondral joint preservation procedures about the hip. In their analysis, the authors found that microfracture was the most commonly used technique. Microfracture had an 89.6% success rate and PROs for all procedures demonstrated statistically significant increases post-operatively [51].

Resection and labral advancement

Some success has been achieved with resection and labral advancement of high-grade rim lesions and report favourable outcomes. The negative of this technique is the risk of iatrogenic acetabular dysplasia and need for resultant PAO. Peters et al could not determine difference in clinical and radiographic outcomes between microfracture, debridement, or resection/labral advancement for high grade rim lesions [52].

Biological treatments and technology

A number of treatments involve harnessing biological technology to encourage chondral healing in full-thickness chondral lesions. Most of these were first utilised in the knee before recently being borrowed for hip pathology and so most have limited data in the hip literature on outcomes.

Stem cells or MSCs augmentation can enhance the healing and quality of the reparative cartilage [53,54]. Bone marrow aspiration concentrate (BMAC) can be harvested and injected into the joint through a needle as an outpatient procedure 6 weeks after a microfracture treatment to augment the biologics of the microfracture healing process and quality of repair cartilage.

Autologous matrix-induced chondroplasty (AMIC) is a single surgery procedure that combines microfracture with application of a porous resorbable type I and III collagen matrix over the defect. This traps the microfracture-induced MSCs within the defect and provides a porous membrane to facilitate stable growth of a cartilage-like tissue. The membrane is held in place by creating a sharp border to the chondral defect and from the pressure of the femoral head; otherwise, the addition of fibrin glue can be helpful for membrane fixation.

Microfragmented adipose tissue transplantation (MATT) with or without microfracture has been suggested as an ideal treatment for delamination lesions [55]. The advantage of microfracture and MATT is that it requires only one surgical intervention and is readily available without pre-operative planning. Jannelli and Fontana [56] report that adipose tissue is chondrogenic, a source of large quantity MSCs comparable to bone marrow aspirate but less invasive and requires simpler preparation.

Matrix-induced autologous chondrocyte implantation (MACI) is a two-stage surgical procedure that first requires biopsy of chondrocytes from the hip or removal of unstable cartilage fragments at time of initial diagnostic scope and chondral debridement [56]. The chondrocytes are then cultured on a matrix that functions as a scaffold and then the matrix, or membrane, is implanted over the defect during a second surgery [55]. Protein and carbohydrate matrices and artificial polymers have all been proposed as the membrane of choice [56]. As confidence in imaging grows and biologic treatment becomes mainstream, one can imagine diagnosing a lesion on MRI and deciding to harvest cartilage from an unaffected joint such as the knee. 3-year follow-up data from Krueger has shown excellent improvement in outcome measures with two clinical failures in 32 study subjects when using traditional injectable autologous chondrocyte implantation (ACI) for full-thickness acetabular defects of >2 cm^2 [57].

Single-stage autologous matrix-enhanced chondrocyte transplantation (AMECT) is a novel technique that involves transplanting the excised cartilage from the femoroplasty into a femoral head or acetabular defect. The graft is mixed with whole blood, BioCartilage (Arthrex, Naples, Florida) and delivered to the chondral defect under dry arthroscopic conditions. The graft is held in place with fibrin glue [58].

Comparing chondral treatment results

There are limited studies in the literature comparing outcomes between treatments for chondral lesions in the hip. Domb et al [59] compared outcomes of FAI patients with chondral lesions treated with and without microfracture after a minimum follow-up period of 2 years. All patients significantly improved but no significant difference between groups was noted. Comparing 5-year results of microfracture versus AMIC treatments for full-thickness acetabular lesions, Fontana et al [60] reported that both did equally well at a year but while results deteriorated in the microfracture group, they were stable in the AMIC group over the following 4 years. Similarly, Fontana also noted improvement up to 3 years after AMIC for grade III and IV acetabular lesions in 201 hips with sustained 40-point improvement in HHS at a mean follow-up of 5 years [61]. When comparing AMIC to MACI, Fontana found similar results with medium-sized lesions but noted the benefit of one surgery with AMIC over the two-stage MACI.

Chondral treatment algorithm

Jannelli and Fontana [56] proposed a treatment algorithm based on their experience and current outcomes studies. They recommended debridement of partial thickness lesions, microfracture with near full chondral thickness lesions but small in diameter (<2 cm^2). MACI or autologous matrix-induced chondrogenesis (AMIC) was recommneded for full-thickness lesions >2 cm². MATT or microfracture with chondrolabral refixation and fibrin glue was suggested for delamination lesions. The advantage of microfracture, AMIC, and MATT is one surgical intervention while MACI requires harvesting chondrocytes and culturing them for a future reimplantation. Furthermore, Jannelli and Fontana [56] cautioned that addressing pathomorphology that caused the cartilage lesions, such as Cam lesions, was necessary for success. Finally, they discouraged chondral treatment in Tönnis grades II or greater due to high failure rates. Dallich and colleagues have also produced an excellent summary chart of the appropriate use of different articular cartilage modalities around the hip joint from multiple sources [62].

Future technology and advancements in chondral repair undoubtedly are on the horizon. Unfortunately, it will take years and large well-designed studies to know what patient and chondral lesion factors will lead to the optimal treatment and outcomes.

Capsular laxity, deficiency, repair, and reconstruction

While failure of early hip arthroscopy was often due to failure to treat the bony deformity of Cam lesions, over the last 15–20 years, knowledge of associated pathomorphology and arthroscopic techniques to address these pathologies has improved. A less common complication has become apparent with respect to hip arthroscopy; capsular instability. As larger bony deformities and labral reconstructions were undertaken, larger capsular portals were required. Interportal capsulotomy and later T-capsulotomy became the workhorses of hip arthroscopy, enabling the surgeon to debride larger Cam lesions and even reconstruct a labrum from gracilis graft. These larger portals were often re-approximated as an afterthought with several stitches that may or not heal completely. Reports of hip dislocations following hip arthroscopy when initially reported was dramatic but by many considered an anomaly in an otherwise minimally invasive surgical movement [63]. However, over time, it became clear that some patients did not improve with arthroscopy despite adequate treatment of labral and Cam pathology and a sense of instability was reported by patients.

Symptomatic instability as either primary or iatrogenic pathology subsequent to arthroscopic treatment of FAI has been described. Myers et al [64] examined the effects of sectioning capsule and labrum in cadavers. They demonstrated with biplane fluoroscopy that defects in the capsule alone and capsule and labrum together, but not labrum alone, lead to increased anteroposterior translation and external rotation in the native hip and are likely culprits in symptomatic hip instability. Attention to capsular closure as an important part of the procedure has been emphasised. In addition to symptoms of instability, it has been shown that there is a distinct pattern of labral and chondral pathology that is straight anterior or lateral with accompanying shallow width of acetabular articular cartilage injury. In addition to symptoms of instability, it has been shown that there is a distinct pattern of labral and chondral pathology that is straight anterior or lateral with accompanying shallow width of acetabular articular cartilage injury. Capsular plication has been suggested by numerous authors to combat iatrogenic or congenital hip joint laxity [65,66].

Prevention: Frank et al [67] noted improved outcomes in both final HOS and failure rate in a cohort of 32 patients treated with hip arthroscopy with complete repair of the T capsulotomy versus a similar cohort of 32 patients with closure of the T but not the interportal capsulotomy.

Repair of capsule: A cadaveric study by Baha et al [68] indicated a near complete restoration of capsular kinematics when complete capsular closure is performed. Krautler et al [69] performed MRI follow-up on 49 hips undergoing arthroscopy for FAI, with 23 hips undergoing capsular repair. The authors found that by 24 weeks after surgery, 83% of the non-repaired capsules had closed and that repair of the capsule for small- to medium-sized interportal capsulotomies may not be necessary. Wylie et al [70] reported on 20 patients who were treated with arthroscopic capsular repair for iatrogenic instability after prior hip arthroscopy including two patients with a dislocation episode. 19 of the 20 patients had improved physical abilities and average HOS-sports improved from 36 to 88 at minimum 2-year follow-up. A more recent study from Philippon et al [71] indicated superior HOSs when the capsulotomy was closed when compared to a matched cohort of unrepaired capsules. Interestingly, there was no difference in the MCID mHHS between the two groups. Another study indicated that capsular closure made no difference in surgical outcomes at 3 years after surgery [72]. Finally, a randomised study by Economopoulos and colleagues [73] found superior PROs in the complete closure group when compared to isolated t-capsulotomy or interportal capsulotomy closure.

Clearly, capsular management with hip arthroscopy is an evolving topic. The current literature, however, has recently tilted in favour of capsular closure with the possible addition of plication in select patients. Whether capsulectomy is advantageous in inflammatory hip conditions, repair necessary in FAI surgery, and whether capsular plication results in improved clinical outcomes over repair in hips prone to instability have been discussed in recent reviews [74–76]. Further studies are needed with PROs at follow-up after these procedures to better understand the rates of complications and demonstrate the ability to optimise outcomes of hip arthroscopy while minimising stiffness and avoiding or resolving symptoms of instability.

EXTRA-ARTICULAR HIP IMPINGEMENT

While there has been much focus on identification and treatment of intra-articular FAI, there is a growing body of evidence describing extra-articular sources of impingement. Subspine impingement (SSI) involves the anterior–inferior iliac spine (AIIS) and proximal femoral neck while ischiofemoral impingement (IFI) involves the ischium and the lesser trochanter.

Anterior–inferior iliac spine impingement

The AIIS has been demonstrated to impinge against the distal femoral neck in certain hips leading to loss of hip flexion and internal rotation resulting in pain and subchondral cystic changes in the distal femoral neck. To further characterise and understand AIIS morphologic variants contributing to impingement, Hetsroni et al [77] evaluated 3D CT reconstructions of 53 hips with impingement. Based upon this study, they classified AIIS by whether there was a normal sulcus between the AIIS and the acetabular rim and whether the AIIS extended to or beyond the rim. Samim et al [78] additionally reported on MRI assessment of SSI with further evaluation of contributing morphologic features beyond the AIIS. Of the 62 patients included for analysis, 32% were identified as having SSI. Patients with SSI were more likely to possess a distal Cam defect, signs of impingement of the distal femoral neck, and superior capsular oedema.

Resection of the AIIS prominence has been shown to improve hip flexion and decrease. A recent retrospective analysis of 10 patients treated with arthroscopic decompression of the AIIS with mean follow-up of 15 months demonstrated an 18° increase in hip flexion as well as a 34-point increase in the HHS [79]. An additional evaluation by Nwachukwu et al [80] reported on 33 females treated with arthroscopic decompression of the AIIS. The authors reported satisfactory clinical improvement in PROs at 1-year follow-up. Additionally, de Sa et al [81] performed a systematic review of extra-articular hip impingement with inclusion of 14 studies and 333 hips. With regards to arthroscopic management of SSI, the authors identified an 18.5° improvement in hip flexion ROM and visual analogue scale (VAS) pain scores as well as the mHHS.

Ischiofemoral impingement

Ischiofemoral impingement is a relatively uncommon diagnosis described as a symptomatic extra-articular impingement between the ischium and proximal femur (most commonly the lesser trochanter). The condition is associated with increased valgus and anteverted femoral morphology resulting in reduced femoral offset or ischiofemoral space (IFS). Impingement occurs with external rotation of the femur in extension resulting in compression of the soft tissue in the space between the lesser trochanter and ischium.

Hatem et al [82] reported on 2-year results in five hips having undergone endoscopic resection of the lesser trochanter. Return to sport averaged 4.4 months and significant improvement in HHS at final follow-up. Patients were treated with endoscopic resection of the lesser trochanter, which resulted in significant improvement HHS at 12 months follow-up. de Sa et al [81] further reported improvement of extra-articular IFI symptoms following open surgical management.

Iliopsoas pain and impingement

The iliopsoas is a powerful hip flexor that passes over the rim of the pelvis at the level of the anteromedial acetabulum with insertion to the lesser trochanter. Iliopsoas pathology including tendonitis, bursitis, labral impingement, and snapping is well described with several studies having evaluated outcomes following iliopsoas release in native hips.

In evaluation of 300 consecutive hip arthroscopies, Nelson and Keene [83] identified a 10% incidence of iliopsoas impingement (ISI) on the acetabular labrum. At 2-year follow-up, patients demonstrated significant improvement in the mHHS with 77% reporting good-to-excellent results. Furthermore, Adib et al performed a retrospective study review of 60 patients having developed post-arthroscopic iliopsoas tendinitis. 32 (53%) patients required iliopsoas tendon sheath injections while seven (12%) patients underwent revision arthroscopy [84]. In their systematic review of extra-articular hip pathology, de Sa et al [81] identified that 88% of patients reported good-to-excellent outcomes and significant improvements in clinical outcome scores following arthroscopic treatment of ISI.

However, the surgeon should understand that release of the iliopsoas tendon is not without consequence. Brandenburg et al [85] compared postoperative iliopsoas muscle volume and seated hip flexion strength in patients having undergone arthroscopic labral repair and iliopsoas tenotomy versus a controls group having undergone isolated arthroscopic labral repair. The authors reported that iliopsoas tenotomy was associated with a 25% volume loss and 19% decrease in seated hip flexion strength. Furthermore, as an important hip stabiliser, Sansone et al [86] were concerned that arthroscopic release of the iliopsoas resulted in the occurrence of two iatrogenic hip dislocations in their series.

PAEDIATRIC HIP DISEASE

Legg–Calvé–Perthes disease

Legg–Calvé–Perthes (LCP) disease is caused by a vascular insult of the hip occurring in skeletally immature children aged 5–9 years old. It is not uncommon for young adults with sequelae of LCP to present with symptoms and radiographic findings consistent with both hip impingement and instability, making surgical decision-making challenging [87,88]. The efficacy of surgical treatment in the early stages of LCP remains a topic of debate. Historically, surgical management has focussed on containment of the femoral head within the acetabulum with the surgical hip dislocation technique expanding treatment options of the post-Perthes hip. This approach allows for femoral head reshaping and treatment of concomitant intra-articular hip pathology with several recent reports identifying improved hip biomechanics and patient outcomes. Modified approaches to surgical hip dislocation involving the development of an extended retinacular flap are being utilised to address complicated morphologic changes of the femoral head [89]. Collectively termed 'femoral head reduction,' these techniques offer the potential for substantial modification of post-Perthes femoral morphology. However, in evaluation of epiphysiodesis or isolated descent of the GT for the management of LCP, Haskel et al [90] demonstrated no difference in neck-shaft angle and abductor strength testing at 6 years post-operatively.

Hip arthroscopy has also been utilised to address chondrolabral pathology, loose bodies, and Cam lesions associated with LCP disease. However, much of LCP pathology is related to proximal femoral deformity associated with acetabular dysplasia. Therefore, further study is warranted to provide a more comprehensive understanding of the appropriate indications for arthroscopic management of LCP disease.

Although the literature consists of many case reports and series, there remains a need for long-term outcome studies with development of surgical algorithms to guide management of the complex deformities associated with LCP.

Slipped capital femoral epiphysis

The aetiology of SCFE is unknown but likely includes factors such as adolescent obesity, mechanical components, and endocrine disorders. SCFE usually occurs around 13 years of age for boys and 11 years of age for girls. A recent natural history review by Matthew and Larson [91] reported a 15–50% risk of avascular necrosis (AVN) following acute, unstable slips. They further identified a 5% risk of THA at 20 years with the history of AVN as the highest independent risk factor.

For the vast majority of acute SCFE in children, in situ pinning is regularly utilised but does not correct the deformity. Some evidence supports favourable outcomes with this approach but it remains difficult to predict which hips will become symptomatic. Although conventional wisdom has held that the majority of hips with mild-to-moderate deformity do well into young adulthood, more recent evidence suggests that even mild slips may lead to FAI, pain, loss of function, and early joint degeneration.

Similar to LCP, surgical hip dislocation has proven valuable for addressing the morphologic abnormalities commonly encountered in more severe slips. For severe slip angles > 45° with an open proximal femoral physis, subcapital realignment via the modified Dunn procedure has proven safe and effective. However, there may be an increased risk of AVN following subcapital realignment in the setting of a closed physis. A recent report has further described improvement in head–neck offset in mostly mild to moderate slips managed arthroscopically [92]. All nine hips treated at a mean of 56 months following in situ pinning demonstrated acetabular cartilage or labral injury at the time of arthroscopy. All but one patient demonstrated improvement in HOS at a mean follow-up of 28.6 months.

In an effort to optimise hip mechanics and articular longevity, Schoenecker et al [93] formulated a surgical algorithm for the varied pathomorphology seen with stable slips. The algorithm considers the pattern of slip to aid in appropriate determination of surgical indications.

IMPLICATIONS FOR EVENTUAL TOTAL HIP ARTHROPLASTY

Not only do some hip conditions have abnormal anatomy to start with, hip preservation sometimes adds deformity or complexity to the soft-tissues and bony structures that further complicate eventual THA. The surgeon may consider the likelihood of hip preservation success weighed against the risk of complicating THA in the future particularly with proximal femoral osteotomies that change the anatomy of the intertrochanteric/subtrochanteric region required for femoral stem broaching and bony fixation. Several groups have found increased rates of blood loss and transfusions, overall rate of revision predominately for aseptic loosening, as well as greater use of modular revision type implants especially on the femoral side in young patients with prior hip preservation surgery undergoing THA. Salvo and colleagues, in a systematic review, found no differences in short- and mid-term outcomes between patients that had prior hip arthroscopy undergoing hip arthroplasty [94]. In another systematic review, this same conclusion was reached by Rosinsky [95]. They, however, could not conclude whether complications were increased in the post-hip arthroscopy cohort compared to the primary arthroplasty group. Finally, Dwyer looked at 20 years follow-up on hip arthroscopy patients treated for labrum tears and chondral flaps. There was a 41% conversion rate to hip arthroplasty in the cohort. Factors that predicted future arthroplasty were age >40 years old and the presence of both femoral and acetabular chondral lesions [96].

On the other hand, it appears that improving acetabular coverage through PAO does not negatively affect future THA; Amanatullah et al [97] demonstrated no difference in complications, revision rates and HHS for THAs in hips that undergone previous PAO compared to a matched cohort of THAs that had not undergone prior PAO.

CONCLUSION

It is now recognised that a variety of hip pathomorphological conditions such as acetabular dysplasia and alteration of normal femoral and acetabular anatomy leading to development of FAI can produce pain and premature OA in young adult and adolescent hips. It is also recognised that the heterogeneous nature of the anatomy and clinical presentation in these patients create substantial difficulty in selecting the correct diagnosis and appropriate treatment. Expansion of knowledge in the areas of disease pathogenesis, disease staging, and surgical treatment has improved surgical outcomes. The diverse nature of hip pathomorphology also complicates design of high-level clinical studies to investigate outcomes. Current literature on hip preservation treatment is most often a small series of variable treatment methods for a spectrum of pathology with intermediate-term outcomes at best. The rapidly expanding field of hip preservation surgery is benefiting from higher-level studies examining the clinical outcomes and basic science in the treatment of hip pathology. Longer term outcomes and the development of 'best practices' will help to standardise the treatment options in the field of hip preservation. Only with this, we will be able to predict outcomes and understand the long-term impact of various hip preservation surgeries on hip joint survivorship.

ACKNOWLEDGEMENTS

The authors would like to thank Lucas A Anderson MD, Frank R Avilucea MD, Christopher E Pelt MD, Jill A Erickson MD, and Christopher L Peters MD for their substantial past contributions to this chapter.

REFERENCES

1. Tannast M, Hanke MS, Zheng G, Steppacher SD, Siebenrock KA. What are the radiographic reference values for acetabular under- and overcoverage? Clin Orthop Relat Res 2015; 473:1234–1246.
2. Parry JA, Swann RP, Erickson JA, et al. Midterm Outcomes of Reverse (Anteverting) Periacetabular Osteotomy in Patients with Hip Impingement Secondary to Acetabular Retroversion. Am J Sports Med 2016; 44:672–676.
3. Heyworth BE, Novais EN, Murray K, et al. Return to play after periacetabular osteotomy for treatment of acetabular dysplasia in adolescent and young adult athletes. Am J Sports Med 2016; 44:1573–1581.
4. Abraham CL, Knight SJ, Peters CL, Weiss JA, Anderson AE. Patient-specific chondrolabral contact mechanics in patients with acetabular dysplasia following treatment with peri-acetabular osteotomy. Osteoarthritis Cartilage 2017; 25:676–684.
5. Knight SJ, Abraham CL, Peters CL, Weiss JA, Anderson AE. Changes in chondrolabral mechanics, coverage, and congruency following peri-acetabular osteotomy for treatment of acetabular retroversion: A patient-specific finite element study. J Orthop Res 2017; 35:2567–2576.
6. Troelsen A, Elmengaard B, Soballe K. Medium-term outcome of periacetabular osteotomy and predictors of conversion to total hip replacement. J Bone Joint Surg Am 2009; 91:2169–2179.
7. Steppacher SD, Tannast M, Ganz R, Siebenrock KA. Mean 20-year follow-up of Bernese periacetabular osteotomy. Clin Orthop Relat Res 2008; 466:1633–1644.
8. Cunningham T, Jessel R, Zurakowski D, Millis MB, Kim YJ. Delayed gadolinium-enhanced magnetic resonance imaging of cartilage to predict early failure of Bernese periacetabular osteotomy for hip dysplasia. J Bone Joint Surg Am 2006; 88:1540–1548.
9. Lerch TD, Steppacher SD, Liechti EF, Tannast M, Siebenrock KA. One-third of Hips After Periacetabular Osteotomy Survive 30 Years with Good Clinical Results, No Progression of Arthritis, or Conversion to THA. Clin Orthop Relat Res 2017; 475:1154–1168.
10. Wells J, Nepple JJ, Crook K, et al. Femoral Morphology in the Dysplastic Hip: Three-dimensional Characterizations with CT. Clin Orthop Relat Res 2017; 475:1045–1054.
11. Redmond JM, Gupta A, Stake CE, Domb BG. The Prevalence of Hip Labral and Chondral Lesions Identified by Method of Detection During Periacetabular Osteotomy: Arthroscopy Versus Arthrotomy. Arthroscopy 2014; 30:382–388.
12. Ginnetti JG, Pelt CE, Erickson JA, Van Dine C, Peters CL. Prevalence and treatment of intra-articular pathology recognized at the time of periacetabular osteotomy for the dysplastic hip. Clin Orthop Relat Res 2013; 471:498–503.

13. Kain MS, Novais EN, Vallim C, Millis MB, Kim YJ. Periacetabular osteotomy after failed hip arthroscopy for labral tears in patients with acetabular dysplasia. J Bone Joint Surg Am 2011; 93:57–61.
14. Siebenrock KA, Schoeniger R, Ganz R. Anterior femoro-acetabular impingement due to acetabular retroversion. Treatment with periacetabular osteotomy. J Bone Joint Surg Am 2003; 85-A:278–286.
15. Peters CL, Anderson LA, Erickson JA, Anderson AE, Weiss JA. An algorithmic approach to surgical decision making in acetabular retroversion. Orthopedics 2011; 34:10.
16. Byrd JW, Jones KS. Hip arthroscopy in the presence of dysplasia. Arthroscopy 2003; 19:1055–1060.
17. Hwang DS, Kang C, Lee JK, et al. The utility of hip arthroscopy for patients with painful borderline hip dysplasia. J Orthop Surg (Hong Kong) 2020; 28:2309499020923162.
18. Beck EC, Drager J, Nwachukwu BU, et al. Patients with Borderline Hip Dysplasia Achieve Clinically Significant Improvement after Arthroscopic Femoroacetabular Impingement Surgery: A Case-Control Study With a Minimum 5-Year Follow-up. Am J Sports Med 2020; 48:1616–1624.
19. Cancienne JM, Beck EC, Kunze KN, et al. Functional and Clinical Outcomes of Patients Undergoing Revision Hip Arthroscopy with Borderline Hip Dysplasia at 2-Year Follow-up. Arthroscopy 2019; 35:3240–3247.
20. Cvetanovich GL, Levy DM, Weber AE, et al. Do Patients with Borderline Dysplasia Have Inferior Outcomes After Hip Arthroscopic Surgery for Femoroacetabular Impingement Compared with Patients with Normal Acetabular Coverage? Am J Sports Med 2017; 45:2116–2124.
21. Zurmuhle CA, Anwander H, Albers CE, et al. Periacetabular Osteotomy Provides Higher Survivorship Than Rim Trimming for Acetabular Retroversion. Clin Orthop Relat Res 2017; 475:1138–1150.
22. Fujii M, Nakashima Y, Noguchi Y, et al. Effect of intra-articular lesions on the outcome of periacetabular osteotomy in patients with symptomatic hip dysplasia. J Bone Joint Surg Brit 2011; 93:1449–1455.
23. Ganz R, Parvizi J, Beck M, et al. Femoroacetabular impingement: a cause for osteoarthritis of the hip. Clin Orthop Relat Res 2003; 417:112–120.
24. Beck M, Kalhor M, Leunig M, Ganz R. Hip morphology influences the pattern of damage to the acetabular cartilage: femoroacetabular impingement as a cause of early osteoarthritis of the hip. J Bone Joint Surg Brit 2005; 87:1012–1018.
25. Clohisy JC, Carlisle JC, Beaule PE, et al. A systematic approach to the plain radiographic evaluation of the young adult hip. J Bone Joint Surg Am 2008; 90:47–66.
26. Nepple JJ, Lehmann CL, Ross JR, Schoenecker PL, Clohisy JC. Coxa profunda is not a useful radiographic parameter for diagnosing pincer-type femoroacetabular impingement. J Bone Joint Surg Am 2013; 95:417–423.
27. Ganz R, Gill TJ, Gautier E, et al. Surgical dislocation of the adult hip a technique with full access to the femoral head and acetabulum without the risk of avascular necrosis. J Bone Joint Surg Brit 2001; 83:1119–1124.
28. Tangtiphaiboontana J, Zhang AL, Pandya NK. Outcomes of intra-articular corticosteroid injections for adolescents with hip pain. J Hip Preserv Surg 2018; 5:54–59.
29. Kraeutler MJ, Garabekyan T, Fioravanti MJ, Young DA, Mei-Dan O. Efficacy of a non-image-guided diagnostic hip injection in patients with clinical and radiographic evidence of intra-articular hip pathology. J Hip Preserv Surg 2018; 5:220–225.
30. Whelan DB, Dwyer T, Ajrawat P, Chahal J, Hoit G. Physiotherapy as an Initial Treatment Option for Femoroacetabular Impingement: A Systematic Review of the Literature and Meta-analysis of 5 Randomized Controlled Trials. Am J Sports Med 2019; 48:2042–2050.
31. Malloy P, Stone AV, Kunze KN, et al. Patients with Unilateral Femoroacetabular Impingement Syndrome Have Asymmetrical Hip Muscle Cross-Sectional Area and Compensatory Muscle Changes Associated with Preoperative Pain Level. Arthroscopy 2019; 35:1445–1453.
32. Espinosa N, Rothenfluh DA, Beck M, Ganz R, Leunig M. Treatment of femoro-acetabular impingement: preliminary results of labral refixation. J Bone Joint Surg Am 2006; 88:925–935.
33. Larson CM, Giveans MR, Stone RM. Arthroscopic debridement versus refixation of the acetabular labrum associated with femoroacetabular impingement: mean 3.5-year follow-up. Am J Sports Med 2012; 40:1015–1021.
34. White BJ, Patterson J, Herzog MM. Bilateral Hip Arthroscopy: Direct Comparison of Primary Acetabular Labral Repair and Primary Acetabular Labral Reconstruction. Arthroscopy 2018; 34: 433–444.
35. Bhatia S, Ellman M, Nho SJ, et al. Bilateral Hip Arthroscopy: Direct Comparison of Primary Acetabular Labral Repair and Primary Acetabular Labral Reconstruction. Arthroscopy 2018; 34:1748–1751.
36. Carreira DS, Kruchten MC, Emmons BR, Martin RL. Arthroscopic Labral Reconstruction Using Fascia Lata Allograft: Shuttle Technique and Minimum Two-Year Results. J Hip Preserv Surg 2018; 5:247-258.
37. White BJ, Stapleford AB, Hawkes TK, Finger MJ, Herzog MM. Allograft Use in Arthroscopic Labral Reconstruction of the Hip with Front-to-Back Fixation Technique: Minimum 2-Year Follow-up. Arthroscopy 2016; 32:26–32.

38. Amar E, Sampson TG, Sharfman ZT, et al. Acetabular labral reconstruction using the indirect head of the rectus femoris tendon significantly improves patient reported outcomes. Knee Surg Sports Traumatol Arthrosc 2017; 26:2512–2518.
39. Locks R, Chahla J, Bolia IK, Briggs KK, Philippon MJ. Outcomes Following Arthroscopic Hip Segmental Labral Reconstruction Using Autologous Capsule Tissue or Indirect Head of Rectus Tendon. J Hip Preserv Surg 2018; 5:73–77.
40. Chandrasekaran S, Darwish N, Close MR, et al. Arthroscopic Reconstruction of Segmental Defects of the Hip Labrum: Results in 22 Patients with Mean 2-Year Follow-Up. Arthroscopy 2017; 33:1685–1693.
41. Maldonado DR, Kyin C, Rosinsky PJ, et al. Circumferential Acetabular Labral Reconstruction for Irreparable Labral tears in the Primary Setting: Minimum Two-Year Outcomes with a Nested Matched-Pair Control. Arthroscopy 2020; 36:2583–2597.
42. Maldonado DR, Lall AC, Walker-Santiago R, et al. Hip Labral Reconstruction: Consensus Study on Indications, Graft Type and Technique Among High-Volume Surgeons. J Hip Preserv Surg 2019; 6:41–49.
43. Atzmon R, Radparvar JR, Sharfman ZT, et al. Graft Choices for Acetabular Labral Reconstruction. J Hip Preserv Surg 2018; 5:329–338.
44. Ilizaliturri VMJr, Byrd JW, Sampson TG, et al. A Geographic Zone Method to Describe Intra-Articular Pathology in Hip Arthroscopy: Cadaveric Study and Preliminary Report. Arthroscopy 2008; 24:534–539.
45. Utsunomiya H, Briggs KK, Dornan GJ, et al. Predicting Severe Cartilage Damage in the Hip: A Model Using Patient-Specific Data From 2,396 Hip Arthroscopies. Arthroscopy 2019; 35:2051–2060.e13.
46. Pascual-Garrido C, Li DJ, Grammatopoulos G, et al. The Pattern of Acetabular Cartilage Wear Is Hip Morphology-dependent and Patient Demographic-dependent. Clin Orthop Relat Res 2019; 477:1021–1033.
47. Mella C, Nunez A, Villalon I. Treatment of acetabular chondral lesions with microfracture technique. SICOT J 2017;3:45.
48. Philippon MJ, Schenker ML, Briggs KK, Maxwell RB. Can microfracture produce repair tissue in acetabular chondral defects? Arthroscopy 2008; 24:46–50.
49. MacDonald AE, Bedi A, Horner NS, et al. Indications and Outcomes for Microfracture as an Adjunct to Hip Arthroscopy for Treatment of Chondral Defects in Patients with Femoroacetabular Impingement: A Systematic Review. Arthroscopy 2016; 32:190–200e192.
50. Levinson C, Naal FD, Salzmann GM. Is There a Scientific Rationale for the Refixation of Delaminated Chondral Flaps in Femoroacetabular Impingement? A Laboratory Study. Clin Orthop Relat Res 2020; 478:854–867.
51. O'Connor M, Minkara AA, Westermann RW, Rosneck J, Lynch TS. Outcomes of Joint Preservation Procedures for Cartilage Injuries in the Hip: A Systematic Review and Meta-Analysis. Orthop J Sports Med 2018; 6:1–11.
52. Peters CL, Anderson LA, Diaz-Ledezma C, Anderson MB, Parvizi J. Does the nature of chondrolabral injury affect the results of open surgery for femoroacetabular impingement? Clin Orthop Relat Res 2015; 473:1342–1348.
53. Strauss EJ, Barker JU, Kercher JS, Cole BJ, Mithoefer K. Augmentation Strategies following the Microfracture Technique for Repair of Focal Chondral Defects. Cartilage 2010; 1:145–152.
54. McIlwraith CW, Frisbie DD, Rodkey WG, et al. Evaluation of intra-articular mesenchymal stem cells to augment healing of microfractured chondral defects. Arthroscopy 2011; 27:1552–1561.
55. Chahla J, LaPrade RF, Mardones R, et al. Biological Therapies for Cartilage Lesions in the Hip: A New Horizon. Orthopedics 2016; 39:e715–723.
56. Jannelli E, Fontana A. Arthroscopic treatment of chondral defects in the hip: AMIC, MACI, micro fragmented adipose tissue transplantation (MATT), and other options. SICOT J 2017; 3:43.
57. Krueger DR, Gesslein M, Schuetz M, Perka C, Schroeder JH. Injectable Autologous Chondrocyte Implantation (ACI) in Acetabular Cartilage Defects—Three-Year Results. J Hip Preserv Surg 2018; 5:386–392.
58. Craig MJ, Maak TG. Single-Stage Arthroscopic Autologous Matrix–Enhanced Chondral Transplantation (AMECT) in the Hip Arthrosc Tech 2020; 9:e399–e403.
59. Domb BG, El Bitar YF, Lindner D, Jackson TJ, Stake CE. Arthroscopic hip surgery with a microfracture procedure of the hip: clinical outcomes with two-year follow-up. Hip Int 2014; 24:448–456.
60. Fontana A, de Girolamo L. Sustained five-year benefit of autologous matrix-induced chondrogenesis for femoral acetabular impingement-induced chondral lesions compared with microfracture treatment. Bone Joint J 2015; 97-B:628–635.
61. Fontana A. Autologous Membrane Induced Chondrogenesis (AMIC) for the treatment of acetabular chondral defect. Muscles Ligaments Tendons J 2016; 6:367–371.
62. Dallich AA, Rath E, Atzmon R, et al. Chondral Lesions in the Hip: a Review of Relevant Anatomy, Imaging, and Treatment Modalities. J Hip Preserv Surg 2019; 6:3–15.

63. Matsuda DK. Acute iatrogenic dislocation following hip impingement arthroscopic surgery. Arthroscopy 2009; 25:400–404.
64. Myers CA, Register BC, Lertwanich P, et al. Role of the acetabular labrum and the iliofemoral ligament in hip stability: an in vitro biplane fluoroscopy study. Am J Sports Med 2011; 39:85S-91S.
65. Shoichi N, Hironobu H, Kensuke H, et al. Arthroscopic Capsular Repair Using Proximal Advancement for Instability Following Hip Arthroscopic Surgery: a Case Report. J Hip Preserv Surg 2019; 6:91–96.
66. Stone AV, Mehta N, Beck EC, et al. Comparable Patient-Reported Outcomes in Females with or without Joint Hypermobility After Hip Arthroscopy and Capsular Plication for Femoroacetabular Impingement Syndrome. J Hip Preserv Surg 2019; 6:33–40.
67. Frank RM, Lee S, Bush-Joseph CA, et al. Improved outcomes after hip arthroscopic surgery in patients undergoing T-capsulotomy with complete repair versus partial repair for femoroacetabular impingement: a comparative matched-pair analysis. Am J Sports Med 2014; 42:2634–2642.
68. Baha P, Burkhart TA, Getgood A, Degen RM. Complete Capsular Repair Restores Native Kinematics After Interportal and T-Capsulotomy. Am J Sports Med 2019; 47:1451–1458.
69. Kraeutler MJ, Strickland CD, Brick MJ, et al. A Multicenter, Double-Blind, Randomized Controlled Trial Comparing Magnetic Resonance Imaging Evaluation of Repaired Versus Unrepaired Interportal Capsulotomy in Patients Undergoing Hip Arthroscopy for Femoroacetabular Impingement. J Hip Preserv Surg 2018; 5:349–356.
70. Wylie JD, Beckmann JT, Maak TG, Aoki SK. Arthroscopic Capsular Repair for Symptomatic Hip Instability After Previous Hip Arthroscopic Surgery. Am J Sports Med 2016; 44:39–45.
71. Bolia IK, Fagotti L, Briggs KK, Philippon MJ. Midterm Outcomes Following Repair of Capsulotomy Versus Nonrepair in Patients Undergoing Hip Arthroscopy for Femoroacetabular Impingement with Labral Repair. Arthroscopy 2019; 35:1828–1834.
72. Atzmon R, Sharfman ZT, Haviv B, et al. Does Capsular Closure Influence Patient-Reported Outcomes in Hip Arthroscopy for Femoroacetabular Impingement and Labral Tear? J Hip Preserv Surg 2019; 6:199–206.
73. Economopoulos KJ, Chhabra A, Kweon C. Prospective Randomized Comparison of Capsular Management Techniques During Hip Arthroscopy. Am J Sports Med 2019; 48:395–402.
74. Bedi A, Galano G, Walsh C, Kelly BT. Capsular management during hip arthroscopy: from femoroacetabular impingement to instability. Arthroscopy 2011; 27:1720–1731.
75. Ekhtiari S, de Sa D, Haldane CE, et al. Hip arthroscopic capsulotomy techniques and capsular management strategies: a systematic review. Knee Surg Sports Traumatol Arthrosc 2017; 25:9–23.
76. Ortiz-Declet V, Mu B, Chen AW, et al. Should the Capsule Be Repaired or Plicated After Hip Arthroscopy for Labral Tears Associated with Femoroacetabular Impingement or Instability? A Systematic Review. Arthroscopy 2018; 34:303–318.
77. Hetsroni I, Poultsides L, Bedi A, Larson CM, Kelly BT. Anterior inferior iliac spine morphology correlates with hip range of motion: a classification system and dynamic model. Clin Orthop Relat Res 2013; 471:2497–2503.
78. Samim M, Walter W, Gyftopoulos S, Poultsides L, Youm T. MRI Assessment of Subspine Impingement: Features Beyond the Anterior Inferior Iliac Spine Morphology. Radiology 2019; 293:412–421.
79. Hetsroni I, Larson CM, Dela Torre K, et al. Anterior inferior iliac spine deformity as an extra-articular source for hip impingement: a series of 10 patients treated with arthroscopic decompression. Arthroscopy 2012; 28:1644–1653.
80. Nwachukwu BU, Chang B, Fields K, et al. Outcomes for Arthroscopic Treatment of Anterior Inferior Iliac Spine (Subspine) Hip Impingement. Orthop J Sports Med 2017; 5:2325967117723109.
81. de Sa D, Alradwan H, Cargnelli S, et al. Extra-articular hip impingement: a systematic review examining operative treatment of psoas, subspine, ischiofemoral, and greater trochanteric/pelvic impingement. Arthroscopy 2014; 30:1026–1041.
82. Hatem MA, Palmer IJ, Martin HD. Diagnosis and 2-year outcomes of endoscopic treatment for ischiofemoral impingement. Arthroscopy 2015; 31:239–246.
83. Nelson IR, Keene JS. Results of labral-level arthroscopic iliopsoas tenotomies for the treatment of labral impingement. Arthroscopy 2014; 30:688–694.
84. Adib F, Johnson AJ, Hennrikus WJ, et al. Iliopsoas Tendonitis After Hip Arthroscopy: Prevalence, Risk Factors and Treatment Algorithm. J Hip Preserv Surg 2018; 5:362–369.
85. Brandenburg JB, Kapron AL, Wylie JD, et al. The Functional and Structural Outcomes of Arthroscopic Iliopsoas Release. Am J Sports Med 2016; 44:1286–1291.
86. Sansone M, Ahlden M, Jonasson P, et al. Total dislocation of the hip joint after arthroscopy and iliopsoas tenotomy. Knee Surg Sports Traumatol Arthrosc 2013; 21:420–423.

87. Anderson LA, Crofoot CD, Erickson JA, Peters CL. Staged surgical dislocation and redirectional periacetabular osteotomy: a report of five cases. J Bone Joint Surg Am 2009; 91:2469–2476.
88. Clohisy JC, Nepple JJ, Ross JR, Pashos G, Schoenecker PL. Do surgical hip dislocation and periacetabular osteotomy improve pain in patients with Perthes-like deformities and acetabular dysplasia? Clin Orthop Relat Res 2015; 473:1370–1377.
89. Siebenrock KA, Anwander H, Zurmuhle CA, et al. Head reduction osteotomy with additional containment surgery improves sphericity and containment and reduces pain in Legg-Calvé-Perthes disease. Clin Orthop Relat Res 2015; 473:1274–1283.
90. Haskel JD, Feder OI, Mijares J, Castañeda P. Isolated Trochanteric Descent and Greater Trochanteric Epiphysiodesis Are Not Effective in the Treatment of Post-Perthes Deformity. Clin Orthop Relat Res 2020; 478:169–175.
91. Matthew SE, Larson AN. Natural history of slipped capital femoral epiphysis. J Pediatr Orthop 2019; 39:S23–S27.
92. Wylie JD, Beckmann JT, Maak TG, Aoki SK. Arthroscopic treatment of mild to moderate deformity after slipped capital femoral epiphysis: intra-operative findings and functional outcomes. Arthroscopy 2015; 31:247–253.
93. Schoenecker PL, Gordon JE, Luhmann SJ, et al. A treatment algorithm for stable slipped capital femoral epiphysis deformity. J Pediatr Orthop 2013; 33:S103–111.
94. Chaudhry ZS, Salem HS, Hammoud S, Salvo JP. Does Prior Hip Arthroscopy Affect Outcomes of Subsequent Hip Arthroplasty? A Systematic Review. Arthroscopy 2019; 35:631–643.
95. Rosinsky PJ, Kyin C, Shapira J, et al. Hip Arthroplasty After Hip Arthroscopy: Are Short-term Outcomes Affected? A Systematic Review of the Literature. J Arthrosc Relat Res 2019; 35:2736–2746.
96. Dwyer MK, Tumpowsky C, Boone A, Lee J, McCarthy JC. What Is the Association Between Articular Cartilage Damage and Subsequent THA 20 Years After Hip Arthroscopy for Labral Tears? Clin Orthop Relat Res 2019; 477:1211–1220.
97. Amanatullah DF, Stryker L, Schoenecker P, et al. Similar clinical outcomes for THAs with and without prior periacetabular osteotomy. Clin Orthop Relat Res 2015; 473:685–691.

Chapter 3

What is new in total hip arthroplasty? Direct anterior approach

Harlan B Levine, Gregg R Klein

INTRODUCTION

In this edition of What is New in Total Hip Arthroplasty (THA), we will take an in-depth look at the recent literature regarding the direct anterior approach. The direct anterior approach continues to gain in popularity in North America and more surgeons are being trained in this technique. Public perception is that this is a better hip replacement and more patients are seeking surgeons who perform the direct anterior approach. As a result, surgeons have shifted towards this procedure in their practices as a result of public pressure. This article will provide a balanced review of the recent literature regarding the direct anterior approach to help surgeons make informed decisions when selecting the best approach for their patients and will address short- and long-term outcomes, the risk or revision, the utility of different stem designs, and the use of fluoroscopy.

SHORT-TERM OUTCOMES

Miller et al [1] studied the influence of surgical approach on outcomes following THA in the first 90 days of the post-operative period. This study compared the anterior approach and posterior approach in primary THA looking at outcomes including pain, severity, narcotic usage, and Harris hip scores as well as postoperative complications. 13 prospective studies, 7 of which were randomised, in which patients were treated with either a direct anterior or posterior THA, were examined. For this meta-analysis, a total of 524 direct anterior hips were identified and a total of 520 posterior hips were identified. Using the data available, the direct anterior approach was statistically significant for a lower pain score, lower narcotic usage, and improved hip function compared to the posterior approach. No differences were observed for rates of dislocation, fracture, haematoma, infection, thromboembolic event, or reoperations. The authors concluded that the direct anterior approach may offer less pain, a lower narcotic demand, and improved hip function, and is

Harlan B Levine MD, Director, Hip and Knee Service, Hackensack University Medical Center, Assistant Professor, Department of Orthopedic Surgery, Hackensack Meridian School of Medicine, Rothman Orthopedic Institute, Paramus, NJ
Email: harlan.levine@rothmanortho.com

Gregg R Klein MD, Vice-Chairman, Department of Orthopedic Surgery, Hackensack University Medical Center, Associate Professor, Department of Orthopedic Surgery, Hackensack Meridian School of Medicine, Rothman Orthopedic Institute, Paramus NJ
Email: gregg.klein@rothmanortho.com

not associated with an increased complication rate compared to the posterior approach in the first 90 postoperative days. The authors state that surgeons should select their surgical approach based on their preferences and experiences while being mindful of anatomical characteristics of the patient.

In 2013, Barrett at al [2] published their results on a prospective randomised study comparing direct anterior versus posterior lateral THA. This study showed that patients with the direct anterior approach appeared to have better results in the immediate postoperative period up to 3 months. No significant differences between the groups were noted at later time points. The authors have performed a concise 5-year follow-up evaluation of these same patients and conclude that both approaches yield good results at an average of 5-year follow-up with respect to survivorship, function, rate of complications, and radiographic analysis [3].

Brismar et al [4] randomised 100 patients to receive either a direct anterior or direct lateral THA and followed them 5 years to assess early gains in pain reduction and hip function as well as assess rates of complications. The authors noted that patients in the direct anterior group had less pain with activity and performed better on early functional tests including the timed up and go test and had higher Harris hip scores and EQ-5D index at 8 weeks post-operatively. The authors did not note any relevant differences between these groups with respect to pain, hip function, or quality of life at 1 or 5 years post-operatively. However, seven complications related to surgical approach were noted in the direct anterior group whereas none were noted in the direct lateral group. The authors note that the early positive results in the direct anterior THA may be the result of a less traumatic approach but caution that later complications are concerning.

Chang et al [5] followed 72 patients randomly assigned to receive either a direct anterior or posterior approach THA performed by two senior surgeons. The patients were evaluated preoperatively as well as at 2 weeks, 6 weeks, and 12 weeks post-operatively. Data showed no difference between the two groups with respect to Western Ontario McMasters Arthritis Index and Oxford Hip Scores. No significant difference was noted in the 10-meter walk test, EuroQoL, and radiographic analysis. Hip flexion activity was favoured in the direct anterior group at 6 weeks. At 12 weeks, a lateral femoral cutaneous femoral nerve neuropraxia was seen in 83% of patients in the direct anterior group and in 0% of patients in the posterior group. The authors conclude that the approaches are comparable, and that the choice of surgical approach should be based on surgeon preference and experience as well as patient factors.

Peters et al [6] reviewed the Dutch arthroplasty register to determine if there was a difference in patient reported outcome measures (PROMs) at 3 months post-operatively between different surgical approaches for THA. The authors identified 12,774 primary THAs for which pre-operative in 3-month post-operative PROMs were available. In this series, there were 7,286 posterolateral THAs, 3,363 direct anterior THAs, 1,052 direct lateral THAs, and 573 anterolateral THAs. The authors note that improvements in PROMs were significant for all four approaches. However, the results of this study indicate a larger improvement in self-reported physical functioning in THAs utilising an anterior or posterolateral approach comparted with the anterolateral and direct lateral approaches. The study also shows better pain relief after 2 months with the posterolateral and anterior approaches. No relevant differences in PROMs were noted between the anterior and posterolateral approaches.

Maldanado et al [7] reviewed prospectively collected data and matched 205 patients who had undergone a direct anterior THA to 205 patients who had undergone a posterolateral THA and assessed for differences in multiple PROMs at a minimum of 2 years follow-up. The results of this study show that the patients in the direct anterior group had higher scores at final follow-up for the VR-12 mental, VR-12 physical, as well as SF-12 physical scores. Both groups had comparable Harris hip scores and FJS-12 scores. The authors conclude that both groups achieved comparable scores from the majority of PROMs; however, the direct anterior group achieved superior quality of life outcomes when compared with a propensity score matched group of posterolateral surgeries.

In a small series of 61 hips, Ozaki et al [8] compared Harris hip scores as well as PROMs between 30 patients who had a direct anterior approach and 31 who had a posterior approach. The authors found that there was no difference in pre-operative or post-operative Harris hip scores between these two groups. They also noted that there was no difference between the Western Ontario and McCaster University Arthritis Index and the Japanese Orthopaedic Association Hip Disease Evaluation Questionnaire, but post-operative Forgotten Joint Score was significantly higher in the direct anterior group than the posterior group.

In the randomised controlled trial, patients were randomly assigned to receive either a direct anterior approach or a posterolateral approach [9]. Upto 60 patients were enrolled into each group. Perioperative and post-operative outcomes were recorded. The direct anterior approach had better functional recovery at 3 months based on Harris hip scores, University of California Los Angeles activity scores, as well as gait analysis. However, by 6 months, functional recovery was similar between these two groups.

INCREASED RISK OF REVISION BY APPROACH

Many studies have used large institutional and registry databases to examine the risk of complications and revisions with different approaches in THA. Aggarwal et al [10] received the 2019 Frank Stinchfield Award for their manuscript looking at the risk of infection between direct anterior approaches and non-direct anterior approaches. Evaluating a consecutive series of 6,086 patients undergoing primary total hip replacement at a single institution between 2013 and 2016, a total of 1,985 patients were identified who had undergone a direct anterior THA and 4,101 patients were identified as having a non-direct anterior THA. The overall infection rate during this time was 0.82% and did reduce from 0.96% in 2013 to 0.53% in 2016. The authors attributed this overall reduction in infection rate to improved infection prevention protocols including the use of aspirin for deep vein thrombosis (DVT) prophylaxis, dilute iodine lavage, vancomycin powder in the wound, and gram-negative coverage when deemed appropriate. Despite these protocols and lower rates of infection, the authors did find that the patients undergoing a direct anterior approach were 2.2 times more likely to develop an infection than those who had undergone a non-anterior approach.

Kuijpers et al [11] noted that the outcomes in younger patients are inferior to those seen in older patients undergoing THA and that younger patients have a greater chance of outliving their implants, and that implant survival at mid- and long-term follow-up is lower in patients <55 years old. Querying the Dutch Arthroplasty Register, the authors looked at the risk of revision in 19,682 THAs performed in patients <55 years old. While the overall rate of revision was very low in this study at 0.89% at 5 years for dislocation, there was noted to be an overall lower rate of revision in the anterior approach as compared to all other approaches including the posterior approach. However, because the overall rate of revision was so low, the authors were unable to determine the effect of factors including surgical approach on the risk of revision due to dislocation as an endpoint. The authors also note that the lower risk of revision of an anterior approach may disappear with longer follow-up.

However, in another study from the same registry, it was found that the highest risk of revision for any reason was the anterior approach, even after excluding the first 150 procedures of a surgeon's experience to minimise the effect of the learning curve. Zijlstra et al [12] examined the effects of femoral head size and surgical approach on the risk of revision for dislocation in THA. In this study, they analysed 166,231 total hip replacements from the Dutch Arthroplasty Register performed between 2007 and 2015. Of these original surgeries, there were 3,754 revisions performed. Revision for dislocation as well as all other causes was calculated, and it was found that the posterior–lateral approach was associated with a higher rate of dislocation but that the risk for revision for all other causes, especially femoral stem loosening, was highest in anterior and anterior–lateral approaches. It is interesting to note that with stratification based on head size, that there was an increased risk of dislocation with the posterior–lateral approach with smaller heads. However, with 36 mm heads, the risk of revision for dislocation was similar among all approaches. The authors also stress that the overall rate of dislocation in this series was quite low at about 1% overall and that the overall rate of revision for dislocation was 0.5–1%. When looking at the risk of revision for all other causes, including femoral loosening and periprosthetic fractures, it was noted that the risk of revision was highest with the direct anterior approach at 2.9% and lowest with the posterior–lateral approach at 2%. The authors hypothesise that the increased rate of revision for aseptic loosening or a fracture was related to the increase in difficulty of femoral exposure in the direct anterior approach.

The increased risk of aseptic loosening and periprosthetic fracture has been found in other studies looking at the rate of revision between direct anterior approaches versus other approaches including posterolateral. Panichkul et al [13] compared 514 THAs performed with the posterior or lateral approach using either an extensively coated cobalt chrome stem or a straight, dual-tapered, proximally porous-coated titanium stem with 594 direct anterior THAs utilising a proximally coated, titanium tapered-wedge stem. In this series, there were no revisions in the posterior or lateral group and five stem revisions in the anterior group for either aseptic loosening or periprosthetic fractures. The increased revision rate in the anterior group was statistically significant.

The increased risk of femoral side failure in direct anterior THA has been noted by other authors as well. Meneghini et al [14] reviewed 478 consecutive early revisions performed within 5 years of the index surgery at three academic centres. Results of this study showed an increased rate of early revision secondary to femoral failure in patients who had undergone a direct anterior THA (50.9% of all revisions in this study) compared to hip replacements performed through a direct lateral (34.8%) or posterior (14.3%) approach. Angerame et al [15] compared the direct anterior approach with the posterior approach to evaluate the incidence of early failure in total arthroplasty stratified by the approach. About 2,431 direct anterior hips and 4,463 posterior hips were compared and a total of 103 revisions were identified. The direct anterior approach had a higher rate of early revision for femoral component loosening compared to the posterior approach. In another study, Eto et al [16] looked at the rate of revision as well as the time to revision between direct anterior and non-anterior approaches. The results of their study showed a significant difference in time to revision between these approaches with a mean duration to revision of 3.0 ± 2.7 years in the direct anterior approach and 3.6 ± 2.8 years in the non-anterior group. Revision for aseptic loosening of the stem was also more common in the direct anterior group (30%) compared to the nonanterior group (8%).

To determine the risk of complications among patients undergoing THAs utilising a direct anterior approach versus lateral and posterior approaches, Pincus et al [17] examined all THAs performed for diagnosis of osteoarthritis in Ontario. Canada over a 5-year period. The authors included a large sample size to make sure that the study was appropriately powered to detect significant differences in rates of complications. The authors acknowledged that surgical techniques have advanced over the years and attempted to look at a modern era of surgery and, therefore, only included procedures performed between 2015 and 2019. They also controlled for potential confounding variables that are known to affect surgical complications including morbid obesity, diabetes, hypertension, congestive heart failure, chronic obstructive pulmonary disease, frailty, low socioeconomic status, and surgeon's experience. Total 30,098 patients were included, out of which 16,079 underwent an anterior approach, 21,248 a lateral approach, and 5,855 a posterior approach in 73 hospitals performed by 298 surgeons. Patients in the anterior approach group were younger, had lower rates of morbid obesity, diabetes, and hypertension, and were treated by higher volume surgeons than those in the lateral and posterior groups. Despite the differences in these potential confounding variables which would lead to a lower rate of complication in the anterior group, patients undergoing surgery with an anterior approach had a statistically significant greater risk of major surgical complication. The authors point out that the anterior approach has a risk profile that is different from that perceived by the public and call for surgeons to have a balanced discussion with patients regarding potential risks of these procedures.

It should be noted that other authors have not found an increased rate of early femoral complications in the direct anterior approach. Cidambi et al [18] reviewed 1,120 consecutive direct anterior THAs and noted a perioperative femoral complication rate of 1% and a femoral loosening rate of 0.55% at 2 years follow-up. They conclude that the anterior approach is safe and offers predictable results when performed by experienced surgeons. Sheth et al [19] reviewed the Kaiser Permanente Total Joint Replacement Registry and identified 42,438 primary THAs. In this cohort of patients, the direct anterior group had an aseptic revision rate of 1.1% whereas the posterior group had an aseptic revision rate of 1.9%. The results of this large database study indicate that the anterior and anterolateral surgical approaches had a lower risk of dislocation without an increased risk of early revision in comparison to other approaches.

INFLUENCE OF STEM DESIGN ON RISK OF COMPLICATIONS

Authors have noted the impact of femoral stem design on the risk of periprosthetic fracture and aseptic loosening in direct anterior THA. In a study of the Dutch Arthroplasty Registry, Janssen et al [20] looked at the effect of stem design on early rates of aseptic loosening of different styles of cementless stems inserted through an anterior or anterolateral approach compared to a posterior approach. They reviewed 63,354 hip arthroplasties. They found that cementless femoral stems with a proximal shoulder have a higher rate of early aseptic loosening when inserted through an anterior or anterolateral approach compared with a posterior approach. They theorise that an anatomically shaped stem may be preferable when an anterior or anterolateral approach is used, although further analysis was suggested. Cidambi et al [18] reviewed 899 patients with 2 years follow-up after direct anterior THA with different stem designs. There were no revisions for aseptic loosening in the collared, fully hydroxyapatite-coated compaction broached, or triple tapered proximal fit and fill stems. The highest rate of revision was noted in short medial lateral tapered stems. Panichkul et al [21] performed a systematic review and meta-analysis to look at the effects of different stem designs on revision rates and postoperative complications in direct anterior THA. Multiple femoral implant designs were examined including collared, collarless, short, and long stems. While the collared and long femoral stems had a decreased overall complication rate compared to the collarless and short stems, there was no difference between the stems with respect to revision rates. The authors conclude that further prospective, randomised controlled studies are needed as the current literature is insufficient to draw conclusions regarding optimal stem design for direct anterior THA.

INTRAOPERATIVE FLUOROSCOPY UTILITY

The use of intraoperative fluoroscopy during direct anterior THA has been seen as a potential benefit as it allows surgeons to confirm implant position during the procedure. However, its use is associated with increased cost and surgical time, may introduce potential contamination from the radiographic arm, and is operator dependent to obtain an accurate image. The contention has been that by using fluoroscopy, the surgeon can ensure that implants are placed in the optimal position to improve hip stability. However, there is limited data demonstrating improved component position with the use of intraoperative fluoroscopy. In a single surgeon series, 42 consecutive hips were performed by the direct anterior approach using intraoperative fluoroscopy and were compared to 42 consecutive hips performed without intraoperative fluoroscopy [22]. In this series, no statistical significant difference was noted in acetabular inclination or restoration of femoral offset. However, a statistically significant but small difference was shown in acetabular anteversion of 13.7° in the fluoroscopy group versus 11.2° in the non-arthroscopy group. In a similar study, Bingham at al [23] retrospectively reviewed 125 patients who had a direct anterior hip using intraoperative fluoroscopy and compared them with 140 patients who underwent a direct anterior hip without intraoperative fluoroscopy. No clinical or statistically significant differences were noted in acetabular inclination, anteversion, or leg length discrepancy between these two groups. It should be noted that each of these groups had surgery by a different surgeon and intraoperative fluoroscopy was used with a fracture table whereas a standard operative table was used in the non-fluoroscopy group. In an earlier study, Jennings et al [24] retrospectively reviewed direct anterior hip replacements performed with fluoroscopy in 98 patients to 101 performed without fluoroscopy. In this single surgeon study, a statistically significant difference in cup abduction was noted but no statistically significant difference in anteversion was seen. However, 80% of implants in the fluoroscopy group compared with 63% of implants in the non-fluoroscopy group were within the combined safe zone. The authors conclude that fluoroscopy may not be necessary for proper anteversion but may increase ideal safe zone placement of the components.

INTRAOPERATIVE FLUOROSCOPY SAFETY

While the utility of intraoperative fluoroscopy is debatable, it remains common place in the operating room for many surgeons performing direct anterior THA. Several studies have looked at the safety of fluoroscopy on both the patient and surgeon. McNabb et al [25] looked at the radiation exposure to both patients and surgeons by placing dosimetry badges at the sternal notch and pubic symphysis of patients as well as outside of the thyroid shield of surgeons during direct anterior THA. For patients, the authors found that the radiation exposure at the thyroid as well as at the gonads was well below the threshold for carcinogenesis, and, in fact, was approximately one-third of that of a standard pelvic radiograph. They also calculated how much radiation surgeons were exposed to on a cumulative basis which was found to be insignificant. The authors concluded that radiation exposure to the patient is negligible per case and, to the surgeon, is negligible on a cumulative basis. In another study, Jinnai et al [26] examined radiation exposure time during direct anterior THA to determine if radiation exposure exceeded safety limits. They concluded that radiation exposure is minimal to the surgeon and that a surgeon would need to perform 45,000 surgeries per year to exceed maximum tissue exposure at the skin, more than 27,000 surgeries annually to exceed safety levels at the eyes, and more than 238,000 surgeries to exceed radiation safety levels at the chest. They conclude that the use of intraoperative fluoroscopy in direct anterior THA is safe with respect to radiation exposure.

REFERENCES

1. Miller LE, Gondusky JS, Bhattacharyya S, et al. Does surgical approach affect outcomes in total hip arthroplasty through 90 days of follow-up? A systematic review with meta-analysis. J Arthroplasty 2018; 33:1296–1302.
2. Barrett WP, Turner SE, Leopold JP. Prospective randomized study of direct anterior vs. posterolateral approach for total hip arthroplasty. J Arthroplasty 2013; 28:1634–1638.
3. Barrett WP, Turner SE, Murphy JA, et al. Prospective, Randomized Study of Direct Anterior Approach vs Posterolateral Approach Total Hip Arthroplasty: A Concise 5-Year Follow-Up Evaluation. J Arthroplasty 2019; 34:1139–1142.
4. Brismar BH, Hallert O, Tedhamre A, et al. Early gain in pain reduction and hip function, but more complications following the direct anterior minimally invasive approach for total hip arthroplasty: a randomized trial of 100 patients with 5 years of follow up. Acta Orthop 2018; 89:484–489.
5. Cheng TE, Wallis JA, Taylor NF, et al. A Prospective Randomized Clinical Trial in Total Hip Arthroplasty-Comparing Early Results Between the Direct Anterior Approach and the Posterior Approach. J Arthroplasty 2017; 32:883–890.
6. Peters RM, van Beers LWAH, van Steenbergen LN, et al. Similar superior patient-reported outcome measures for anterior and posterolateral approaches after total hip arthroplasty: postoperative patient-reported outcome measure improvement after 3 months in 12,774 primary total hip arthroplasties using the anterior, anterolateral, straight lateral, or posterolateral approach. J Arthroplasty 2018; 33:1786–1793.
7. Maldonado DR, Kyin C, Walker-Santiago R, et al. Direct anterior approach versus posterior approach in primary total hip replacement: comparison of minimum 2-year outcomes. Hip Int 2019; 31:166–173.
8. Ozaki Y, Baba T, Homma Y, et al. Posterior versus direct anterior approach in total hip arthroplasty: difference in patient-reported outcomes measured with the Forgotten Joint Score-12. Sicot J 2018; 4:54.
9. Zhao HY, Kang PD, Xia YY, et al. Comparison of early functional recovery after total hip arthroplasty using a direct anterior or posterolateral approach: a randomized controlled trial. J Arthroplasty 2017; 32:3421–3428.
10. Aggarwal VK, Weintraub S, Klock J, et al. 2019 Frank Stinchfield Award: A comparison of prosthetic joint infection rates between direct anterior and non-anterior approach total hip arthroplasty. Bone Joint J 2019; 101-B:2–8.

11. Kuijpers MFL, Hannink G, Vehmeijer SBW, et al. The risk of revision after total hip arthroplasty in young patients depends on surgical approach, femoral head size and bearing type; an analysis of 19,682 operations in the Dutch arthroplasty register. BMC Musculoskelet Disord 2019; 20:385.

12. Zijlstra WP, De Hartog B, Van Steenbergen LN, et al. Effect of femoral head size and surgical approach on risk of revision for dislocation after total hip arthroplasty. Acta Orthop 2017; 88:395–401.

13. Panichkul P, Parks N, Ho H, et al. New approach and stem increased femoral revision rate in total hip arthroplasty. Orthopedics 2015; 31:1–7.

14. Meneghini RM, Elston AS, Chen AF, et al. Direct anterior approach: risk factor for early femoral failure of cementless total hip arthroplasty: a multicenter study. J Bone Joint Surg Am 2017; 99:99–105.

15. Angerame MR, Fehring TK, Masonis JL, et al. Early failure of primary total hip arthroplasty: is surgical approach a risk factor? J Arthroplasty 2018; 33:1780–1785.

16. Eto S, Hwang K, Huddleston JI, et al. The direct anterior approach is associated with early revision total hip arthroplasty. J Arthroplasty 2017; 32:1001–1005.

17. Pincus D, Jenkinson R, Paterson M, et al. Association between surgical approach and major surgical complications in patients undergoing total hip arthroplasty. JAMA 2020; 323:1070–1076.

18. Cidambi KR, Barnett SL, Mallette PR, et al. Impact of femoral stem design on failure after anterior approach total hip arthroplasty. J Arthroplasty 2018; 33:800–804.

19. Sheth D, Cafri G, Inacio MC, et al. Anterior and anterolateral approaches for THA are associated with lower dislocation risk without higher revision risk. Clin Orthop Relat Res 2015; 473:3401–3408.

20. Janssen L, Wijnands KAP, Janssen D, et al. Do stem design and surgical approach influence early aseptic loosening in cementless THA? Clin Orthop Relat Res 2018; 476:1212–1220.

21. Panichkul P, Bavonratanavech S, Arirachakaran A, et al. Comparative outcomes between collared versus collarless and short versus long stem of direct anterior approach total hip arthroplasty: a systematic review and indirect meta-analysis. Eur J Orthop Surg Traumatol 2019; 29:1693–1704.

22. Holst DC, Levy DL, Angerame MR, Yang CC. Does the use of intraoperative fluoroscopy improve postoperative radiographic component positioning and implant size in total hip arthroplasty utilizing a direct anterior approach? Arthroplast Today 2019; 6:94–98.

23. Bingham JS, Spangehl MJ, Hines JT, et al. Does intraoperative fluoroscopy improve limb-length discrepancy and acetabular component positioning during direct anterior total hip arthroplasty? J Arthroplasty 2018; 33:2927.

24. Jennings JD, Iorio J, Kleiner MT, et al. Intraoperative fluoroscopy improves component position during anterior hip arthroplasty. Orthopedics 2015; 38:e970–e975.

25. McNabb DC, Jennings JM, Levy DL, et al. Direct anterior hip replacement does not pose undue radiation exposure risk to the patient or surgeon. J Bone Joint Surg Am 2020; 99:2020–2025.

26. Jinnai Y, Baba T, Zhuang X. Does a fluoro-assisted direct anterior approach for total hip arthroplasty pose an excessive risk of radiation exposure to the surgeon? SICOT J 2020; 6:6.

Chapter 4

What is new in total hip arthroplasty? A Latin-American Perspective in 2020

Claudio Diaz-Ledezma, Cristián Morales Huircaman

INTRODUCTION

During the last century, in Latin America and particularly in Chile, we have followed international trends in orthopaedics, by adapting experiences from the United States and Europe to our own patient population. In the year 2020, with a pandemic affecting orthopaedic practices all over the world, we have incorporated, faster than ever, some of the technologies that are changing patients' care.

In this chapter, we will describe some of the most important current concepts related to the management of total hip arthroplasty (THA) demand and efficiency, from the perspective of two Latin American surgeons practicing both in public and private hospitals in a country considerably affected by the novel coronavirus disease 2019 (COVID-19) crisis.

THE IMPACT OF THE COVID-19 CRISIS ON ELECTIVE AND EMERGENCY (FRACTURE-RELATED) THA

Since the arrival of the coronavirus to Latin America on February 25, 2020 [1,2], the measures adopted by the different governments have failed to stop the spread of the pandemic. According to the latest reports from the World Health Organization, Latin America concentrates 40% of new cases worldwide [3].

The current COVID-19 crisis has caused an unprecedented global economic recession, the worst since 1870 [4,5]. Considering that we, as a region, represent only 8% of global gross domestic product (GDP) [6], we should expect a social impact even more substantial than in other world regions.

Specifically, in the area of orthopaedics, the consequences may be dramatic. Chile and the rest of the countries in the region do not have national arthroplasty registries [7], so the magnitude of the impact is still unknown. However, the policies adopted have not been different from those of the United States and Europe, where all kinds of elective arthroplasties,

Claudio Diaz-Ledezma MD, Clinica Las Condes & Hospital El Carmen de Maipú. Santiago, Chile
Email: claudioadiaz@gmail.com

Cristián Morales Huircaman MD, Hospital El Carmen de Maipú & Clinica Red Salud Santiago, Santiago, Chile
Email: crmorale@gmail.com

including revision surgeries, were cancelled at some point [8–10]. While we are writing this chapter, we are still not allowed to resume elective surgery by our government authorities.

Orthopaedic services have had to be restructured. The number of emergency trauma cases decreased due to social isolation; however, in a recent report, the incidence of osteoporotic hip fractures in older adults has surprisingly remained stable [11]. This group of patients represents a population particularly vulnerable to COVID-19 given their older age and underlying comorbidities, with a reported mortality of between 13 and 20% in those over 80 years of age [12].

A recent multicenter study shows the complexity of these patients' prognosis, with a mortality of 30.4% for older adults with a hip fracture and confirmation of COVID-19 by polymerase chain reaction (PCR) test [13]. Notwithstanding these numbers, surgical resolution, especially hip arthroplasty, contributes to the management of COVID patients by allowing early mobilisation and improving respiratory mechanics [14].

In Chile, by June 2020, we have not yet reached the peak of the COVID-projected cases. Hip replacement surgery in patients with hip fractures remains an emergency. Our challenge is to determine if the present protocols will translate into better results for our patients.

INNOVATIONS TO IMPROVE SURGICAL PRACTICES

The crisis of Latin American health systems in times of COVID may favour the implementation of emerging technologies. From this perspective, the concept of *Disruptive Innovation* popularised in 1995 by Clayton Christensen [15] offers a framework for developing tactics to improve the quality of care while controlling costs [16]. In the field of orthopaedics, we believe that telemedicine, telerehabilitation, and the widespread use of artificial intelligence are the disruptive innovations that have had the most impact during this pandemic.

Telemedicine is defined as the remote diagnosis and treatment of patients through telecommunications technology [17]. Its implementation has allowed delivering quality medical care while complying with the rules of social distancing, preventing virus transmission, and protecting healthcare workers [18]. Its explosive use in the US is reflected in a recent study, where 83% of the 106 institutions consulted reported the current pandemic as the reason for implementing telemedicine [19]. In the particular field of adult reconstruction, telemedicine, before the COVID scenario, has demonstrated to decrease the number of unscheduled consultations with no compromise on patient satisfaction [20]. In Chile, telemedicine began its development in 1993 [21]. It has been proven that orthopaedic telemedicine is applicable in our country [22]. Our group started with telemedicine and telerehabilitation in 2019 using the Physitrack platform. However, as in leading countries, it is not until these days that it was vertiginously implemented in the field of orthopaedics.

Machine learning is a branch of artificial intelligence [23] that builds computer algorithms ('machines') to identify ('learn') patterns and characteristics contained within a database [24]. Its aim is to create predictive algorithms [24]. Its development in the health area is linked to the immense and growing number of data ('Big Data') collected over an extended period of time [25]. Specifically, in the field of adult reconstruction, the application of these new technologies has allowed to predict hospital stays and generate payment models according to pre-operative risk [26], to develop predictive models for prolonged use of opioids [27], among others.

Aiming to follow the same standards of the leading countries [28], our group developed the first predictive model for length of stay in patients undergoing THA, by using machine learning. We are working with a public database of hospital discharges (>1,000,000) from the Ministry of Health. Such is the interest in this project that we have been awarded and funded by the Chilean Society of Orthopaedics and Traumatology [29].

In regards to the use of robotics in THA, some groups have been gaining experience in our country, with no published data to the best of our knowledge. We are completely in agreement with some of the most pre-eminent American surgeons who, in the case of robotics and arthroplasty, have declared that – 'In the era of value-based healthcare, new innovations should improve the quality of arthroplasty care to justify their increased cost to the healthcare system' [30].

RATE OF UTILISATION AND DISPARITIES IN TOTAL HIP ARTHROPLASTY ACCESS

According to the US National Institute of Health (NIH), health disparities are the differences in the incidence, prevalence, mortality, and burden of diseases and other adverse health conditions that exist among specific population groups [31]. The disparity in access to THA is a significant and complex problem in some countries and includes factors such as access to specialist care, patient characteristics, and insurance [32–36]. In Chile, since 2006, the law guarantees access to surgical treatment of severe hip osteoarthritis for those patients who are >65 years of age. However, it is unknown if our health policies have an impact on egalitarian access to THA.

A recent study from our group (in review) calculated a mean utilisation rate of THA in Region Metropolitana between 2016 and 2018, which was 144/100,000 for patients 65 years of age and older. Our mean utilisation rate is low, even under the 2011 Organisation for Economic Co-operation and Development (OECD) average (164/100,000 patients 65 years of age and older) [37]. We were able to demonstrate that poverty rate at the patient's living area and type of insurance were two factors that correlate with mean utilisation rate in Region Metropolitana (a geographical area with 6,061,185 inhabitants, equivalent to 40.1% of the national population). The higher the poverty rate, the lower the access measured as mean utilisation rate. In areas of low-poverty rate (<10%), the 51% of the cases were operated under private insurance, with a statistically significant difference compared to areas where the poverty rate is higher than 30%, where only 4.5% of the cases were operated under private insurance.

We believe that the first step to resolve inequalities is to recognise them. Thus, our next step, as a country, will be to create a strategy to overcome this significant issue that affects our patients, especially when elective surgeries are resumed.

FOLLOWING THE AMERICAN TRENDS TO IMPROVE QUALITY

We expect that the demand for total hip replacement in our region will increase after the COVID crisis. A recent survey among American Association of Hip and Knee Surgeons (AAHKS) international members (in which 37 of the 99 participants were Latin American surgeons) showed that the total number of arthroplasty cases deferred by each surgeon was, on average, 81 (range: 4–2000) [8].

The above-mentioned fact imposes us a challenge: to improve the operating room efficiency. A recent study in our country showed that the use of operating rooms is far from ideal. It was estimated that increasing the surgical volume by 27%, with respect to the current volume, has an additional cost of only 7%. Increasing the volume by 106% may have an additional cost of <50% [38]. In this regard, we consider that the overlapping surgery strategy could be an excellent alternative in our setting. It has been proven that overlapping arthroplasty surgeries do not compromise patients' safety nor increase readmissions or complications [39]. Also, this tactic improves the efficiency and revenues for the systems [40]. In Latin America, overlapping surgery in elective total joint arthroplasty is undoubtedly a strategy that should be implemented.

Performing outpatient surgery has already proven to be a reproducible alternative in our setting [41]. We hope that it will be incorporated more massively, as we are convinced it reflects the success and excellence in perioperative care [41].

Similarly, we believe that the incorporation of value-based arthroplasty concepts [42] and bundled-payment models will help to improve the quality of our care [43]. Consequently, it can help to evaluate how hospitals and surgeons perform [44]. Our group, in particular, has already incorporated the Surgeons' Scorecard system [45] because we consider it useful in improving performance. Eventually, with the correct methodology, the creation of performance comparison rankings among institutions should be a contribution to our region.

IMPROVING THE VALUE IN TOTAL HIP ARTHROPLASTY

The numerator of the value equation: Acting on patient-reported outcome measures

Decision support tools have a role in our daily practice as arthroplasty surgeons [46,47]. The Arthroplasty Candidacy Help Engine (ACHE) tool allows informing the patient what to expect in terms of post-operative functional improvement [48], using the Oxford Hip Score. This same score has been proven to be useful to predict who is not a good candidate for THA by Masri in his practice [49]. We believe this approach contributes to improve the visualisation of patient-reported outcome measures (PROMs) from the patient's own perspective, and consequently, to enhance the numerator in the value equation.

Regarding the impact of delayed surgical access and its relevance on patients' outcome [50], we must consider that a significant proportion of our population depends on government-funded healthcare to undergo THA. This fact results in many patients being on a 'waiting list' for the procedure. In our country, a universal approach has not been proposed to prioritise patients, so management is 'first come, first serve', which is not only inefficient [51] but may also leave patients relegated more than necessary [21]. Eventually, the 'worse than death' phenomenon may occur, as reported by Scott and cols [52] in the UK. Our group has adopted the Sampietro–Colom score [53] intending to make the prioritisation process auditable and science-based.

To optimise surgical referrals from primary care, we have demonstrated the usefulness of the American Academy of Orthopaedic Surgeons (AAOS) – appropriate use criteria tool [54], which in the hands of primary care physicians performs not inferiorly than formal online education (article in review).

The denominator of the value equation: Costs

Time-driven activity-based cost calculation has recently been shown to be a methodology that better reflects the expenses incurred during the joint arthroplasty episode of care [55,56]. Thus, we believe it should be adopted in our region.

Among the tactics to reduce the costs in joint arthroplasty, bundled payments have demonstrated to succeed [57,58]. However, there are still concerns about the costs of post-discharge care [59], which are difficult to control. We expect that telerehabilitation platforms massification, in agreement with the current evidence [60–62], will spread the word that formal physical therapy for all patients is not an absolute requirement.

Regarding implant costs, which are the most significant proportion of the episode of care [63], we believe that the preferred vendor alternative, as Boylan and Cols demonstrated [64], is a fantastic idea to reduce costs, thus it should be established in our region.

As we have no locally produced data to predict outcomes in our patients, we still rely on calculators produced in the US to predict possible complications [65,66]. To our knowledge, it has not been determined who are the patients that can successfully participate in bundled payment models and who will become 'bundled busters' [67,68] in our region. We hope our initiative [29] will open a door for this type of research by using orthopaedic data science and artificial intelligence in our country.

CONCLUSION

The COVID-19 crisis has imposed enormous challenges on the practice of joint reconstruction surgeons, considering that the vast majority of the procedures we perform are elective. The adventure of innovating in crisis times will be successful if our actions meet the established goals. We firmly believe that the trend towards efficiency, cost containment, 'open innovation' [69], and value creation around THA is the path that Latin America has to follow.

REFERENCES

1. Rodriguez-Morales AJ, Gallego V, et al. COVID-19 in Latin America: The implications of the first confirmed case in Brazil. Travel Med Infect Dis 2020; 35:101613.
2. Burki T. COVID-19 in Latin America. Lancet Infect Dis 2020; 20:547–548.
3. WHO. Coronavirus Disease Situation Report n.d. https://www.who.int/docs/default-source/coronaviruse/situation-reports/20200612-covid-19-sitrep-144.pdf?sfvrsn=66ff9f4f_2 [Last accessed 01 May 2022].
4. The World Bank. The Global Economic Outlook During the COVID-19 Pandemic: A Changed World n.d. https://www.worldbank.org/en/news/feature/2020/06/08/the-global-economic-outlook-during-the-covid-19-pandemic-a-changed-world# [Last accessed 01 May 2022].
5. The World Bank. Impact of COVID-19 on global poverty. World Bank. n.d. https://blogs.worldbank.org/opendata/updated-estimates-impact-covid-19-global-poverty [Last accessed 01 May 2022.]
6. Comisión Económica para América Latina y el Caribe (CEPAL). Programa de Comparación Internacional (PCI) n.d. https://www.cepal.org/es/comunicados/america-latina-caribe-representa-8-pib-global-la-poblacion-mundial-segun-nuevo-informe [Last accessed 01 May 2022].
7. Figueroa D, Figueroa F, Calvo R, et al. Trends in Total Knee Arthroplasty in a Developing Region: A Survey of Latin American Orthopaedic Surgeons. J Am Acad Orth Surg 2020; 28:189–193.
8. Athey AG, Cao L, Okazaki K, et al. Survey of AAHKS International Members on the Impact of COVID-19 on Hip and Knee Arthroplasty Practices. J Arthroplasty 2020; 35:S89–S94.
9. Bedard NA, Elkins JM, Brown TS. Effect of COVID-19 on Hip and Knee Arthroplasty Surgical Volume in the United States. J Arthroplasty 2020; 35:S45–S48.

10. Thaler M, Khosravi I, Hirschmann MT, et al. Disruption of joint arthroplasty services in Europe during the COVID-19 pandemic: an online survey within the European Hip Society (EHS) and the European Knee Associates (EKA). Knee Surg Sports Traumatol Arthrosc 2020; 28:1712–1719.

11. Nuñez JH, Sallent A, Lakhani K, et al. Impact of the COVID-19 Pandemic on an Emergency Traumatology Service: Experience at a Tertiary Trauma Centre in Spain. Injury 2020; 51: 1414–1418.

12. Our World In Data. Mortality Risk of COVID-19 n.d. https://ourworldindata.org/mortality-risk-covid#the-current-case-fatality-rate-of-covid-19 [Last accessed 01 May 2022].

13. Muñoz Vives JM, Jornet-Gibert M, et al. Mortality Rates of Patients with Proximal Femoral Fracture in a Worldwide Pandemic: Preliminary Results of the Spanish HIP-COVID Observational Study*. J Bone Joint Surg 2020; 02:e69.

14. Catellani F, Coscione A, D'Ambrosi R, et al. Treatment of Proximal Femoral Fragility Fractures in Patients with COVID-19 During the SARS-CoV-2 Outbreak in Northern Italy. J Bone Joint Surg 2020.

15. Harvard Business Review. What Is Disruptive Innovation? Harvard Business Review. n.d. https://hbr.org/2015/12/what-is-disruptive-innovation [Last accessed 01 May 2022].

16. Hansen E, Bozic KJ. The Impact of Disruptive Innovations in Orthopaedics. Clin Orthop Relat Res 2009; 467:2512–2520.

17. Bashshur RL, Shannon GW, Krupinski EA, et al. National Telemedicine Initiatives: Essential to Healthcare Reform. Telemed E Health 2009; 15:600–610.

18. Loeb AE, Rao SS, Ficke JR, et al. Departmental Experience and Lessons Learned With Accelerated Introduction of Telemedicine During the COVID-19 Crisis. J Am Acad Orthop Surg 2020; 28:e469–e476.

19. Parisien RL, Shin M, Constant M, et al. Telehealth Utilization in Response to the Novel Coronavirus (COVID-19) Pandemic in Orthopaedic Surgery. J Am Acad Orthop Surg 2020; 28:e487–92.

20. Sharareh B, Schwarzkopf R. Effectiveness of Telemedical Applications in Postoperative Follow-Up After Total Joint Arthroplasty. J Arthroplasty 2014; 29:918–922.e1.

21. Programa Nacional de Telesalud n.d. https://www.minsal.cl/wp-content/uploads/2018/03/Programa-Nacional-de-Telesalud.pdf [Last accessed 01 May 2022].

22. Prada C, Izquierdo N, Traipe R, Figueroa C. Results of a New Telemedicine Strategy in Traumatology and Orthopedics. Telemed J E Health 2019; 99:2020–2025.

23. Myers TG, Ramkumar PN, Ricciardi BF, et al. Artificial Intelligence and Orthopaedics: An Introduction for Clinicians. J Bone Joint Surg 2020; 102:830–840.

24. Bayliss L, Jones LD. The role of artificial intelligence and machine learning in predicting orthopaedic outcomes. Bone Joint J 2019; 101-B:1476–1478.

25. Shaha SH, Sayeed Z, Anoushiravani AA, El-Othmani MM, Saleh KJ. Big Data, Big Problems. Orthop Clin N Am 2016; 47:725–732.

26. Ramkumar PN, Navarro SM, Haeberle HS, et al. Development and Validation of a Machine Learning Algorithm After Primary Total Hip Arthroplasty: Applications to Length of Stay and Payment Models. J Arthroplasty 2019; 34:632–637.

27. Karhade AV, Schwab JH, Bedair HS. Development of Machine Learning Algorithms for Prediction of Sustained Postoperative Opioid Prescriptions After Total Hip Arthroplasty. J Arthroplasty 2019; 34:2272–2277.e1.

28. Diaz Ledezma C, Radovic I. What's new in hip arthroplasty? South American perspective. Recent Advances in Orthopedics-2. New Delhi: Jaypee Brothers Medical Publishers (P) Ltd.; 2018.

29. Díaz-Ledezma C, Díaz-Solís D, Muñoz-Reyes R, Castro JT. Premio de Investigación SCHOT 2020: desarrollo y validación de un modelo multivariables de predicción de estadía hospitalaria en pacientes mayores de 65 años sometidos artroplastia total de cadera electiva en Chile utilizando aprendizaje de máquinas. Revista Chilena de Ortopedia y Traumatología 2021; 62:e180–192.

30. Booth RE, Sharkey PF, Parvizi J. Robotics in Hip and Knee Arthroplasty: Real Innovation or Marketing Ruse. J Arthroplasty 2019; 34:2197–2198.

31. National Heart, Lung, and Blood Institute, National Institutes of Health. Health Disparities, NHLBI, NIH. https://www.nhlbi.nih.gov/health/educational/healthdisp/#source1 [Last accessed 01 May 2022].

32. Ibrahim SA. Racial and ethnic disparities in hip and knee joint replacement: a review of research in the Veterans Affairs Health Care System. J Am Acad Orthop Surg 2007; 15:S87–S94.

33. Morgan RC, Slover J. Breakout session: Ethnic and racial disparities in joint arthroplasty. Clin Orthop Relat Res 2011; 469:1886–1890.

34. Wang Y, Simpson JA, Wluka AE, et al. Reduced rates of primary joint replacement for osteoarthritis in Italian and Greek migrants to Australia: the Melbourne Collaborative Cohort Study. Arthritis Res Ther 2009; 11:R86.

35. Martin CT, Callaghan JJ, Liu SS, Gao Y, Johnston RC. Disparity in preoperative patient factors between insurance types in total joint arthroplasty. Orthopedics 2012; 35:e1798–1803.
36. Dunlop DD, Manheim LM, Song J, et al. Age and racial/ethnic disparities in arthritis-related hip and knee surgeries. Med Care 2008; 46:200–208.
37. Pabinger C, Geissler A. Utilization rates of hip arthroplasty in OECD countries. Osteoarthritis Cartilage 2014; 22:734–741.
38. Comisión Nacional de Productividad | Estudio "Eficiencia en Pabellones y priorización de pacientes para cirugía electiva" n.d. https://www.comisiondeproductividad.cl/estudios/estudios-finalizados-mandatados-por-el-gobierno-de-chile/eficiencia-en-pabellones-y-priorizacion-de-pacientes-para-cirugia-electiva/ [Last accessed 01 May 2022].
39. Suarez JC, Al-Mansoori AA, Borroto WJ, Villa JM, Patel PD. The Practice of Overlapping Surgery Is Safe in Total Knee and Hip Arthroplasty. JB JS Open Access 2018; 3:e0004.
40. Zachwieja E, Yayac M, Wills BW, et al. Overlapping Surgery Increases Operating Room Efficiency Without Adversely Affecting Outcomes in Total Hip and Knee Arthroplasty. J Arthroplasty 2020; 35:1529–1533.e1.
41. Paredes O, Ñuñez R, Klaber I. Successful initial experience with a novel outpatient total hip arthroplasty program in a public health system in Chile. Int Orthop 2018; 42:1783–1787.
42. Schwartz AJ, Bozic KJ, Etzioni DA. Value-based Total Hip and Knee Arthroplasty: A Framework for Understanding the Literature. J Am Acad Orthop Surg 2019; 27:1–11.
43. Preston JS, Caccavale D, Smith A, et al. Bundled Payments for Care Improvement in the Private Sector: A Win for Everyone. J Arthroplasty 2018; 33:2362–2367.
44. van Schie P, van Steenbergen LN, van Bodegom-Vos L, Nelissen RGHH, Marang-van de Mheen PJ. Between-Hospital Variation in Revision Rates After Total Hip and Knee Arthroplasty in the Netherlands: Directing Quality-Improvement Initiatives. J Bone Joint Surg Am 2020; 102:315–324.
45. Winegar AL, Jackson LW, Sambare TD, et al. A Surgeon Scorecard Is Associated with Improved Value in Elective Primary Hip and Knee Arthroplasty. J Bone Joint Surg Am 2019; 101:152–159.
46. Quintana JM, Bilbao A, Escobar A, Azkarate J, Goenaga JI. Decision trees for indication of total hip replacement on patients with osteoarthritis. Rheumatology (Oxford) 2009; 48:1402–1409.
47. Harris AHS, Kuo AC, Weng Y, et al. Can Machine Learning Methods Produce Accurate and Easy-to-use Prediction Models of 30-day Complications and Mortality After Knee or Hip Arthroplasty? Clin Orthop Relat Res 2019; 477:452–460.
48. Price A, Smith J, Dakin H, et al. The Arthroplasty Candidacy Help Engine tool to select candidates for hip and knee replacement surgery: development and economic modelling. Health Technol Assess 2019; 23:1–216.
49. Neufeld ME, Masri BA. Can the Oxford Knee and Hip Score identify patients who do not require total knee or hip arthroplasty? Bone Joint J 2019; 101-B:23–30.
50. Garbuz DS, Xu M, Duncan CP, Masri BA, Sobolev B. Delays worsen quality of life outcome of primary total hip arthroplasty. Clin Orthop Relat Res 2006; 447:79–84.
51. Fielden JM, Cumming JM, Horne JG, et al. Waiting for hip arthroplasty: economic costs and health outcomes. J Arthroplasty 2005; 20:990–997.
52. Scott CEH, MacDonald DJ, Howie CR. "Worse than death" and waiting for a joint arthroplasty. Bone Joint J 2019; 101-B:941–950.
53. Sampietro-Colom L, Espallargues M, Rodríguez E, Comas M, Alonso J, Castells X, et al. Wide social participation in prioritizing patients on waiting lists for joint replacement: a conjoint analysis. Med Decis Making 2008; 28:554–566.
54. Rees HW. Management of Osteoarthritis of the Hip. J Am Acad Orthop Surg 2020; 28:e288.
55. Akhavan S, Ward L, Bozic KJ. Time-driven Activity-based Costing More Accurately Reflects Costs in Arthroplasty Surgery. Clin Orthop Relat Res 2016; 474:8–15.
56. Palsis JA, Brehmer TS, Pellegrini VD, Drew JM, Sachs BL. The Cost of Joint Replacement: Comparing Two Approaches to Evaluating Costs of Total Hip and Knee Arthroplasty. J Bone Joint Surg Am 2018; 100:326–333.
57. Siddiqi A, White PB, Mistry JB, et al. Effect of Bundled Payments and Health Care Reform as Alternative Payment Models in Total Joint Arthroplasty: A Clinical Review. J Arthroplasty 2017; 32:2590–2597.
58. Murphy WS, Siddiqi A, Cheng T, et al. 2018 John Charnley Award: Analysis of US Hip Replacement Bundled Payments: Physician-initiated Episodes Outperform Hospital-initiated Episodes. Clin Orthop Relat Res 2019; 477:271–280.
59. Slover JD. You Want a Successful Bundle: What About Post-discharge Care? J Arthroplasty 2016; 31:936–937.
60. Klement MR, Rondon AJ, McEntee RM, Kheir M, Austin MS. Web-Based, Self-Directed Physical Therapy After Total Hip Arthroplasty Is Safe and Effective for Most, but Not All, Patients. J Arthroplasty 2019; 34:513–516.

61. Austin MS, Urbani BT, Fleischman AN, et al. Formal Physical Therapy After Total Hip Arthroplasty Is Not Required: A Randomized Controlled Trial. J Bone Joint Surg Am 2017; 99:648–655.

62. Kuether J, Moore A, Kahan J, et al. Telerehabilitation for Total Hip and Knee Arthroplasty Patients: A Pilot Series with High Patient Satisfaction. HSS J 2019; 15:221–225.

63. Carducci MP, Gasbarro G, Menendez ME, et al. Variation in the Cost of Care for Different Types of Joint Arthroplasty. J Bone Joint Surg Am 2020; 102:404–409.

64. Boylan MR, Chadda A, Slover JD, et al. Preferred Single-Vendor Program for Total Joint Arthroplasty Implants: Surgeon Adoption, Outcomes, and Cost Savings. J Bone Joint Surg Am 2019; 101:1381–3187.

65. Pugely AJ, Callaghan JJ, Martin CT, Cram P, Gao Y. Incidence of and risk factors for 30-day readmission following elective primary total joint arthroplasty: analysis from the ACS-NSQIP. J Arthroplasty 2013; 28:1499–1504.

66. Edelstein AI, Kwasny MJ, Suleiman LI, et al. Can the American College of Surgeons Risk Calculator Predict 30-Day Complications After Knee and Hip Arthroplasty? J Arthroplasty 2015; 30:5–10.

67. Luzzi AJ, Fleischman AN, Matthews CN, et al. The "Bundle Busters": Incidence and Costs of Postacute Complications Following Total Joint Arthroplasty. J Arthroplasty 2018; 33:2734–2739.

68. Wodowski AJ, Pelt CE, Erickson JA, et al. "Bundle busters": who is at risk of exceeding the target payment and can they be optimized? Bone Joint J 2019; 101-B:64–69.

69. Dahlander L, Wallin M. Why Now Is the Time for "Open Innovation." Harvard Business Review 2020. https://hbr.org/2020/06/why-now-is-the-time-for-open-innovation [Last accessed 01 May, 2022].

Chapter 5

What is new in total knee arthroplasty? In klein/courtney recent advances in orthopaedics

Chad A Krueger, Jess H Lonner

INTRODUCTION

Total knee arthroplasty (TKA) is one of the most widely performed procedures within the United States and has consistently been shown to be a cost-effective treatment of degenerative and post-traumatic osteoarthritis [1]. Most TKA components have an expected survival rate of over 95% at 10 years post-operatively [2]. Therefore, if the proper patient is selected and the procedure is well-performed, the majority of patients should greatly benefit from TKA. In this chapter, we will summarise some of the recent literature related to TKA in order to assist in optimising patient outcomes from this impactful intervention.

PATIENT SELECTION (TABLE 5.1)

Ensuring that each patient is properly indicated for TKA is the first step to a good outcome. While older patients tend to have more medical comorbidities compared to younger patients, when those comorbidities are controlled for, older patients have similar patient-reported outcomes [3]. Therefore, patient age, in and of itself, should not be considered a contraindication for a TKA. On the other hand, performing a TKA in a very young and active may put the implants at risk for early failure, despite excellent short-term functional outcomes [4]. More critical than the issue of older age, per se, is the physiological age and presence of comorbidities. While there are many medical comorbidities and behaviours that have been shown to increase the risk of complications after TKA (i.e., diabetes, heart disease, renal disease, liver failure, smoking, etc.), many of the complications related to these medical comorbidities can be decreased by properly managing the patients in the perioperative period. Such management, however, may not decrease the complications associated with some patient comorbidity characteristics. Christensen et al have found that

Chad A Krueger MD, Rothman Orthopaedic Institute, Assistant Professor, Orthopaedic Surgery Sidney Kimmel Medical College, Philadelphia, USA
Email: Chad.krueger@rothmanortho.com

Jess H Lonner MD, Rothman Orthopaedic Institute, Professor of Orthopaedic Surgery, Sidney Kimmel Medical College at Thomas Jefferson University, Philadelphia, USA
Email: Jess.lonner@rothmanortho.com

Table 5.1 A table listing some of the modifiable and nonmodifiable risk factors associated with complications after total knee arthroplasty	
Patient risk factors for complications	
Modifiable	Non-modifiable
Oral health	Advanced age
Glycaemic control	Gender
Malnutrition	Socioeconomic status
Smoking	Haemodialysis
Immunosuppressive or immunomodulating medications	Dementia
Obesity	Previous cerebrovascular or cardiac event
Colonisation with *Staphylococcus aureus*	Previous surgery on ipsilateral joint
Anaemia	Height
Alcohol abuse	
Depression/anxiety	

increased patient body mass index (BMI), body surface area, and height are all associated with increased rates of revision, aseptic loosening, and other complications after TKA [5]. While a patients BMI can be decreased with weight loss, body surface area and height are much harder to modify. In addition, a patient's nutritional status should be optimised preoperatively. While screening for malnourishment is not common in some practices, there is a growing body of literature showing that malnourished patients, no matter their weight, are more likely to have complications after TKA [6]. This is likely secondary to the important role that nutrition plays in wound healing.

It is also important to consider a patient's prior procedures when counselling them preoperatively. Patients undergoing a TKA for post-traumatic osteoarthritis may be at an increased risk for arthrofibrosis and complications overall [7]. A retrospective study by Watters et al also showed that the risk of reoperation for patients undergoing TKA after having a previous anterior cruciate ligament (ACL) reconstruction was five times higher than those undergoing a TKA without a prior reconstruction [8]. However, Chalmers et al found that patients do very well with a TKA procedure after a previous high-tibial osteotomy [9]. Lastly, if there is a question as to whether the patient may be a better candidate for a unicompartmental knee arthroplasty (UKA) or a TKA, surgeons should take solace in the results of the TOPKAT study. In this large, randomised controlled trial (RCT) evaluating which intervention (UKA or TKA) may be best for patients with predominantly unicompartmental arthrosis, the authors found that both procedures offered similar outcomes, complications, and rates of reoperation [10].

BEARING DESIGN

There is no recent data showing the superiority of posterior stabilised (PS), ultracongruent (UC), or cruciate retaining (CR) knees in relationship to each other in terms of revision rates or patient outcomes [11]. However, there continues to be data demonstrating that PS TKAs generally have superior range of motion to CR TKAs [12]. In terms of fixed or mobile-bearing tibial surfaces, Abdel et al did not find any differences in outcomes or revision rates at 10 years postoperatively [13]. Further, there were no measurable differences found in clinical outcomes between TKAs performed with highly cross-linked polyethylene or conventional polyethylene in several recent large analyses [14,15]. Furthermore, when it comes to polyethylene, it is likely that many of the patient's preoperative factors will determine the polyethylene thickness and there is no difference in short-term patient outcomes for thicker polyethylene sizes compared to thinner sizes, provided soft tissue balancing is appropriate, tibial bone quality is reasonable, and joint line restored [16].

In terms of recent data evaluating various TKA designs, a study by Dowesey et al found that medial stabilised implants had similar short-term functional scores when compared to CR and PS designs. Interestingly, the patients in that study who received a medial stabilised knee also reported greater satisfaction at 6 month follow-up compared to patients who received either CR and PS designs [17]. There has also been a renewed interest in cementless TKA designs and a large, prospective, RCT showed equivalent short-term outcomes for both cemented and cementless components of the same design [18]. Such outcomes may make cementless implants more attractive for use in younger patients or those with good bone quality.

LIMB ALIGNMENT AND COMPONENT POSITION

If a surgeon is going to aim for a mechanically aligned knee, the ideal component positioning would, theoretically, leave the limb with neutral alignment in the coronal plane. However, Abdel et al demonstrated that postoperative alignment with up to 3° of variance from neutral alignment conferred no functional or survival benefit for TKA compared to those TKAs that were placed outside of this limit, as long as soft tissues are adequately balanced [19]. These findings are important to consider for two reasons. First, even high-volume surgeons can have mispositioned components in up to 3% of their TKAs and these knees are not necessarily at an increased risk of failure [20]. Second, the notion of kinematic alignment, which aligns the components with respect to the native distal femur and proximal tibia angles while keeping their native soft tissue balance as opposed to mechanically aligned limbs in which the knee joint is reconstructed to be aligned and balanced with the mechanical axis of the entire lower extremity, has yielded excellent clinical outcomes and durability [21]. Third, many new technologies have an explicit aim to help surgeons achieve accurate component placement and good outcomes even if the limb is not perfectly aligned mechanically. However, if there is no clear benefit in terms of modern implant survival or patient outcomes when the components are placed with precise neutral alignment compared to when they are not, alignment may not be the optimal surrogate measure of success and questions the role of popular advanced technologies. Such technologies should also be focussed on improving the balancing the soft tissues, surgical efficiencies, surgical ergonomics, the reduction of inventory and cost-efficacy.

In addition to the coronal alignment of TKA components, it is also important that surgeons aim to optimise the proper axial rotation of femoral and tibial components. While many surgeons use either the transepicondylar axis, Whiteside's line, or reference off of the posterior condylar axis in order to determine femoral rotation, a study by Jang et al showed how difficult it is for surgeons to reliably use any of these measures in isolation to accurately position the femoral component. In their CT-based study involving over 2,000 patients, they found that a combination of all three commonly used methods for femoral component rotation (3° of external rotation from the posterior condyle axis, the Whiteside line, and the anatomic transepicondylar axis) is needed to ensure accurate placement of the femoral component [22]. Furthermore, combining these methods with a soft tissue balancing algorithm is critical for optimising kinematics, stability, and performance.

SOFT-TISSUE BALANCING

While there has been a renewed interest in considering kinematic alignment for TKAs in comparison to mechanical alignment, there is no clear data to support the superiority of one technique over another [23]. While mechanical alignment is the most commonly method used, there are data suggesting that kinematically aligned TKAs have a more normal gait pattern, along with similar survivorship and function compared to mechanically aligned TKA [24]. In terms of measured resection technique versus gap balancing, there is some data suggesting that gap balancing yields superior radiographic and clinical outcomes compared to measured-resection techniques [25], whereas another study found no functional or patient outcome differences when comparing a gap balancing to a measured resection technique when looking at 5 year outcomes for TKAs [26].

PATELLA RESURFACING

While a recent RCT suggests that patella resurfacing leads to improved short-term outcomes after TKA compared to those treated without resurfacing, irrespective of whether there is significant patellar arthritis [27], other studies have found that selectively not resurfacing patellae that are devoid of lateral patellar facet arthritis can produce comparable, or even better, results than resurfacing [28]. In addition, patella resurfacing may not improve the tracking, pain, or revision rate for TKA procedures [28]. A randomised study by Roberts et al that compared patella resurfacing to non-resurfacing in patients without exposed bone on the patella found no clinically significant differences in outcomes at an average follow-up of 7.8 years [29]. There is also conflicting data from the registries from Australia and New Zealand in terms of whether or not routinely resurfacing the patella leads to a higher risk of patella revision [30,31]. Zmistowski et al found that patella resurfacing is not cost-effective in patients in which there was minimal patella arthritis [32]. When considering the severity of complications that can occur from patellar resurfacing (fracture, avascular necrosis, and extensor mechanism disruption), and the inadequacies of their treatments, selective patellar resurfacing, rather than routine resurfacing or not resurfacing, may be a reasonable approach. No matter how the patella is handled intra-operatively, Budhiparama et al demonstrated that there was no additional benefit provided to patients by circumferential patella denervation [33].

Whether the patella is resurfaced or not, it is imperative that the patella track well to ensure an optimal outcome after TKA [34]. Verma et al compared the vertical patella test to the towel clip test in order to see which test may better predict patella tracking intraoperatively. The vertical patella test is performed by everting the patella 90° and translating medially across the femur. If the vertical patella is able to be translated medially enough so that it is at least half way across the trochlea groove, the test is 'positive' and the patella should track well postoperatively, without the need for further releases. The towel clip test is performed by using a towel clip to approximate the medial retinaculum and the vastus medialis intraoperatively and assessing how the patella tracks during knee flexion while the trial or final TKA components are in place. The authors found that the vertical patella test performed as well as the towel clip test at predicting patella tracking while being faster and easier to perform [34].

ROBOTICS

There is growing adoption of robotic-assisted TKA [35], especially as more literature becomes available for surgeons to reference with regard to implementing such technology into their practices and workflow [36,37]. While several studies support the use of robotic assistance in order to more accurately position components [38,39], there are few studies that have looked at the impact of robots on functional outcomes and durability. While Kim et al found no difference in 10 year outcomes between robotic-assisted and conventional TKAs [38], other studies have started to show improved outcomes with robotic-assisted TKAs. In one recent study, a meta-analysis by Agarwal et al demonstrated that robotic-assisted TKA leads to improved Hospital for Special Surgery, Western Ontario and McMaster University scores when compared to conventional TKAs [40]. In addition, Kayani et al found that robotic-assisted TKA patients had increased short-term functional scores and decreased hospital stays compared to conventional TKAs [41]. These improved short-term outcomes seem to be supported by other recent studies as well [42,43].

TOURNIQUET USE

One of the theoretic advantages for using a tourniquet for a TKA is that having a tourniquet in place allows for better cement penetration into the bone during the cementation of components. However, Herndon et al showed that the cement penetration was just as effective when no tourniquet is applied if tranexamic acid (TXA) is used prior to the incision than if a tourniquet was used [44]. Critics of tourniquet use during TKA have suggested that the tourniquet may cause muscle weakness and increased pain postoperatively. However, a prospective, randomised trial comparing TKAs with and without tourniquet use found that there were no differences between groups in terms of short-term function or complications after TKA [24].

INFECTION PREVENTION

Two studies have recently looked at the effect of povidone iodine irrigation during the closure of primary TKAs, with contradictory findings on its effect on decreasing infection risk. One, a retrospective study from the Mayo Clinic found that the addition of povidone iodine did not lead to decreased risks of infection in the 1st year after TKA [45]. The other, a prospective study out of Ottawa did show that the inclusion of a povidone iodine lavage prior to wound closure did lead to a decrease in infections [46]. Recent literature has also made it clear that patients should wait at least 3 months after getting a hyaluronic acid or corticosteroid injection into their knee prior to undergoing a TKA secondary to an increased risk of infection if the injection is given sooner than this time interval [47].

PAIN MANAGEMENT (TABLE 5.2)

The effective management of pain after TKA can impact both short- and long-term outcomes of the procedure [48]. There are myriad methods by which pain can be controlled

Table 5.2 Different analgesia options for various parts of the total knee arthroplasty surgical pathway

Pre-operative	Intra-operative	Post-operative
Nonsteroidal anti-inflammatory drugs	Periarticular injections	Regional blocks
Acetaminophen	Haemostasis	Nonsteroidal anti-inflammatory drugs
Gabapentinoids	Surgeon administered regional blocks	Short-acting opioids
	Corticosteroids	Ice
		Corticosteroids
		Acetaminophen
		Gabapentinoids

after TKA [regional or spinal anaesthesia, periarticular injections, opioids, nonsteroidal anti-inflammatory drugs (NSAIDs), etc.]. In an era of recognition regarding the ills of opioid consumption, if narcotic medications are to be utilised in the treatment of perioperative pain, using the lowest amount possible to control the pain is recommended, and alternative non-opioid medications should be used in concert to reduce opioid requirements. Hannon et al demonstrated that patients used fewer narcotics when they are prescribed 30 immediate release oxycodone pill postoperatively when compared to 90 [49]. In addition, patients should be educated on the proper disposal methods of these medications and a clear plan for opioid use and reduction should be utilised [50].

There have been multiple studies showing that peri-articular injections during and after TKA have similar efficacy to that of epidural anaesthesia and regional blocks [28]. Compared to plain bupivacaine or ropivacaine, periarticular injection with liposomal bupivacaine, is far more expensive and provides equivalent pain control [51,52]. Spinal anaesthesia, while highly effective, increases the risk of urinary retention in men. In that regard, Mahan et al found that spinal anaesthesia with mepivacaine led to a fivefold reduction in urinary retention compared to bupivacaine [53]. Adductor canal blockade (ACB) can be administered in isolation or in conjunction with periarticular injections, with proven reduction in postoperative pain after TKA, without motor blockade [54]. A recent RCT study by Greenky et al found that intra-articular administration of ACB can be performed by the surgical team from within the joint at the time of TKA, with equal efficacy and safety as conventional ACB, but with lower cost [55].

BLOOD AND VENOUS THROMBOEMBOLIC EVENT MANAGEMENT

Multiple studies have demonstrated the efficacy and safety of TXA in reducing bleeding and its consequences after TKA [56]. While many studies have tried to determine an optimal dosing, timing, and route of administration of this drug, almost all of these trials have found the various routes of TXA administration to be equally effective [57]. It also appears that TXA administration is safe for use in patients considered hypercoagulable or previously considered at increased risk of venous thromboembolic events (VTEs), such as those with coagulopathies, cancer history, ischaemic heart disease, or previous venous thromboembolism [58].

The rates of pulmonary embolism (PE) have remained relatively constant in TKA over the past 15 years, despite aggressive forms of thromboprophylaxis [59]. The use of aspirin as a VTE agent has become mainstream for standard risk patients, in part because of studies like that performed by Anderson et al. In their prospective RCT involving 815 total joint arthroplasty patients, they found that there was no difference between aspirin and rivaroxaban in terms of efficacy in preventing VTE postoperatively without any differences in bleeding complications [60]. Furthermore, it appears that aspirin is safe to use as a VTE prophylaxis agent in patients that are at 'high risk' for a postoperative VTE as well, such as patients with hypercoagulability, metastatic cancer, chronic obstructive pulmonary disease, and those with a prior history of stroke [61]. When considering the balance between safety and efficacy, as well as the cost benefits of aspirin compared to other VTE agents [62], it becomes clear why aspirin use for VTE prophylaxis continues to grow [63].

COMPLICATIONS

There are many potential causes of failure for a TKA and learning how to properly evaluate a painful TKA is the first step determining what has gone wrong [64]. One of the most common complications after TKA, idiopathic stiffness, occurs in about 4% of TKA patients. Risk factors for this condition include preoperative stiffness, female gender, and obesity [65]. Manipulation under anaesthesia (MUA) will be required for about 1% of all TKAs and Bozic et al found that about 3.5% of patients who undergo an MUA will end up requiring a revision TKA within 9 months of the procedure for a variety of reasons [66]. Despite improvements in techniques, results of revision for arthrofibrosis remain inferior to those for other reasons, with residual stiffness and functional limitations common [67]. Flexion instability is another relatively common cause of TKA failure with about 10–25% of all revision TKAs being performed for flexion instability [68]. Restoring the patient's posterior condyle offset, ensuring an accurate tibial slope, joint line preservation, and component rotation of all components can help to decrease the risk of flexion instability during a TKA. It is also important to consider that – even when controlling for preoperative factors, patients who are discharged to a rehabilitation facility after TKA have a higher risk of complications, such as infection, and readmission than those discharged to home [69].

REHABILITATION

There is a growing body of literature suggesting that formal physical therapy may not be needed for all patients undergoing TKA and that virtual physical therapy may be equally effective in terms of function, knee motion, and costs [70,71]. In terms of driving after TKA, the most recent data suggests that most patients will regain the ability to drive at the 4-week interval [72] but that some patients may be able to drive sooner than that, particularly after left TKA.

CONCLUSION

In summary, although we continue to refine surgical techniques and perioperative management of our TKA patients, numerous philosophies, care protocols, surgical techniques, and designs may be considered without detriment to the patient, but also sometimes without clear benefit. The field of TKA is ever-changing. What is new in 2020 may seem archaic in 2025, but it is important that sound principles are followed, with the goal always of optimising safe care of our TKA patients [73].

REFERENCES

1. Kamaruzaman H, Kinghorn P, Oppong R. Cost-effectiveness of surgical interventions for the management of osteoarthritis: a systematic review of the literature. BMC Musculoskelet Disord 2017; 18:183.

2. Abdel MP, Ledford CK, Kobic A, Taunton MJ, Hanssen AD. Contemporary failur aetiologies of primary, posterior-stabilised total knee arthroplasty. Bone Joint J 2017; 99-B:647–652.

3. Joly DA, Ludwig T, Mahdavi S, et al. Does Age Influence Patient-Reported Outcomes in Unilateral Primary Total Hip and Knee Arthroplasty? J Arthroplasty 2020; 35:1800–1805.

4. Karas V, Calkins TE, Bryan AJ, et al. Total Knee Arthroplasty in Patients Less Than 50 Years of Age: Results at a Mean of 13 Years. J Arthroplasty 2019; 34:2392–2397.

5. Christensen TC, Wagner ER, Harmsen WS, Schleck CD, Berry DJ. Effect of Physical Parameters on Outcomes of Total Knee Arthroplasty. J Bone Joint Surg Am 2018; 100:1829–1837.

6. Kishawi D, Schwarzman G, Mejia A, Hussain AK, Gonzalez MH. Low Preoperative Albumin Levels Predict Adverse Outcomes After Total Joint Arthroplasty. J Bone Joint Surg Am 2020; 102:889–895.

7. Pinter Z, Jha AJ, McGee A, et al. Outcomes of knee replacement in patients with posttraumatic arthritis due to previous tibial plateau fracture. Eur J Orthop Surg Traumatol 2019; 30:323–328.

8. Watters TS, Zhen Y, Martin JR, et al. Total Knee Arthroplasty After Anterior Cruciate Ligament Reconstruction: Not Just a Routine Primary Arthroplasty. J Bone Joint Surg Am 2017; 99:185–189.

9. Chalmers BP, Limberg AK, Tibbo ME, et al. Total Knee Arthroplasty After High Tibial Osteotomy Results in Excellent Long-Term Survivorship and Clinical Outcomes. J Bone Joint Surg Am 2019; 101:970–978.

10. Beard DJ, Davies LJ, Cook JA, et al. The clinical and cost-effectiveness of total versus partial knee replacement in patients with medial compartment osteoarthritis (TOPKAT): 5-year outcomes of a randomised controlled trial. The Lancet 2019; 394:746–756.

11. Rajgopal A, Aggarwal K, Khurana A, et al. Gait parameters and functional outcomes after total knee arthroplasty using persona knee system with cruciate retaining and ultracongruent knee inserts. J Arthroplasty 2017; 32:87–91..

12. Singleton N, Nicholas B, Gormack N, Stokes A. Differences in outcome after cruciate retaining and posterior stabilized total knee arthroplasty. J Orthop Surg 2019; 27:1–8.

13. Abdel MP, Tibbo ME, Stuart MJ, et al. A randomized controlled trial of fixed- versus mobile-bearing total knee arthroplasty. Bone Joint J 2018; 100-B:925–9.

14. Partridge TCJ, Baker PN, Jameson SS, et al. Conventional Versus Highligh Cross-Linked Polyethylene in Primary Total Knee Replacement: A Comparison of Revision Rates Using Data From the National Joint Registry for England, Wales and Northern Ireland. J Bone Joint Surg Am 2020; 102:119–127.

15. Takemura S, Minoda Y, Sugama R, et al. Comparison of a vitamin E-infused highly crosslinked polyethelene insert and a conventional polyethylene insert for primary total knee arthroplasty at two years postoperatively. Bone Joint J 2019; 101-B:559–564.

16. Garceau SP, Warschawski YS, Tang A, et al. The Effect of Polyethylene Liner Thickness on Patient Outcomes and Failure After Primary Total Knee Arthroplasty. J Arthroplasty 2020; 35:2072–2075.

17. Dowsey MM, Gould DJ, Spelman T, Pandy MG, Choong PF. A Randomized Controlled Trial Comparing a Medial Stabilized Total Knee Prosthesis to a Cruciate Retaining and Posterior Stabilized Design: A Report of the Clinical and Functional Outcomes Following Total Knee Replacement. J Arthroplasty 2020; 35:1583–1590.e2.

18. Nam D, Lawrie CL, Salih R, et al. Cemented Versus Cementless Total Knee Arthroplasty of the Same Modern Design: A Prospective, Randomized Trial. J Bone Joint Surg Am 2019; 101:1185–1192.

19. Abdel MP, Ollivier M, Parratte S, et al. Effect of Postoperative Mechanical Axis Alignment on Survival and Functional Outcomes of Modern Total Knee Arthroplasties with Cement: A Concise Follow-up at 20 Years. J Bone Joint Surg Am 2018; 100:472–478.

20. Kazarian GS, Lawrie CM, Barrack TN, et al. The Impact of Surgeon Volume and Training Status on Implant Alignment in Total Knee Arthroplasty. J Bone Joint Surg Am 2019; 101:1713–1723.

21. Young SW, Sullivan NPT, Walker ML, et al. No Difference in 5-year Clinical or Radiographic Outcomes Between Kinematic and Mechanical Alignment in TKA: A Randomized Controlled Trial. Clin Orthop Relat Res 2020; 478:1271–1279.

22. Jang ES, Connors-Ehlert R, LiArno S, et al. Accuracy of Reference Axes for Femoral Component Rotation in Total Knee Arthroplasty: Computed Tomography-Based Study of 2,128 Femora. J Bone Joint Surg Am 2019; 101:e125.

23. Young SW, Walker ML, Bayan A, et al. The Chitranjan S. Ranawat Award: No difference in 2-year functional outcomes using kinematic versus mechanical alignment in TKA: a randomized controlled clinical trial. Clin Orthop Relat Res 2017; 475:9–20.

24. Goel R, Rondon AJ, Snydor K, et al. Tourniquet Use Does Not Affect Functional Outcomes or Pain After Total Knee Arthroplasty: A Prospective, Double-Blinded, Randomized Controlled Trial. J Bone Joint Surg Am 2019; 101:1821–1828.

25. Huang T, Long Y, George D, Wang W. Meta-analysis of gap balancing versus measured resection techniques in total knee arthroplasty. Bone Joint J 2017; 99-B:151–158.

26. Babazadeh S, Dowsey MM, Vasimalla MG, Stoney JD, Choong PFM. Gap balancing sacrifices joint-line maintenance to improve gap symmetry: 5-year followup of a randomized controlled trial. J Arthroplasty 2018; 33:75–78.

27. Odgaard A, Madsen F, Kristensen PW, Kappel A, Fabrin J. The Mark Coventry Award: patellofemoral arthroplasty results in better range of movement and early patient-reported outcomes than TKA. Clin Orthop Relat Res 2018; 476:87–100.

28. van der M, Michiel J, Mastel MS. Controversial Topics in Total Knee Arthroplasty. JAAOS: Global Research and Reviews 2020; 4:e19.00047.

29. Roberts DW, Hayes TD, Tate CT, Lesko JP. Selective Patellar Resurfacing in Total Knee Arthroplasty: A Prospective, Randomized, Double-Blind Study. J Arthroplasty 2015; 30:216–220.

30. Vertullo CJ, Graves SE, Cuthbert AR, Lewis PL. The Effect of Surgeon Preference for Selective Patellar Resurfacing on Revision Risk in Total Knee Replacement: An Instrumental Variable Analysis of 136,116 Procedures from the Australian Orthopaedic Association National Joint Replacement Registry. J Bone Joint Surg Am 2019; 101:1261–1270.

31. Maney AJ, Koh CK, Frampton CM, Young SW. Usually, Selectively, or Rarely Resurfacing the Patella During Primary Total Knee Arthroplasty: Determining the Best Strategy. J Bone Joint Surg Am 2019; 101:412–420.

32. Zmistowski BM, Fillingham YA, Salmons HI, et al. Routine Patellar Resurfacing During Total Knee Arthroplasty Is Not Cost-Effective in Patients Without Patellar Arthritis. J Arthroplasty 2019; 34:1963–1968.

33. Budhiparama NC, Hidayat H, Novito K, et al. Does Circumferential Patellar Denervation Result in Decreased Knee Pain and Improved Patient-reported Outcomes in Patients Undergoing Non-resurfaced, Simultaneous Bilateral Total Knee Arthroplasty? Clin Orthop Relat Res 2019; 478:2020–2033.

34. Verma A, Lalchandani R. Prospective comparative study of intraoperative "Towel clip test" and "Vertical patella test" assessing lateral retinaculum tightness in patients undergoing TKA. J Clin Orthop Trauma 2019; 10:995–998.

35. Boylan M, Suchman K, Vigdorchik J, Slover J, Bosco J. Technology-Assisted Hip and Knee Arthroplasties: An Analysis of Utilization Trends. J Arthroplasty 2018; 33:1019–1023.

36. Grau L, Lingamfelter M, Ponzio D, et al. Robotic arm assisted total knee arthroplasty workflow optimization, operative times and learning curve. Arthroplast Today 2019; 5:465–470.

37. Lonner JH, Fillingham YA. Pros and Cons: A Balanced View of Robotics in Knee Arthroplasty. J Arthroplasty 2018; 33:2007–2013.

38. Kim YH, Yoon SH, Park JW. Does Robotic-assisted TKA Result in Better Outcome Scores or Long-Term Survivorship Than Conventional TKA? A Randomized, Controlled Trial. Clin Orthop Relat Res 2020; 478:266–275.

39. Gilmour A, MacLean AD, Rowe PJ, et al. Robotic-Arm-Assisted vs Conventional Unicompartmental Knee Arthroplasty. The 2-Year Clinical Outcomes of a Randomized Controlled Trial. J Arthroplasty 2018; 33:S109–115.

40. Agarwal N, To K, McDonnell S, Khan W. Clinical and Radiological Outcomes in Robotic-Assisted Total Knee Arthroplasty: A Systematic Review and Meta-Analysis. J Arthroplasty 2020; 35:3393–3409.e2.

41. Kayani B, Konan S, Tahmassebi J, Pietrzak JRT, Haddad FS. Robotic-arm assisted total knee arthroplasty is associated with improved early functional recovery and reduced time to hospital discharge compared with conventional jig-based total knee arthroplasty: a prospective cohort study. Bone Joint J 2018; 100-B:930–937.

42. Khlopas A, Sodhi N, Hozack WJ, et al. Patient-Reported Functional and Satisfaction Outcomes after Robotic-Arm-Assisted Total Knee Arthroplasty: Early Results of a Prospective Multicenter Investigation. J Knee Surg 2019.

43. Malkani AL, Roche MW, Kolisek FR, et al. New Technology for Total Knee Arthroplasty Provides Excellent Patient-Reported Outcomes: A Minimum Two-Year Analysis. Surg Technol Int 2019; 36:276–280.

44. Herndon CL, Grosso MJ, Sarpong NO, et al. Tibial cement mantle thickness is not affected by tourniquetless total knee arthroplasty when performed with tranexamic acid. Knee Surg Sports Traumatol Arthrosc 2020; 28:1526–1531.

45. Hernandez NM, Hart A, Tauton MJ, et al. Use of Povidone-Iodine Irrigation Prior to Wound Closure in Primary Total Hip and Knee Arthroplasty: An Analysis of 11,738 Cases. J Bone Joint Surg Am 2019; 101:1144–1150.

46. Slullitel PA, Dobransky JS, Bali K, et al. Is There a Role for Preclosure Dilute Betadine Irrigation in the Prevention of Postoperative Infection Following Total Joint Arthroplasty? J Arthroplasty 2020; 35:1374–1378.

47. Richardson SS, Schairer WW, Sculco TP, Sculco PK. Comparison of Infection Risk with Corticosteroid or Hyaluronic Acid Injection Prior to Total Knee Arthroplasty. J Bone Joint Surg Am 2019; 101:112–118.

48. Summers S, Mohile N, McNamara C, et al. Analgesia in Total Knee Arthroplasty: Current Pain Control Modalities and Outcomes. J Bone Joint Surg Am 2020; 102:719–727.

49. Hannon CP, Calkins TE, Li J, et al. The James A Rand Young Investigator's Award: Large Opiod Presriptions Are Unnecessary After Total Joint Arthroplasty: A Randomized Controlled Trial. J Arthroplasty 2019; 34:S4–S10.

50. Nahhas CR, Hannon CP, Yang J, et al. Education Increases Disposal of Unused Opioids After Total Joint Arthroplasty: A Cluser-Randomized Controlled Trial. J Bone Joint Surg Am 2020. Epub ahead of print.

51. Amundson AW, Johnson RL, Abdel MP, et al. A three-arm randomized clinical trial comparing continuous femoral plus single-injection sciatic peripheral nerve blocks versus periarticular injection with ropivacaine or liposomal bupivacaine for patients undergoing total knee arthroplasty. Anesthesiology 2017; 126:1139–1150.

52. Smith EB, Kazarian GS, Maltenfort MG, et al. Periarticular Liposomal Bupivacaine Injection Versus Intra-Articular Bupivacaine Infusion Catheter for Analgesia After Total Knee Arthroplasty: A Double-Blinded, Randomized Controlled. J Bone Joint Surg Am 2017; 99A:1337–1344.

53. Mahan MC, Jildeh TR, Tenbrunsel TN, Davis JJ. Mepivacaine spinal anesthesia facilitates rapid recovery in total knee arthroplasty compared to bupivacaine. J Arthroplasty 2018; 33:1699–1704.

54. Goytizolo EA, Lin Y, Kim DH, et al. Addition of Adductor Canal Block to Periarticular Injection for Total Knee Replacement: A Radomized Trial. J Bone Joint Surg Am 2019; 101:812–820.

55. Greenky MR, McGarth ME, Levicoff EA, et al. Intraoperative Surgeon Administered Adductor Canal Blockade Is Not Inferior to Anethesiologist Administered Adductor Canal Blockade: A Prosepective Randomized Trial. J Arthroplasty 2020; 35:1228–1232.

56. Abdel MP, Chalmers BP, Taunton MJ, et al. Intravenous versus topical tranexamic acid in total knee arthroplasty: both effective in a randomized clinical trial of 640 patients. J Bone Joint Surg Am 2018; 100:1023–1029.

57. Fillingham YA, Darrith B, Calkins TE, et al. Hip Society Research Group. 2019 Mark Coventry Award: a multicentre randomized clinical trial of tranexamic acid in revision total knee arthroplasty: does the dosing regimen matter? Bone Joint J 2019; 101-B:10.

58. Sabbag OD, Abdel MP, Amundson AW, Larson DR, Pagnano MW. Tranexamic Acid Was Safe in Arthroplasty Patients With a History of Venous Thromboembolism: A Matched Outcome Study. J Arthroplasty 2017; 32:S246–S250.

59. Warren JA, Sundaram K, Anis HK, et al. Have Venous Thromboembolism Rates Decreased In Total Hip and Knee Arthroplasty. J Arthroplasty 2020; 35:259–264.

60. Anderson DR, Dunbar M, Murnaghan J, et al. Aspirin or rivaroxaban for VTE prophylaxis after hip or knee arthroplasty. N Engl J Med 2018; 378:699–707.

61. Tan TL, Foltz C, Huang R, et al. Potent Anticoagulation Does Not Reduce Venous Thromboembolism in High-Risk Patients. J Bone Joint Surg Am 2019; 101:589–599.

62. Gutowski CJ, ZZmistowski BM, Lonner JH, Purtill JJ, Parvizi J. Direct Costs of Aspirin versus Warfarin for Venous Thromboembolism Prophylaxis after Total Knee or Hip Arthroplasty. J Arthroplasty 2015; 30:36–38.

63. Bawa H, Weick JW, Dirschl DR, Luu HH. Trends in Deep Vein Thrombosis Prophylaxis and Deep Vein Thrombosis Rates After Total Hip and Knee Arthroplasty. J Am Acad Orthop Surg 2018; 26:698–705.

64. Flierl MA, Sobh AH, Culp BM, Baker EA, Sporer SM. Evaluation of the Painful Total Knee Arthroplasty. J Am Acad Orthop Surg 2019; 27:743–751.

65. Tibbo ME, Limberg AK, Salib CG, et al. Acquired Idiopathic Stiffness After Total Knee Arthroplasty: A Systematic Review and Meta-Analysis. J Bone Joint Surg Am 2019; 101:1320–1330.

66. Bozic KJ, Brigati DP, Huddleston JI, et al. Manipulation Under Anesthesia After Total Knee: Who Still Requires a Revision Arthroplasty? J Arthroplasty 2020; 35:S348–S351.

67. Bingham JS, Bukowski BR, Wyles CC, et al. Rotating-Hinge Revision Total Knee Arthroplasty for Treatment of Severe Arthrofibrosis. J Arthroplasty 2019; 34:S271–S276.

68. Stambough JB, Edwards PK, Mannen EM, et al. Flexion Instability After Total Knee Arthroplasty. J Am Acad Orthop Surg 2019; 27:642–651.

69. McLawhorn AS, Fu MC, Schairer WW, et al. Continued inpatient care after primary total knee arthroplasty increases 30-day postdischarge complications: a propensity score-adjusted analysis. J Arthroplasty 2017; 32:S113–S118.

70. Prvu Bettger J, Green CL, Homes DN, et al. Effects of Virtual Exercise Rehabilitation In-Home Therapy Compared with Traditional Care After Total Knee Arthroplasty: VERITAS, a Randomized Controlled Trial. J Bone Joint Surg Am 2020; 102:101–109.
71. Jansson MM, Rantala A, Miettunen J, Puhto AP, Pikkarainen. The effects and safety of telerehabilitation in patients with lower-limb joint replacement: A systematic review and narrative synthesis. J Telemed Telecare 2020; 1357633X20917868.
72. van der Velden CA, Tolk JJ, Janssen RPA, Reijman M. When is it safe to resume driving after total hip and total knee arthroplasty? A meta-analysis of literature on post-operative brake reaction times. Bone Joint J 2017; 99-B:566–576.
73. Matar HE, Platt SR, Gollish JD, Cameron HU. Overview of Randomized Controlled Trials in Total Knee Arthroplasty (47,675 Patients): What Have We Learnt? J Arthroplasty 2020; 35:1729–1736.e1.

Chapter 6

What is new in knee arthroplasty? European perspective

Tanvir Khan, Andrew Price, Abtin Alvand, William Jackson

INTRODUCTION

Knee arthroplasty is one of the most commonly performed and cost-effective surgical interventions. Europe has had the benefit of having both the first national (Swedish Arthroplasty Register) and largest (National Joint Registry of England and Wales) joint registries in the world. This has enabled a better understanding of both the need and effectiveness of these total knee arthroplasty (TKA). Data from arthroplasty registries indicate that the incidence of both primary and revision knee arthroplasty continues to rise worldwide [1,2]. Despite the overall success, there are a significant proportion of patients who remain dissatisfied following primary arthroplasty [3]. Furthermore, there is an increasing revision burden which is at least partly explained by the increasing numbers of primary arthroplasties being performed, widening indications, and the rising risk of failure with time from implantation.

This chapter focusses on topical developments in the field of knee arthroplasty from a European perspective. It includes changing alignment philosophies, novel implants, surgical techniques, perioperative management, and the increasing revision burden.

EPIDEMIOLOGY

The number of knee replacements performed is increasing worldwide. According to the National Joint Registry (NJR), >100,000 knee replacements are now performed in the

Tanvir Khan PhD, FRCS(Tr&Orth), Senior Knee Fellow, Nuffield Orthopaedic Centre, Windmill Road, Headington, Oxford, UK
Email: Tanvirkhan@doctors.net.uk

Andrew Price PhD, FRCS(Tr&Orth), Professor of Orthopaedic Surgery, Nuffield Orthopaedic Centre and University of Oxford, Windmill Road, Headington, Oxford, UK
Email: andrew.price@ndorms.ox.ac.uk

Abtin Alvand PhD, FRCS(Tr&Orth), Consultant Orthopaedic Surgeon and Senior Clinical Lecturer, Nuffield Orthopaedic Centre and University of Oxford, Nuffield Orthopaedic Centre , Windmill Road, Headington, Oxford, UK
Email: abtin.alvand@ndorms.ox.ac.uk

William Jackson FRCS(Tr&Orth), Consultant Orthopaedic Surgeon, Nuffield Orthopaedic Centre, Windmill Road, Headington, Oxford, UK
Email: william.jackson@ouh.nhs.uk

England and Wales annually. Other European registries have indicated rising annual incidence of primary knee arthroplasty. In the USA, a similar rise has been demonstrated with total procedures in excess of 700,000 per year. Modelling based on data from the UK Clinical Research Practice Datalink database estimated that at the age of 50, the lifetime risk of undergoing TKA is 10.8% for women and 8.1% for men [4]. There are greater numbers of patients under the age of 60 undergoing TKA in the US [5] and these patients are globally at higher risk of revision with a lifetime revision risk of 35% for men and 20% for women [6]. The information is useful when consenting younger patients for their knee surgery but also suggests a projected rise in overall revision rates.

TECHNOLOGICAL ADVANCES IN KNEE ARTHROPLASTY

Total knee replacement design

Posterior cruciate retaining (CR) and posterior cruciate sacrificing (PS) designs continue to be the most commonly used condylar total knee replacement (TKR) options and there remains some debate regarding the superiority of one over the other. A Cochrane review analysed 17 randomised controlled trials (RCTs) including 1,810 patients and 2,206 TKAs. The authors demonstrated a 3.4° higher flexion in patients with posterior stabilised TKAs. Despite the statistically significant difference, it was concluded that the difference would not be clinically relevant. There were no differences found between the groups in terms of patient-reported outcome measures (PROMs), radiological and other clinical outcomes such as pain [7]. In terms of comparative survivorship of PS and CR designs, there have been conflicting reports. The Mayo clinic reported higher survivorship of CR designs in their single-centre series of TKRs performed between 1988 and 1998 (15-year survival 90% for CR and 77% for PS, $p < 0.001$) [8]. More recently, a systematic review and meta-analysis, which included eight RCTs, demonstrated no difference in survivorship between the two designs [9].

Medial pivot designs

Within Europe, there has been greater interest in medial pivot TKA designs which aim to restore kinematics closer to the native knee joint. The medial compartment in the native knee is relatively congruent compared to the lateral side, which translates anteroposteriorly and 'pivots' around the medial compartment during joint motion. Medial pivot TKA designs, which provide greater femoral rollback in the lateral compartment and a relative pivot on the medial side, are thought to increase the contact area and improve kinematics. It has been suggested that patients with bilateral TKAs tend to prefer the side with a medial pivot design compared to the contralateral PS or CR TKA in terms of stability and a more 'normal' feel [10]. Despite this, there is little difference in terms of objective outcomes such as range of motion and PROMs [11]. A systematic review of 1,146 TKAs using the Advance Medial-Pivot system suggested a superior survivorship at 4, 5, and 6 years compared to the NJR published results for unconstrained mobile bearings, PS mobile bearings, constrained condylar bearings, and PS fixed bearings [12]. Other studies have failed to show any significant superiority in terms of survivorship [13].

Alignment philosophies

The standard approach to implantation of TKA has been to achieve neutral mechanical alignment with the anticipation of providing an even distribution of load across the implant surfaces and thus reduce shear forces, reduce potential wear and loosening. Critics of this approach suggest that this largely ignores the native anatomy of the knee and the origin and insertion of soft tissues traversing the joint. There is some evidence from recent studies that only around 5% of individuals have a natural neutral mechanical alignment, which suggests the knee is artificially forced into mechanical alignment during TKR resulting in significant changes to pre-disease knee kinematics post-operatively. This has been suggested as a contributing factor in the dissatisfaction, stiffness, and instability that we see in 15–20% of patient after TKA [3].

Kinematic alignment, a term first coined by Howell, has been suggested as an alternative method, with the aim of placing implants such that the knee's native pre-disease joint line and alignment are restored [14] (**Figure 6.1**). This was initially achieved using patient-specific cutting blocks developed using an MRI scan of the native knee [15]. Computer software would then be used to produce an estimate of the pre-arthritic tibiofemoral articulation. This would allow creation of the cutting blocks, which would allow implantation of the prostheses in the position determined by the software. The technique then progressed to enable the surgeon to use intraoperative landmarks to determine the

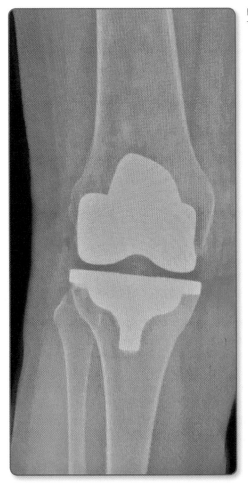

Figure 6.1 Radiograph of a kinematically aligned TKA. TKA, total knee arthroplasty.

bony cuts without the need for patient-specific cutting blocks [16]. Recently published 10-year outcomes data suggests good survivorship of kinematically aligned TKAs [17]. There is also an evidence that kinematically aligned TKAs more closely match native knee kinematics including medial pivot movement and femoral roll back when compared to TKAs which are aligned to the mechanical axis [18,19].

Modified or hybrid versions of the kinematic alignment technique include TKA with functional alignment. Functional alignment techniques aim to achieve a kinematic alignment but within a 'safe' range of coronal alignment of 0 to ±3° [20,21]. This is achieved using a combination of measured resection and gap-balancing strategies. Implant positioning can be modified to account for the native knee's kinematic alignment by modifying the varus-valgus alignment as well as rotation of the implants while also balancing smaller or larger medial/lateral flexion and extension gaps. Functional and hybrid alignment techniques, unlike the kinematic approach, allow minor soft tissue releases where necessary [20–22].

In Europe, there is increasing interest and debate about the use of alternative (non-mechanical) alignment techniques for TKA. Many surgeons believe that a more personalised knee arthroplasty may be one of the strategies for improving outcomes and patient satisfaction after joint arthroplasty.

Robotics

In recent years, there has been a global increasing interest in robotic surgery and this has been seen throughout Europe, particularly in privately funded healthcare systems where cost-effectiveness of treatments has a less impact on adoption of newer technologies (**Figure 6.2**). Knee arthroplasty lends itself well to the possibilities of robotic assistance. It relies on 3D pre-operative imaging of the knee, which uses specialised software to allow planning which optimises individualised bone cuts, implant positioning, and alignment. This pre-operative plan can then be accurately implemented using a robotic device. The technology allows more objective assessment of intraoperative 'knee balance' and can make fine adjustments to the pre-operative plan to optimise the surgery. The first robotic TKA was performed at the Imperial College, London, UK in 1988 using the ACROBOT robotic system (Imperial College, UK) [23]. There are now a number of robotic TKA systems available, which typically either perform all steps of the bony resection (fully active) or allow the surgeon to complete the appropriate cuts as determined by the pre-operative plan (semi-active).

There is some evidence for better accuracy with robotic TKA systems in achieving the planned component positioning, joint line restoration, alignment, and tibial slope when compared with TKA with the traditional jig-based systems [24,25]. In an RCT of 100 TKA patients, Song et al demonstrated superior accuracy in terms of achieving the planned alignment with robotic compared with manual TKA [25,26]. Bellemans reported accuracy to within 1° in all three planes in 25 robotic TKA cases [27]. Recent studies have indicated the learning curve for operative times are 6–20 cases but there was no learning curve demonstrated for implantation of components in the planned positions [28,29].

Optical motion data captured in robotic TKA provides information on alignment, range of motion, flexion/extension gaps, component position, and laxity. Kayani et al demonstrated that robotic TKA resulted in less inadvertent soft tissue injury and trauma to the cut bony surface compared to jig-based TKA in a comparative cohort study of 60 TKAs [30].

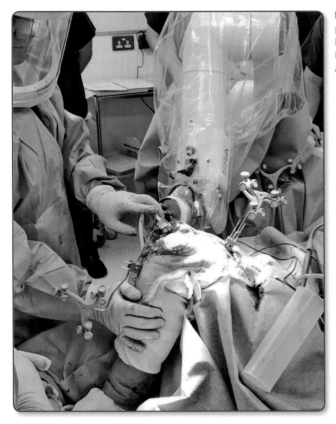

Figure 6.2 Intraoperative photograph of TKA using ROSA Robotic Knee System (Zimmer Biomet, USA). TKA, total knee arthroplasty.

The same group compared early post-operative recovery following robotic TKA with patients undergoing manual unicompartmental knee arthroplasty (UKA) [31,32]. They reported reduced post-operative swelling, lower analgesia requirements, decreased time to straight leg raise, and better knee range of motion at discharge in the robotic TKA group [32]. In terms of PROMs at 6 months post-TKA, Marchand demonstrated better pain, patient satisfaction, and physical function scores in a cohort of robotic TKA patients compared with a matched jig-based TKA cohort [33].

Studies reporting medium- and long-term results of robotic TKA have failed to show any significant improvement in functional outcomes compared to conventional jig-based TKA. At 2 years, both Song et al [25,26] and Liow et al [34] showed no significant difference in functional outcomes scored between robotic TKA and conventional jig-based TKA. Yang et al published a 10-year comparative outcomes which also demonstrated no difference between the groups [35].

Cost associated with robotic knee arthroplasty is one of the main reasons for the slower uptake in usage at present. In addition, there are still some concerns reported by users of instances of soft-tissue injury and intra-operative technical issues requiring a need to revert to conventional jig-based instrumentation [36]. However, within Europe, it looks like this technology is here to stay. We envisage that if this technology can be married with the more personalised alignment philosophies, it could allow surgeons to achieve better functional outcomes and long-term survival of implants.

UNICOMPARTMENTAL KNEE ARTHROPLASTY

At present, global as well as European data shows that most patients requiring knee arthroplasty undergo TKA. In the UK, approximately 8% of primary knee arthroplasties are UKAs and this figure has remained relatively static [37]. It has been estimated that 25–47% of patients who are eligible for knee arthroplasty have single compartment disease and, therefore, would be candidates for both TKA and UKA [38]. The relative low proportion of UKA is a due to a combination of a higher perceived risk of revision, which is supported by global joint registry data, and surgeon/unit experience [39,40]. NJR data in 2017 demonstrated that only 38% of surgeons that reported performing TKA to the registry also performed UKA [37]. The debate around TKA versus UKA for patients who are suitable for both continues.

The TOPKAT study, which was conducted in the UK, is the largest multicentre RCT comparing TKA and UKA for patients with isolated medial compartment disease and the 5-year outcomes were recently published [41]. The study demonstrated a modest clinical benefit of UKA over TKA [41]. This was supported by superior Oxford Knee Scores and patient satisfaction, as well as perceived improvement post-surgery and willingness to have the operation again. In contrast to arthroplasty registry data, there was no difference in re-operations and revision rate between UKA and TKA. The study also suggested that UKA was more cost-effective than TKA, assuming equal implant costs, within the UK healthcare model. A systematic review of patient relevant outcomes from the Oxford group demonstrated shorter operating times, reduced length of stay and fewer early complications, and lower mortality after UKA compared with TKA [42].

A number of authors have investigated the use of patient-specific instrumentation (PSI) and robotics in UKA. Currently, the evidence suggests largely equivalent results to standard instrumentation with no significant improvement in alignment with PSI [43,44]. However, there may be some benefits in PSI's ability to provide reproducibility of a pre-operative plan which has training implications [45]. With regards to robot-assisted UKA, there are a few recent studies which suggest benefits in terms of improved component positioning compared to standard instrumentation as well as equivalent survivorship [46–49].

Lateral UKA is performed less often than medial UKA as the medial compartment has a higher incidence of disease. It is also technically more challenging due partly to the difference in anatomy and kinematics between the compartments as well as implant design. There are conflicting reports of the difference in revision rate after medial and lateral UKA. An earlier study suggested an almost 10-times higher revision rate after lateral compared with medial UKA [50]. More recent studies including a meta-analysis have demonstrated no significant difference in survivorship between medial and lateral UKA [51,52].

The recent published evidence has led to renewed interest in UKA and a steady increase in the proportion of UKAs within Europe. In Denmark, over 20% of all knee arthroplasties are now partial replacements [53].

ENHANCED RECOVERY AND OUTPATIENT KNEE ARTHROPLASTY

Enhanced recovery in knee arthroplasty relies on a multimodal approach with the aim of improving the patient pathway and clinical outcome. The US has really led the way in introducing these pathways, particularly around provision of outpatient arthroplasty pathways. The key factors incorporated in enhanced recovery programmes can be grouped into the pre-operative optimisation of patients, patient education, perioperative anaesthesia, surgical techniques, and post-operative rehabilitation [54]. There is now an increasing volume of evidence that such programmes improve knee arthroplasty outcomes. A reduction in the risk of stroke, myocardial infarction, acute renal failure, and thromboembolism has been demonstrated in addition to health economic benefits [55–57].

A significant element of enhanced recovery programmes is standardised anaesthetic method including spinal and regional anaesthesia which has been shown to result in a reduction in morbidity, length of stay, and to improve the speed of functional recovery [58]. The use of local anaesthetic infiltration intraoperatively is also a useful adjunct within the anaesthetic protocols [59]. The reduction in blood loss using tranexamic acid has also been adopted in enhanced recovery programmes and is effective in decreasing the need for blood transfusions [60]. In terms of lowering the risk of thromboembolism, although low-molecular weight heparin (LMWH) is widely used, newer evidence suggests that aspirin is a feasible option and has additional health economic benefits [61].

There has been increasing interest in outpatient knee arthroplasty for select patient groups and currently account for approximately 5% of TKAs [62]. Gromov [63] reported criteria for same day discharge which included:

- Less than 500 mL blood loss
- Patient back on ward by 3 PM post-surgery
- Physiotherapy review and clearance according to standard protocols
- No clinical symptoms of signs of anaemia
- Pain <3/10 at rest and <5/10 on mobilisation
- Spontaneous urination
- Post-operative check radiograph reviewed and cleared
- Availability of relative or friend to stay with patient for >24 hours
- Motivated patient who accepts same-day discharge

Rodriguez–Merchan summarised the key elements for successful outpatient knee arthroplasty which included careful patient selection, pre-operative education, family and professional outpatient support, clinical expertise, institutional experience, standardised pain management protocols, and recovery programmes [62].

A number of studies have assessed the safety and efficacy of outpatient TKA. Although some papers have suggested higher rates of post-operative complications following discharge [64,65], more recent studies have shown no difference in readmission rates and complications compared to impatient TKA [66]. For UKA, the evidence similarly points to the requirement for standardised protocols with patient selection being a key factor. Bradley reported that the most common reasons for failure of same day discharge were either logistical in nature (late operation in the day), insufficient pain control, and leaking wound. The authors reported no readmissions and a high level of patient satisfaction [67]. Europe is still a little way behind widespread adoption of outpatient arthroplasty. There are many reasons for this including different healthcare systems and structures for reimbursement. The huge demand for joint replacement and the clear benefits in cost-effectiveness of enhanced recovery programs are recognised and several units around Europe have successfully implemented outpatient arthroplasty programs [68]. The recent COVID-19 pandemic is likely to result in an increase in the uptake of interest in outpatient knee arthroplasty as patients and care providers will be keen to reduce the length of time patients remain in hospital following joint replacement.

REVISION KNEE ARTHROPLASTY

Periprosthetic joint infection (PJI) remains the leading cause of early revision following TKA. Data from the Swedish, New Zealand, and Australian registries suggest an increase in incidence of early revision due to infection [54]. In England and Wales, the number of revision operations has increased by more than threefold between 2005 and 2013 [69]. It has been suggested that an increase in the proportion of patients with diabetes, obesity, and severe systemic disease undergoing TKA is a contributory factor in the increasing incidence of PJI [69]. Recent studies have focussed on improving the diagnosis of PJI as well as the management strategies including DAIR (Debridement, Antibiotics, and Implant Retention), single and two-stage revision arthroplasty.

Improving outcomes of revision knee arthroplasty

Survival rates for revision TKA are estimated at around 80% at 10 years [36] and with the widening age criteria for primary TKA, re-revision TKA is likely to increase. According to the NJR, 80% of surgeons performing revision knee arthroplasty undertake <10 revisions per year [37]. There is evidence from Germany that institutions which carry out a high volume of procedures within a subspecialist area have better outcomes [70,71]. Therefore, directing revision work to specialist centres is an important issue which faces many European Healthcare systems. In the UK, development of regional revision networks has been proposed and piloted in the form of a hub and spoke models. The British Association of Surgery of the Knee (BASK) has announced a large pilot which aims to create a pathway for low-volume centres to refer cases to high-volume centres [70]. There are challenges, however, including identification of surgeons and specialist centres and determining what constitutes high volume. Nonetheless, the future model of care of patients requiring revision knee arthroplasty within a nationalised healthcare service is likely to involve a degree of centralisation to specialist centres.

REFERENCES

1. Kurtz S, Ong K, Lau E, Mowat F, Halpern M. Projections of primary and revision hip and knee arthroplasty in the United States from 2005 to 2030. J Bone Joint Surg Am 2007; 89:780–785.
2. Patel A, Pavlou G, Mujica-Mota RE, Toms AD. The epidemiology of revision total knee and hip arthroplasty in England and Wales: a comparative analysis with projections for the United States. A study using the National Joint Registry dataset. Bone Joint J 2015; 97-B:1076–1081.
3. 3.Beswick AD, Wylde V, Gooberman-Hill R, Blom A, Dieppe P. What proportion of patients report long-term pain after total hip or knee replacement for osteoarthritis? A systematic review of prospective studies in unselected patients. BMJ Open 2012; 2:e000435.
4. Culliford DJ, Maskell J, Kiran A, et al. The lifetime risk of total hip and knee arthroplasty: results from the UK general practice research database. Osteoarthritis Cartilage 2012; 20:519–524.
5. Pabinger C, Lothaller H, Geissler A. Utilization rates of knee-arthroplasty in OECD countries. Osteoarthritis Cartilage 2015; 23:1664–1673.
6. Bayliss LE, Culliford D, Monk AP, et al. The effect of patient age at intervention on risk of implant revision after total replacement of the hip or knee: a population-based cohort study. Lancet 2017; 389:1424–1430.
7. Verra WC, van den Boom LG, Jacobs W, et al. Retention versus sacrifice of the posterior cruciate ligament in total knee arthroplasty for treating osteoarthritis. Cochrane Database Syst Rev 2013; CD004803.

8. Abdel MP, Morrey ME, Jensen MR, Morrey BF. Increased long-term survival of posterior cruciate-retaining versus posterior cruciate-stabilizing total knee replacements. J Bone Joint Surg Am 2011; 93:2072–2078.
9. Li N, Tan Y, Deng Y, Chen L. Posterior cruciate-retaining versus posterior stabilized total knee arthroplasty: a meta-analysis of randomized controlled trials. Knee Surg Sports Traumatol Arthrosc 2014; 22:556–564.
10. Atzori F, Salama W, Sabatini L, Mousa S, Khalefa A. Medial pivot knee in primary total knee arthroplasty. Ann Transl Med 2016; 4:6.
11. Bae DK, Cho SD, Im SK, Song SJ. Comparison of Midterm Clinical and Radiographic Results Between Total Knee Arthroplasties Using Medial Pivot and Posterior-Stabilized Prosthesis-A Matched Pair Analysis. J Arthroplasty 2016; 31:419–424.
12. Fitch DA, Sedacki K, Yang Y. Mid- to long-term outcomes of a medial-pivot system for primary total knee replacement: a systematic review and meta-analysis. Bone Joint Res 2014; 3:297–304.
13. Bordini B, Ancarani C, Fitch DA. Long-term survivorship of a medial-pivot total knee system compared with other cemented designs in an arthroplasty registry. J Orthop Surg Res 2016; 11:44.
14. Howell SM, Howell SJ, Kuznik KT, Cohen J, Hull ML. Does a kinematically aligned total knee arthroplasty restore function without failure regardless of alignment category? Clin Orthop Relat Res 2013; 471:1000–1007.
15. Kim KK, Howell SM, Won YY. Kinematically Aligned Total Knee Arthroplasty with Patient-Specific Instrument. Yonsei Med J 2020; 61:201–209.
16. Howell SM, Papadopoulos S, Kuznik KT, Hull ML. Accurate alignment and high function after kinematically aligned TKA performed with generic instruments. Knee Surg Sports Traumatol Arthrosc 2013; 21:2271–2280.
17. Howell SM, Shelton TJ, Hull ML. Implant Survival and Function Ten Years After Kinematically Aligned Total Knee Arthroplasty. J Arthroplasty 2018; 33:3678–3684.
18. Ishikawa M, Kuriyama S, Ito H, et al. Kinematic alignment produces near-normal knee motion but increases contact stress after total knee arthroplasty: A case study on a single implant design. Knee 2015; 22:206–212.
19. Matsumoto T, Takayama K, Ishida K, et al. Radiological and clinical comparison of kinematically versus mechanically aligned total knee arthroplasty. Bone Joint J 2017; 99-B:640–646.
20. Kayani B, Konan S, Tahmassebi J, et al. A prospective double-blinded randomised control trial comparing robotic arm-assisted functionally aligned total knee arthroplasty versus robotic arm-assisted mechanically aligned total knee arthroplasty. Trials 2020; 21:194.
21. Oussedik S, Abdel MP, Victor J, Pagnano MW, Haddad FS. Alignment in total knee arthroplasty. Bone Joint J 2020; 102-B:276–279.
22. Riviere C, Lazic S, Boughton O, et al. Current concepts for aligning knee implants: patient-specific or systematic? EFORT Open Rev 2018; 3:1–6.
23. Jakopec M, Harris SJ, Rodriguez y Baena F, et al. The first clinical application of a "hands-on" robotic knee surgery system. Comput Aided Surg 2001; 6:329–339.
24. Moon YW, Ha CW, Do KH, et al. Comparison of robot-assisted and conventional total knee arthroplasty: a controlled cadaver study using multiparameter quantitative three-dimensional CT assessment of alignment. Comput Aided Surg 2012; 17:86–95.
25. Song EK, Seon JK, Yim JH, Netravali NA, Bargar WL. Robotic-assisted TKA reduces postoperative alignment outliers and improves gap balance compared to conventional TKA. Clin Orthop Relat Res 2013; 471:118–126.
26. Song EK, Seon JK, Park SJ, et al. Simultaneous bilateral total knee arthroplasty with robotic and conventional techniques: a prospective, randomized study. Knee Surg Sports Traumatol Arthrosc 2011; 19:1069–1076.
27. Bellemans J, Vandenneucker H, Vanlauwe J. Robot-assisted total knee arthroplasty. Clin Orthop Relat Res 2007; 464:111–116.
28. Kayani B, Konan S, Huq SS, Tahmassebi J, Haddad FS. Robotic-arm assisted total knee arthroplasty has a learning curve of seven cases for integration into the surgical workflow but no learning curve effect for accuracy of implant positioning. Knee Surg Sports Traumatol Arthrosc 2019; 27:1132–1141.
29. Sodhi N, Khlopas A, Piuzzi NS, et al. The Learning Curve Associated with Robotic Total Knee Arthroplasty. J Knee Surg 2018; 31:17–21.
30. Kayani B, Konan S, Pietrzak JRT, Haddad FS. Iatrogenic Bone and Soft Tissue Trauma in Robotic-Arm Assisted Total Knee Arthroplasty Compared With Conventional Jig-Based Total Knee Arthroplasty: A Prospective Cohort Study and Validation of a New Classification System. J Arthroplasty 2018; 33:2496–2501.
31. Kayani B, Konan S, Tahmassebi J, Pietrzak JRT, Haddad FS. Robotic-arm assisted total knee arthroplasty is associated with improved early functional recovery and reduced time to hospital discharge compared with conventional jig-based total knee arthroplasty: a prospective cohort study. Bone Joint J 2018; 100-B:930–937.

32. Kayani B, Konan S, Tahmassebi J, Rowan FE, Haddad FS. An assessment of early functional rehabilitation and hospital discharge in conventional versus robotic-arm assisted unicompartmental knee arthroplasty: a prospective cohort study. Bone Joint J 2019; 101-B:24–33.

33. Marchand RC, Sodhi N, Khlopas A, et al. Patient Satisfaction Outcomes after Robotic Arm-Assisted Total Knee Arthroplasty: A Short-Term Evaluation. J Knee Surg 2017; 30:849–853.

34. Liow MHL, Goh GS, Wong MK, et al. Robotic-assisted total knee arthroplasty may lead to improvement in quality-of-life measures: a 2-year follow-up of a prospective randomized trial. Knee Surg Sports Traumatol Arthrosc 2017; 25:2942–2951.

35. Yang HY, Seon JK, Shin YJ, Lim HA, Song EK. Robotic Total Knee Arthroplasty with a Cruciate-Retaining Implant: A 10-Year Follow-up Study. Clin Orthop Surg 2017; 9:169–176.

36. Khan M, Osman K, Green G, Haddad FS. The epidemiology of failure in total knee arthroplasty: avoiding your next revision. Bone Joint J 2016; 98-B:105–112.

37. NJR. National Joint Registry 15th Annual Report. http://wwwnjrreportsorguk/Portals/0/PDFdownloads/ NJR 15th Annual Report 2018pdf [Last accessed 01 May, 2022.]

38. Willis-Owen CA, Brust K, Alsop H, Miraldo M, Cobb JP. Unicondylar knee arthroplasty in the UK National Health Service: an analysis of candidacy, outcome and cost efficacy. Knee 2009; 16:473–478.

39. Chawla H, Ghomrawi HM, van der List JP, et al. Establishing Age-Specific Cost-Effective Annual Revision Rates for Unicompartmental Knee Arthroplasty: A Meta-Analysis. J Arthroplasty 2017; 32:326–335.

40. Chawla H, van der List JP, Christ AB, et al. Annual revision rates of partial versus total knee arthroplasty: A comparative meta-analysis. Knee 2017; 24:179–190.

41. Beard DJ, Davies LJ, Cook JA, et al. The clinical and cost-effectiveness of total versus partial knee replacement in patients with medial compartment osteoarthritis (TOPKAT): 5-year outcomes of a randomised controlled trial. Lancet 2019; 394:746–756.

42. Wilson HA, Middleton R, Abram SGF, et al. Patient relevant outcomes of unicompartmental versus total knee replacement: systematic review and meta-analysis. BMJ 2019; 364:l352.

43. Alvand A, Khan T, Jenkins C, et al. The impact of patient-specific instrumentation on unicompartmental knee arthroplasty: a prospective randomised controlled study. Knee Surg Sports Traumatol Arthrosc 2018; 26:1662–1670.

44. Ollivier M, Parratte S, Lunebourg A, Viehweger E, Argenson JN. The John Insall Award: No Functional Benefit After Unicompartmental Knee Arthroplasty Performed With Patient-specific Instrumentation: A Randomized Trial. Clin Orthop Relat Res 2016; 474:60–68.

45. Ng CTJ, Newman S, Harris S, Clarke S, Cobb J. Patient-specific instrumentation improves alignment of lateral unicompartmental knee replacements by novice surgeons. Int Orthop 2017; 41:1379–1385.

46. Bell SW, Anthony I, Jones B, et al. Improved Accuracy of Component Positioning with Robotic-Assisted Unicompartmental Knee Arthroplasty: Data from a Prospective, Randomized Controlled Study. J Bone Joint Surg Am 2016; 98:627–635.

47. Gaudiani MA, Nwachukwu BU, Baviskar JV, Sharma M, Ranawat AS. Optimization of sagittal and coronal planes with robotic-assisted unicompartmental knee arthroplasty. Knee 2017; 24:837–43.

48. Gaudiani MA, Samuel LT, Kamath AF, Courtney PM, Lee GC. Robotic-Assisted versus Manual Unicompartmental Knee Arthroplasty: Contemporary Systematic Review and Meta-analysis of Early Functional Outcomes. J Knee Surg 2020; 34:1048–1056.

49. Pearle AD, van der List JP, Lee L, et al. Survivorship and patient satisfaction of robotic-assisted medial unicompartmental knee arthroplasty at a minimum two-year follow-up. Knee 2017; 24:419–428.

50. Heyse TJ, Khefacha A, Peersman G, Cartier P. Survivorship of UKA in the middle-aged. Knee 2012; 19:585–591.

51. Han SB, Lee SS, Kim KH, et al. Survival of medial versus lateral unicompartmental knee arthroplasty: A meta-analysis. PLoS One 2020; 15:e0228150.

52. van der List JP, McDonald LS, Pearle AD. Systematic review of medial versus lateral survivorship in unicompartmental knee arthroplasty. Knee 2015; 22:454–460.

53. Henkel C, Mikkelsen M, Pedersen AB, et al. Medial unicompartmental knee arthroplasty: increasingly uniform patient demographics despite differences in surgical volume and usage-a descriptive study of 8,501 cases from the Danish Knee Arthroplasty Registry. Acta Orthop 2019; 90:354–359.

54. Price AJ, Alvand A, Troelsen A, et al. Knee replacement. Lancet 2018; 392:1672–1682.

55. Duncan CM, Hall Long K, Warner DO, Hebl JR. The economic implications of a multimodal analgesic regimen for patients undergoing major orthopedic surgery: a comparative study of direct costs. Reg Anesth Pain Med 2009; 34:301–307.

56. Malviya A, Martin K, Harper I, et al. Enhanced recovery program for hip and knee replacement reduces death rate. Acta Orthop 2011; 82:577–581.

57. Savaridas T, Serrano-Pedraza I, Khan SK, et al. Reduced medium-term mortality following primary total hip and knee arthroplasty with an enhanced recovery program. A study of 4,500 consecutive procedures. Acta Orthop 2013; 84:40–43.
58. Johnson RL, Kopp SL, Burkle CM, et al. Neuraxial vs general anaesthesia for total hip and total knee arthroplasty: a systematic review of comparative-effectiveness research. Br J Anaesth 2016; 116:163–176.
59. Hu B, Lin T, Yan SG, et al. Local Infiltration Analgesia Versus Regional Blockade for Postoperative Analgesia in Total Knee Arthroplasty: A Meta-analysis of Randomized Controlled Trials. Pain Physician 2016; 19:205–214.
60. Chen TP, Chen YM, Jiao JB, et al. Comparison of the effectiveness and safety of topical versus intravenous tranexamic acid in primary total knee arthroplasty: a meta-analysis of randomized controlled trials. J Orthop Surg Res 2017; 12:11.
61. NICE. Venous thromboembolism in over 16s: reducing the risk of hospital-acquired deep vein thrombosis or pulmonary embolism. London: NICE, 2018. https://www.nice.org.uk/guidance/ng89 [Last accessed 01 May, 2022.]
62. Carlos Rodriguez-Merchan E. Outpatient total knee arthroplasty: is it worth considering? EFORT Open Rev 2020; 5:172–179.
63. Gromov K, Kjaersgaard-Andersen P, Revald P, Kehlet H, Husted H. Feasibility of outpatient total hip and knee arthroplasty in unselected patients. Acta Orthop 2017; 88:516–521.
64. 64.Arshi A, Leong NL, D'Oro A, et al. Outpatient Total Knee Arthroplasty Is Associated with Higher Risk of Perioperative Complications. J Bone Joint Surg Am 2017; 99:1978–1986.
65. Lovecchio F, Alvi H, Sahota S, Beal M, Manning D. Is Outpatient Arthroplasty as Safe as Fast-Track Inpatient Arthroplasty? A Propensity Score Matched Analysis. J Arthroplasty 2016; 31:197–201.
66. Crawford DA, Adams JB, Berend KR, Lombardi AV Jr. Low complication rates in outpatient total knee arthroplasty. Knee Surg Sports Traumatol Arthrosc 2020; 28:1458–1464.
67. Bradley B, Middleton S, Davis N, et al. Discharge on the day of surgery following unicompartmental knee arthroplasty within the United Kingdom NHS. Bone Joint J 2017; 99-B:788–792.
68. Jenkins C, Jackson W, Bottomley N, et al. Introduction of an innovative day surgery pathway for unicompartmental knee replacement: no need for early knee flexion. Physiotherapy 2019; 105:46–52.
69. Lenguerrand E, Whitehouse MR, Beswick AD, et al. Risk factors associated with revision for prosthetic joint infection following knee replacement: an observational cohort study from England and Wales. Lancet Infect Dis 2019; 19:589–600.
70. Ahmed SS, Haddad FS. Networks in orthopaedics. Bone Joint J 2020; 102-B:273-275.
71. Halder AM, Gehrke T, Gunster C, et al. Low Hospital Volume Increases Re-Revision Rate Following Aseptic Revision Total Knee Arthroplasty: An Analysis of 23,644 Cases. J Arthroplasty 2020; 35:1054–1059.

Chapter 7

Revision total hip and knee replacement

Ari Seidenstein

INTRODUCTION

Although primary total hip and knee replacements are widely known to be hugely successful procedures, the frequency of revision total joint arthroplasty (TJA) is increasing at a rapid pace. The most common indications for revision hip surgery include dislocation, mechanical loosening, and infection. Other less common aetiologies of revision total hip arthroplasty (THA) include implant failure, peri-prosthetic fracture, osteolysis and bearing surface wear [1]. The most common aetiologies of revision total knee arthroplasty (TKA) are infection as well as mechanical loosening. Less frequent reasons for revision knee surgery include instability, poly wear, peri-prosthetic fracture and osteolysis [2]. Given the current era of bundled payment programmes and pay-for-performance based care combined with the increased costs of revision implants and longer hospital stays associated with these procedures, these challenging operations pose a significant economic burden on the healthcare system. In this section, we provide updates from the literature published in the last few years on the most recent advances in revision total hip and knee replacement with regard to identifying risk, enhancing outcomes, and improving surgical techniques and implant design.

RISK FACTORS

Revision total joint replacement is inherently fraught with higher complication rates when compared to primary procedures. Several patient risk factors exist that can lead to poor outcomes and complications following revision surgery. In order to minimise these complications, reduce costs and improve outcomes, particular attention has recently been focussed on eliminating modifiable risk factors and optimising other non-modifiable risk factors.

Smoking prior to revision TJA increases the risk of any wound complication, deep infection and re-operation of any kind. Moreover, smoking increases the risk of these complications in revision TKA more so than with primary TKA [3,4]. Smoking cessation

Ari Seidenstein MD, Associations – Rothman Orthopaedic Institute, Assistant Professor, Orthopaedic Surgery, Hackensack Meridian School of Medicine, Chief of Orthopaedic Surgery, Holy Name Medical Center, US
Email: aseidenstein@gmail.com

programmes should be implemented for revision arthroplasty patients prior to surgery whenever possible.

Morbid obesity, defined as body mass index (BMI) > 40 kg/m^2, is another modifiable risk factor of TJA patients. Patients who are morbidly obese have a significantly greater risk of lower functional and clinical outcome scores as well as higher risk of re-operation and re-revision [5,6]. Although certain revision scenarios can be considered urgent, weight loss should be encouraged, if possible, prior to surgery.

Patients with chronic obstructive pulmonary disease (COPD) undergoing revision TKA have a greater risk for post-operatively developing wound dehiscence, pneumonia, re-intubation, renal insufficiency and renal failure complications than those without COPD [7]. Surgeons should counsell patients that their COPD status significantly increases post-operative complication risk and these patients should be as medically optimised as possible.

Pre-operative vitamin D levels should also be considered a modifiable risk factor in revision joint arthroplasty. Low vitamin D was found to be associated with an increased risk of 90-day complications as well as peri-prosthetic joint infection (PJI) and should be considered to be part of the pre-operative testing [8].

Higher levels of pre-operative red cell distribution width (RDW), pre-operative anaemia and hyponatraemia are also associated with less optimal outcomes after TJA revision including effects on mortality, post-operative complications, length of stay, and re-admission [9–11]. Although RDW, Hgb and Na$^+$ are already included in the complete blood count (CBC) and "Basic Metabolic Panel" as part of pre-admission testing, these values can be used to counsel patients regarding risk of post-operative outcomes.

BLOOD MANAGEMENT AND VENOUS THROMBOEMBOLISM PROPHYLAXIS

Revision TJA carries with it a higher risk of bleeding compared to primary surgeries. That being said, the use and dosing of peri-operative tranexamic acid (TXA) as well as the type of post-operative chemical anti-coagulation used are of obvious concern in this patient population.

The pre-operative use of intravenous TXA in revision total joint replacement has been shown to reduce both allogeneic blood transfusions and peri-operative blood loss without increasing the risk of venous thromboembolism (VTE) [12–15]. Furthermore, studies show that despite the higher risk of blood loss in revision TJA, surgeons should still use the lowest effective dose as well as the least costly TXA regimen [16].

Although revision surgery has been shown to be an independent risk factor for wound drainage, it has not been shown to be an independent risk factor for VTE [17]. Having said that, aspirin is as effective as other chemoprophylactic agents without the increased risk of bleeding and should still be considered for VTE prophylaxis in low-risk patients [18,19].

All in all, there have recent substantial decreases in the incidence of blood transfusions following revision TJA. These reductions have been attributed to multiple changes, including the use of novel pharmaceuticals and devices for bleeding control and blood management, the use of aspirin as an anti-coagulant, as well as more stringent transfusion-trigger guidelines [20].

PERI-PROSTHETIC JOINT INFECTION

Peri-prosthetic joint infection occurs in approximately 1–2% of primary total joint arthroplasties and up to 3–10% of revision arthroplasties. Patients undergoing treatment for PJI have a two-fold increase in in-hospital mortality for each surgical admission compared to aseptic revisions [21]. As the volume of both primary and revision arthroplasties performed on an annual basis continue to rise, the incidence of PJIs is purported to grow considerably as well. In 2018, Parvizi et al presented the first validated, evidence-based criteria for diagnosing PJI after hip and knee arthroplasty [22] (**Tables 7.1** to **7.3**). Despite the scoring system, diagnosis in some patients remains uncertain. These patients may benefit from the use of novel techniques such as next-generation sequencing [23]. More recently, plasma fibrinogen, a coagulation-related indicator, has shown promise as

Table 7.1 Major criteria

Major criteria	Decision
Two positive cultures of the same organism	Infected
Sinus tract with evidence of communication to the joint or visualisation of the prosthesis	Infected

Table 7.2 Preoperative diagnosis

Minor Criteria	Score	Decision
Serum		
Elevated C-reactive protein (CRP) or D-dimer	2	
Elevated erythrocyte sedimentation rate (ESR)	1	≥6 infected
Synovial		
Elevated synovial white blood cell count (WBC) or leukocyte esterase (LE)	3	2–5 possibly infected*
Positive alpha-defensin	3	
Elevated synovial polymorphonuclear (PMN) %	2	0–1 not infected
Elevated synovial CRP	1	

*For patients with inconclusive minor criteria, intraoperative criteria can also be used to fulfill the definition of PJI

Table 7.3 Intraoperative diagnosis

Criteria	Score	Decision
Preoperative score	As calculated preoperatively	≥6 infected
Positive histology	3	4–5 inconclusive*
Positive purulence	3	
Single positive culture	2	≤3 not infected

*Consider further molecular diagnostics such as next-generation sequencing

another diagnostic marker of PJI, with both good sensitivity and specificity [24]. Leucocyte esterase strips have also been found to be a reliable diagnostic marker, even in the setting of antibiotic administration, and can be used both pre-operatively or intra-operatively for diagnosis [25,26]. It has also been suggested by Rothenberg et al that sonication cultures be performed of explanted components in revision surgery for aseptic loosening as there may be a percentage of these patients that are infected [27].

In the setting of acute peri-prosthetic joint infection (APJI), irrigation and debridement with exchange of modular components while retaining the fixed components has been the gold standard for treatment due to overall decreased patient morbidity. Unfortunately, some studies have reported failure rates as high as 60–84%. It has been shown that there is a much higher rate for failure for acute haematogenous infections when compared to acute post-surgical infections as well [28]. Discrepancies in success rates have also been attributed to variable time of symptom onset to surgery, overall patient health, organism virulence as well as differences in surgical technique. In a recent study, Chung et al reported a higher likelihood of infection control with a two-stage debridement with prosthesis retention [29]. During the first stage of this technique, modular pieces are removed, sterilised and re-inserted, a through debridement is performed, and high-dose antibiotic-impregnated cement beads are placed in the joint. At the time of the second stage, the beads are removed, another irrigation and debridement is performed and new modular components are inserted.

Two-stage exchange arthroplasty remains the current gold standard for chronic PJIs in the United States (US). Infection eradication rates range from 75% to 100% with this technique. One question often asked by surgeons in this setting is when re-implantation should occur and whether delaying the second stage confers a higher rate of treatment success. Rezaie et al showed no improvement in results with delaying time to re-implantation. Moreover, there was a general trend towards higher failure rates in those with wait times >26 weeks [30]. The potential for emergence of resistant organisms between the stages of a two-stage revision is also of potential concern [31]. Patients with co-morbidities, low pre-operative haemoglobin levels and a high BMI should be carefully managed and observed as these patients are at higher risk for acute kidney injury after the first-stage revision surgery. Surgeons may consider using lower doses of powdered antibiotics in these patients [32,33]. The patient co-morbidity index was significantly associated with treatment outcome highlighting the importance of host optimisation and risk stratification prior to re-implantation. A single positive bacterial culture during re-implantation has also been shown to be independently associated with subsequent failure and revision of the antibiotic-laden cement spacer should be considered in this situation [34]. Della Valle et al have shown that the addition of 3 months of oral antibiotics after re-implantation improves infection-free survival [35].

Although two-stage revision is still the gold standard for the treatment of chronic PJI, recent studies have shown that a single-stage exchange arthroplasty can be successful. Contraindications for this approach include a severely immunocompromised patient, significant bone and/or soft-tissue compromise, concurrent acute sepsis, multi-drug resistant or atypical organisms, and a fungal infection [36,37]. These patients have also been shown to have markedly improved health-related quality of life and patient-reported function [38]. There is also an associated cost reduction when comparing a single-stage revision with a two-stage revision [39].

In a large cohort study, Kheir et al were able to identify risk factors and their relative weight for predicting PJI treatment failure [40]. Given that some of those risk factors are modifiable, scores can be improved upon and should be addressed before treating a patient for PJI. Risk of hip and knee PJI recurrence is increased in female patients, those with heart disease and/or psychiatric disorders as well as the presence of a sinus tract pre-operatively [41,42]. Patients with PJI of the hip and with heart disease are at higher risk of infection persistence. Early re-infections after two-stage revisions are usually associated with resistant bacterial pathogens whereas late failures involved new pathogens [43]. Either way, failure rates are considerably higher when undergoing a second two-stage revision and patients should be counselled as such [44,45].

Fungal PJIs are a rare occurrence, accounting for <1% of all PJIs. Having said that, there is a substantial associated rate of morbidity and mortality. Kuo et al showed that fungal PJI patients are older, have more co-morbidities, have had significantly more revision surgery on the index joint, and have a failure rate almost twice that of nonfungal PJI patients [46]. *Candida* species was also found to be the most common fungal pathogen responsible for PJI. Diagnosing fungal PJI can be challenging as well. Serum and synovial markers are significantly reduced in fungal PJIs, most probably due to the weakened immune systems in this patient cohort. Two-stage exchange arthroplasty appears to have a higher treatment success when compared to both irrigation and debridement and one-stage revision. Patients should receive a prolonged period of anti-fungal therapy. However, addition of anti-fungal agents to bone cement spacers remains controversial and further research is needed.

REVISION TOTAL HIP REPLACEMENT

Direct anterior approach

The direct anterior approach (DAA) has established itself as a standard approach for primary THA. That being said, the approach is often criticised as an approach that is limited to primary arthroplasty. This is due to the location of the muscular conjunction of the rectus femoris and vastus lateralis muscles at the level of the lesser trochanter and the nerve branches of the femoral nerve, which cross the area from the medial to the lateral side. The vastus lateralis is innervated by branches of the femoral nerve that cross the interval distally and laterally to the lesser trochanter. If the DAA is extended to the bone distal to the lesser trochanter by splitting the conjunction between the rectus and vastus lateralis, it would destroy these nerve branches and consequently cause muscular degeneration.

Nogler et al have proposed an alternate distal extension of the DAA to reach the femur at the posterior border of the vastus lateralis and incorporating the lateral approach to the femoral diaphysis [47]. Here the iliotibial band is split through its anterior border and retracted laterally, thus opening the interval to the lateral-posterior aspect of the vastus muscle. This alternate extension technique preserves all neurovascular structures.

Proximal extension of the DAA for revision THA allows for access to the anterior column of the acetabulum. A novel surgical technique has been developed for augmentation of the anterior column using highly porous metal augments with this approach allowing for increased stability of the acetabulum component [48].

The DAA represents a viable option in acetabulum-only revision with good medium-term results and a low complication rates, particularly in relation to dislocation [49].

In the same breath, due to the learning curve, the DAA and any of its extensions should only be used in revision THA by those with sufficient experience with the approach in primary THA.

Instability and dual mobility

Instability remains one of the most concerning complications following revision total hip replacement. Although acetabular component position remains an important variable in decreasing the risk of dislocation, patients undergoing revision THA often have abductor dysfunction or greater trochanteric osteolysis which may compromise the abductor mechanism and make the patient more prone to post-operative instability [50]. Dealing with this issue is challenging and several strategies exist such as the use of large femoral heads, the use of constrained liners, and the use of tripolar liners. Recently, the advent of the dual mobility articulation has presented itself as another solution to this problem. The dual mobility articulation includes an outer highly cross-linked polyethylene liner and a smaller ceramic or cobalt-chrome femoral head. The outer polyethylene liner articulates with the metal cup or liner and the inner femoral head. This construct allows for a larger effective head size leading to increased stability and decreased impingement [51].

Early and mid-term results demonstrate dual mobility articulations to have superior survivorship and lower dislocation rates compared to fixed-bearing implants with large diameter heads (40 mm) [52–57]. Even though the use of the dual mobility implants themselves may be more costly, there is a greater payer savings associated with their utilisation secondary to the lower absolute risk of re-intervention [58]. Recurrent dislocations seen in patients revised with dual mobility constructs were mostly seen in those patients with polyethylene outer diameter ≤ 38 mm [59].

When revising an acetabular component due to recurrent instability, a dual mobility construct may be favourable to a constrained liner because it puts less force on the prosthesis. The undue force put on the acetabular component with a constrained line [secondary to impingement because of restricted range of motion (ROM)] could theoretically increase the risk of aseptic loosening of the acetabular component. Furthermore, the ability to close reduce a dual mobility construct is a distinct advantage over constrained liners. Recurrent instability seen after implantation of a constrained liner has also been noted to be successfully treated with conversion to a dual mobility construct [60].

Hip resurfacing arthroplasties can also be successfully converted to a THA using dual mobility components. In the setting of a well-fixed and appropriately positioned hip resurfacing acetabular component, this technique avoids the morbidity of acetabular revision while also decreasing metal ion levels and increasing functional outcomes compared to both component revisions [61]. That being said, it should be confirmed that the retained cup does not have significant existing damage to the articular surface [62]. Caution should be used when applying this technique to younger, more active patients whom may be adversely affected by increased prosthesis wear in the long term.

Unstable hemi-arthroplasties have been seen to be successfully treated with revision THA using a dual mobility construct as well [63]. Utilising the dual mobility construct allows the surgeon to reproduce the large effective head size of a hip hemi-arthroplasty, thereby increasing the stability of the hip.

Dual mobility cups do generate increased levels of nickel ions in the blood that are comparable to those seen with the use of certain spine implants [64]. The clinical consequences of these are unknown. Having said that, elevated chromium and cobalt ion levels have not been seen in patients with dual mobility constructs [65]. Although new acetabular components with a metal articulation (non-modular or modular) can be implanted, good results have also been seen when cementing dual mobility liners into already well-fixed acetabular components with only a comparatively marginal release of metal ions [66,67].

There are potential concerns associated with the routine use of dual mobility constructs in the revision setting. One rare complication that is specific to dual mobility constructs is the potential risk of intra-prosthetic dislocation. This is most often seen when attempting a closed reduction of a dislocated dual mobility construct. These intra-prosthetic dislocations were mostly seen in older models and when using smaller diameter (22 mm) heads. Having said that, it should be recommended to reduce these dislocations under fluoroscopic guidance so as not to impinge the outer polyethylene liner from the smaller diameter head while doing so [68].

Head-neck taper corrosion

Head-neck taper corrosion, also known as trunnionosis, is a wear process caused by mechanical corrosion. It occurs most commonly in metal-on-polyethylene (MOP) implants and accounts for 0.7–3 % of all THA revisions [69]. Patients may present with delayed onset groin, buttock or thigh pain. Trunnionosis may lead to aseptic loosening and/or osteolysis from the local release of metal debris as well, possibly causing its true incidence to be under-reported [70]. More serious cases may lead to local tissue necrosis, destruction of the abductor muscles and/or a pseudo-tumour [71]. The mean time to presentation is 5 years from the index procedure.

Implant factors thought to be related to increased risk of trunnionosis include large femoral head size (36 mm and above) as well as smaller diameter and shorter tapers on femoral stems. Femoral stems that are manufactured from stiffer alloys (titanium and cobalt-chrome) are more likely to resist corrosion damage. In regard to surgical technique, coaxial impaction of the femoral head onto a clean trunnion has been proposed to increase construct stability and pull-off strength while subsequently increasing resistance to corrosion. Length of time from implantation, higher BMI, and increased patient activity are all associated with increased mechanical stress and higher corrosion [69,70].

Metal-on-polyethylene trunnionosis has been characterised by a specific pattern of elevated serum metal ions. These patients have a much higher serum cobalt/chrome ratio (5:1) compared to that seen in metallosis in metal-on-metal THAs (1:1 or 2:1) [69,70]. Moreover, a synovial cobalt-to-chrome ratio is >1.4 ng/mL as a test threshold has a 95% sensitivity [72,73]. Metal artefact reduction sequence MRI remains the gold standard to clearly visualise the extent of any adverse local tissue reaction (ALTR) as well as the presence of a pseudo-tumour [74].

Evidence-based treatment guidelines for trunnionosis patients are currently lacking. It has been suggested that patients with mild and transient symptom who also have inconclusive metal ions and negative MRI findings can be placed observed with serial evaluations. These patients should also be told to abstain from high impact activities. For those patients that have more severe symptoms and/or have a confirmed laboratory or image-based diagnosis, the most appropriate treatment would be revision THA. Pre-operatively, the surgeon should be aware of the implants to be revised and, more specifically, the angle and type of taper of the femoral stem. All necrotic tissue should be excised. The acetabulum component can be retained as long as it is well fixed and well aligned. Degree of damage to the trunnion should be carefully examined. It has been suggested in multiple studies to use ceramic heads with titanium sleeves to both avoid the risk of recurrent trunnionosis while preventing crack or fracture of the ceramic head from the damaged trunnion [75]. In cases of gross trunnion damage, the femoral component may need to be revised in its entirety [76]. Liner exchange has been recommended to prevent further metallosis or ALTR from metal debris that could not otherwise be removed.

Symptomatic mechanically assisted crevice corrosion is a potentially devastating diagnosis due to decreased soft-tissue viability and bone stock associate with ALTR. This leads to a high early major complication rate following revision surgery, more commonly dislocation, deep infection and aseptic loosening [77]. Patients should be made aware of the increased risk prior to surgery. Pre-revision MRI findings of solid lesions with abductor deficiency and intra-operative tissue damage are risk factors associate with the occurrence of a complication after revision surgery [78]. In the presence of extensive tissue damage, a constrained liner or dual mobility construct should be considered [79]. That being said, if a patient does avoid a major complication, improvement from revision surgery is measurable and precipitous. Furthermore, a significant reduction in serum metal ion levels can be seen within 3 months of revision surgery [80].

Revision of metal on metal total hip arthroplasties

Numerous metal-on-metal hip arthroplasties (MoMHAs) have been implanted in the recent past, either in the form of hip resurfacing arthroplasty or THA. MoMHAs have been shown to have high early failure rates secondary to adverse reactions to metal debris (ARMD) in addition to other conventional modes of failure (i.e. infection, dislocation, loosening, etc.) seen in THAs with other bearing surfaces. This mode of failure is different from others given the associated soft-tissue problems, the potentially destructive and progressive nature of the disease, as well as its occurrence in otherwise asymptomatic and well-functioning MoMHAs. Although it is clear that symptomatic patients with pseudo-tumours should be revised in a timely fashion and asymptomatic patients with normal investigations should undergo routine surveillance, historically there have been an abundance of patients where proper management remained unclear. Early studies observed MoMHA revisions performed for ARMD had a high risk of re-revision, poor patient-reported outcomes, and inferior results compared with non-ARMD revisions.

Consequently, surgeons and worldwide regulatory authorities widely recommended early revision for ARMD associated with a lower surgical threshold [81]. Moreover, revisions of failed MoMHAs have been occurring with a high volume now for more than a decade [82]. To that effect, whether it be due to increased surgeon experience or lower thresholds to perform revision surgery, the clinical post-operative results and patient-reported outcomes have improved [83,84]. Recently, it has been shown that synovial fluid cobalt has the highest correlation with an ALTR with a threshold of 19.75 ng/mL and a specificity of 89% [72]. This test, as well as others, is only one piece of information, and although useful, should not be used in a vacuum to make the decision to operate.

Matharu et al observed that patients undergoing MoMHA revision for ARMD had approximately half the risk of re-revision and death compared with matched patients undergoing non-ARMD revision surgery [85]. However, infected MoMHA revisions were responsible for this increased mortality risk observed after non-ARMD revision which can also be seen in non-MoMHA revision surgery. Non-ARMD revision performed for infection and dislocation had the lowest implant survival. Contrary to other bearing surfaces in which infected revisions occur early, the revision risk for infection continues to increase with time since implantation in MoMHAs. This is of particular concern given that many MoMHRs may undergo future revision for infection and the reported associated poor prognosis. Although dislocation is an uncommon mode of failure after MoMHA, the re-revision rates are high after revision surgery for this indication. Intuitively, this could be partially associated with the reduction in femoral head size at the time of revision. 19% of the re-revisions performed in this study were for ARMD. Reasons for re-revisions for ARMD are speculated to be incomplete ARMD lesion debridement, revision to a construct that may include a MoM junction (i.e. trunnionosis), or possible misdiagnosis of the initial revision indication. Although research is needed to refine the thresholds for performing ARMD revision surgery, it is believed that the thresholds need not be lowered any further because of the potential for surgical risk to outweigh any benefits.

REVISION TOTAL KNEE REPLACEMENT

Revision for stiffness

Stiffness after TKA can have numerous aetiologies including primary arthrofibrosis, patella baja, malrotation, component overstuffing, instability and coronal malalignment. Generally speaking, revision TKA is reserved for those patients who failed to improve with physical therapy, manipulation under anaesthesia, and/or arthroscopic or open lysis of adhesions. Revision surgery is thought to be the most effective for the correction of surgical errors, including problems with sizing and positioning of components, patella thickness and joint-line level. Revision of all components offers the largest improvements in motion and function in these properly selected patients [86].

Lysis of adhesions may be more appropriate for those patients with primary arthro-fibrosis. Although these patients have been shown to have improvement in their pain level, the post-operative ROM generally does not get better.

Van Rensch et al reported that all indications except severe stiffness for revision TKA had a similar clinical outcome which was maintained up to 7.5-year follow-up. The severe stiffness group had worse outcomes and deteriorated slightly at a longer follow-up [87].

Generally speaking, revision TKA for a primary indication of stiffness does substantially increase ROM, with a mean improvement of 30°, and improves pre-operative flexion contractures. Revision surgery can also be associated with significant improvement in Knee Society Scores (KSSs). That being said, these patients, on average, are not achieving "functional" ROM post-operatively, with a mean flexion of 67–98°. Consequently, the most common complication is persistent stiffness [88]. Rutherford et al reported that 30% of patients had a decrease in one or more component of the KSS or a net decrease in ROM [89].

Hermans et al reported better results at 2 years follow-up when implanting a rotating hinged knee (RHK) implant compared to a constrained condylar knee device. The RHK group demonstrated significantly better knee function scores, knee function improvement, knee pain improvement, and greater maximal flexion and extension [90].

Stem size and fixation method

Considering the presence of bone defects and compromised soft-tissues, achieving lasting fixation in revision TKA can be especially challenging. Having said that, the ideal method of fixation and stem design for revision knee components is still not known. Fixation of modular stems can be achieved either by full-length cementation or with a press-fit hybrid technique wherein cement is placed on the undersurface of the component as well as the metaphyseal portion of the components up until the junction with the stem.

Although excellent mechanical survival has been reported with both techniques, there is concern over the difficulty of removing a fully cemented stem. That being said, Maslaris et al reported this can be minimised by using a conical stem rather than a cylindrical stem [91].

Fleischman et al recently showed, in the largest comparative study to date, that both methods provide a viable solution for obtaining durable mid-term to long-term stem fixation in revision TKA [92]. It was also reported that for hybrid fixation risk of mechanical failure was reduced by 41.2% for every 10% increase in the canal filling ratio. Surgeons should attempt to maximise canal filling by reaming appropriately and obtaining a solid press-fit.

Ettinger et al revealed that small femoral stems (50 mm) resulted on average in about 3° more of hyperextension when compared to longer stems (100 mm, 150 mm) [93]. This caused a greater amount of sagittal malalignment and subsequent decreased posterior condylar offset (PCO) ratio. Previous studies have shown PCO ratio to be an independent outcome predictor in revision TKA.

While there were no differences between the cemented and hybrid fixation groups in post-operative American Knee Society Score (AKSS) clinical evaluation indices and the SF-36 health index, Gomez–Vallejo et al did report higher WOMAC scores for hybrid fixation revision TKA patients [94]. Fleischman et al also reported better alignment obtained with that ideal mechanical alignment is achieved more reliably with press-fit stems from improved diaphyseal engagement [95]. In light of these findings and the inherent risk of further loosening, hybrid fixation was suggested as a preferred technique in both studies.

Metaphyseal sleeves and cones

Revision TKA is a challenging operation for many reasons. Reconstruction of bony defects in the distal end of the femur and proximal end of the tibia remains a difficult problem. Use of porous-coated metaphyseal sleeves or porous tantalum metaphyseal cones in order to address bone deficiency also enables restoration of mechanical stability and can help to augment lasting fixation. These implants are both indicated for Anderson Orthopaedic Research Institute type 2B and type 3 defects [96]. They provide both long-term biologic fixations to the native bone while also offering a stable construct for cemented fixation [97]. Additionally, these implants allow for joint reconstruction near anatomic level.

Zanirato et al showed excellent mid-term aseptic survivorship for both, 97.3% at a mean follow-up of 3.6 years for cones and 97.8% at 4.5 years for sleeves [98]. Ihekweazu et al have reported that sufficient fixation can be achieved with only limited amounts of bone ongrowth (14.7% in tibial sleeves and 21.3% in femoral sleeves) [99]. Similarly, Fedorka et al also showed excellent radiographic ingrowth and short-term stable fixation [100]. Additionally, Bonanzinga et al reported metaphyseal sleeves to have a low septic loosening rate, low intra-operative fracture rate, and good-to-excellent clinical outcomes [101]. Wirries et al reported stable fixation of metaphyseal sleeves at a mean follow-up of 5.0 years with a survival rate of 98% [102].

Burastero et al observed tantalum cones to be considered as a safe and effective option in the management of massive bone defects in septic knee revision surgery. Excellent clinical and radiographic mid-term outcomes were achieved with a low complication rate [103]. Klim et al reported similar results for the use of metaphyseal sleeves used in septic revision TKAs. This study showed promising mid-term results regarding clinical scores, osseointegration, and aseptic loosening [104].

Fink et al communicated a novel distraction technique, utilising trabecular metal cones, to stabilise peri-prosthetic metaphyseal fractures of knee. Although the study group was small, this technique displayed reproducibly good results [105].

REFERENCES

1. Gwam CU, Mistry JB, Mohamed NS, et al. Current Epidemiology of Revision Total Hip Arthroplasty in the United States: National Inpatient Sample 2009 to 2013. J Arthroplasty 2017; 32:2088–2092.
2. Delanois RE, Mistry JB, Gwam CU, et al. Current Epidemiology of Revision Total Knee Arthroplasty in the United States. J Arthroplasty 2017; 32:2663–2668.
3. Bedard NA, Dowdle SB, Wilkinson BG, et al. What is the Impact of Smoking on Revision Total Knee Arthroplasty? J Arthroplasty 2018; 33:S172–S176.
4. Bedard NA, Dowdle SB, Owens JM, et al. What is the Impact of Smoking on Revision Total Hip Arthroplasty? J Arthroplasty 2019; 33:S182–S185.
5. Hanna SA, McCalden RW, Somerville L, et al. Morbid Obesity is a Significant Risk of Failure Following Revision Total Hip Arthroplasty. J Arthroplasty 2017; 32:3098–3101.
6. Sisko ZW, Vasarhelyi EM, Somerville LE, et al. Morbid Obesity in Revision Total Knee Arthroplasty: A Significant Risk Factor of Re-Operation. J Arthroplasty 2019; 34:932–938.
7. Gu A, Wei C, Maybee CM, et al. The Impact of Chronic Obstructive Pulmonary Disease on Postoperative Outcomes in Patients Undergoing Revision Total Knee Arthroplasty. J Arthroplasty 2018; 33:2956–2960.
8. Traven SA, Chiaramonti AM, Barfield WR, et al. Fewer Complications Following Revision Hip and Knee Arthroplasty in Patients with Normal Vitamin D Levels. J Arthroplasty 2017; 32:S193–S196.
9. Aali-rezaie A, Alijanipour P, Shohat N, et al. Red Cell Distribution Width: An Unacknowledged Predictor of Mortality and Adverse Outcomes Following Revision Arthroplasty. J Arthroplasty 2018; 33:3514–3519.
10. Lu M, Sing DC, Kuo AC, Hansen EN. Preoperative Anemia Independently Predicts 30-Day Complications After Aseptic and Septic Revision Total Joint Arthroplasty. J Arthroplasty 2017; 32:S197–S201.
11. Gu A, Chen FR, Chen AZ, et al. Preoperative Hyponatremia is an Independent Risk Factor for Postoperative Complications in Aseptic Revision Hip and Knee Arthroplasty. J Orthopaedics 2020; 20:224–227.
12. Reichel F, Peter C, Ewerbeck V, Egermann M. Reducing Blood Loss in Revision Total Hip and Knee Arthroplasty: Tranexamic Acid is Effective in Aseptic Revisions and in Second-Stage Reimplantations for Periprosthetic Infection. BioMed Res Int 2018; 1–9.
13. Kuo F, Lin P, Wang J, et al. Intravenous Tranexamic Acid Use in Revision Total Joint Arthroplasty: A Meta-Analysis. Drug Des Devel Ther 2018; 12:3163–3170.
14. Peck J, Kepecs DM, Mei B, et al. The Effect of Preoperative Administration of Intravenous Tranexamic Acid During Revision Hip Arthroplasty: A Retrospective Study. J Bone Joint Surg Am 2018; 100:1509–1516.
15. Hines JT, Hernandez NM, Amundson AW, et al.. Intravenous Tranexamic Acid Safely and Effectively Reduces Transfusion Rates in Revision Total Hip Arthroplasty. Bone Joint J 2019; 101-B:104–109.
16. Fillingham YA, Darrith B, Calkins TE, et al. 2019 Mark Coventry Award: A Multicentre Randomized Clinical Trial of Tranexamic Acid in Revision Total Knee Arthroplasty: Does the Dosing Regimen Matter? Bone Joint J 2019; 101-B:10–16.
17. Courtney PM, Boniello AJ, Levine BR, Sheth NP, Paprosky WG. Are Revision Arthroplasty Patients at Higher Risk for Venous Thromboembolic Events than Primary Hip Arthroplasty Patients? J Arthroplasty 2017; 32:3752–3756.
18. Bautista M, Muskus M, Tafur D, et al. Thromboprophylaxis for Hip Revision Arthroplasty: Can We Use the Recommendations for Primary Hip Surgery? A Cohort Study. Clin Appl Thromb/Hemost 2019; 25:1–7.
19. Manista GC, Batko BD, Sexton AC, et al. Anticoagulation in Revision Total Joint Arthroplasty: A Retrospective Review of 1917 Cases. Orthopedics 2019; 42:323–329.
20. Burnett RA, Bedard NA, Demik DE, et al. Recent Trends in Blood Utilization After Revision Hip and Knee Arthroplasty. J Arthroplasty 2017.
21. Shahi A, Tan TL, Chen AF, Maltenfort MG, Parvizi J. In-Hospital Mortality in Patients with Periprosthetic Joint Infection. J Arthroplasty 2017; 32:948–952.

22. Parvizi J, Tan TL, Goswami K, et al. The 2018 Definition of Periprosthetic Hip and Knee Infection: An Evidence-Based and Validated Criteria. J Arthroplasty 2018; 33:1309–1314.

23. Tarabichi M, Shohat N, Goswami K, et al. Diagnosis of periprosthetic joint infection: the potential of next-generation sequencing. J Bone Joint Surg Am 2018; 100:147–154.

24. Li R, Shao H, Hao L, et al. Plasma Fibrinogen Exhibits Better Performance than Plasma D-Dimer in the Diagnosis of Periprosthetic joint Infection: A Multicenter Retrospective Study. J Bone Joint Surg Am 2019; 101:613–619.

25. Zagra L, Villa F, Cappelletti L, et al. Can Leucocyte Esterase Replace Frozen Sections in the Intraoperative Diagnosis of Prosthetic Hip Infection? Bone Joint J 2019; 101-B:372–377.

26. Shahi A, Alvand A, Ghanem E, Restrepo C, Parvizi J. The Lukocyte Esterase Test for Periprosthetic Joint Infection is not Affected by Prior Antibiotic Administration. J Bone Joint Surg Am 2019; 101:739–744.

27. Rothenberg AC, Wilson AE, Hayes JP, O'Malley MJ, Klatt BA. Sonication of Arthroplasty Implants Improves Accuracy of Periprosthetic Joint Infection Cultures. Clin Orthop Relat Res 2017; 475:1827–1836.

28. Shohat N, Goswami K, Tan TL, Fillingham Y, Parvizi J. Increased Failure After Irrigation and Debridement for Acute Hematogenous Periprosthetic Joint Infection. J Bone Joint Surg Am 2019; 101:696–703.

29. Chung AS, Niesen MC, Graber TJ, et al. Two-stage Debridement with Prosthesis Retention for Acute Periprosthetic Joint Infections. J Arthroplasty 2019; 34:1207–1213.

30. Rezaie AA, Goswami K, Shohat N, et al. Time to Reimplantation: Waiting Longer Confers No Added Benefit. J Arthroplasty 2018; 33:1850–1854.

31. George J, Newman JM, Klika AK, et al. Changes in Antibiotic Susceptibility of Staphylococcus aureus Between the Stages of 2-Stage Revision Arthroplasty. J Arthroplasty 2018; 33:1844–1849.

32. Edelstein AI, Okroj KT, Rogers T, Della Valle CJ, Sporer SM. Nephrotoxicity After the Treatment of Periprosthetic Joint Infection with Antibiotic-Loaded Cement Spacers. J Arthroplasty 2018; 33:2225–2229.

33. Geller JA, Cunn G, Herschmiller T, Murtaugh T, Chen A. Acute Kidney Injury After First-Stage Joint Revision for Infection: Risk Factors and the Impact of Antibiotic Dosing. J Arthroplasty 2017; 32:3120–3125.

34. Akgun D, Muller M, Perka C, Winkler T. A Positive Bacterial Culture During Re-Implantation is Associated with a Poor Outcome in Two-Stage Exchange Arthroplasty for Deep Infection. Bone Joint J 2017; 99-B:1490–1495.

35. Frank JM, Kayupov E, Moric M, et al. The Mark Coventry Award: Oral Antibiotics Reduce Reinfection After Two-Stage Exchange: A Multicenter, Randomized Controlled Trial. Clin Orthop Relat Res 2017; 475:56–61.

36. Thakrar RR, Horriat S, Kayani B, Haddad FS. Indications for a Single-Stage Exchange Arthroplasty for Chronic Prosthetic Joint Infection. Bone Joint J 2018; 101-B:374.

37. Negus JJ, Gifford PB, Haddad FS. Single-Stage Revision Arthroplasty for Infection-An Underutilized Treatment Strategy. J Arthroplasty 2017; 32:2051–2055.

38. Pulsen NR, Mechlenburg I, Soballe K, Troelsen A, Lange J. Improved Patient-Reported Quality of Life and Hip Function After Cementless 1-Stage Revision for Chronic Periprosthetic Infection. J Arthroplasty 2019; 34:2763–2769.

39. Bori G, Navarro G, Morata L, et al. Preliminary Results Changing from Two-Stage to One-Stage Revision Arthroplasty Protocol Using Cementless Arthroplasty for Chronic Infected Hip Replacements. J Arthroplasty 2018; 33:527–532.

40. Kheir MM, Tan TL, George J, et al. Development and Evaluation of a Prognostic Calculator for the Surgical Treatment of Periprosthetic Joint Infection. J Arthroplasty 2018; 33:2986–2992.

41. Triantafyllopoulos GK, Memtsoudis SG, Zhang W, et al. Periprosthetic Infection Recurrence After 2-Stage Exchange Arthroplasty: Failure or Fate? J Arthroplasty 2017; 32:526–531.

42. Xu C, Wang Q, Kuo F, et al. The Presence of Sinus Tract Adversely Affects the Outcome of Treatment of Periprosthetic Joint Infections. J Arthroplasty 2019; 34:1227–1232.

43. Garvin KL, Miller RE, Gilbert TM, White AM, Lyden ER. Late Reinfection May Recur More than 5 Years After Reimplantation of THA and TKA: Analysis of Pathogen Factors. Clin Orthop Relat Res 2018; 476:345–352.

44. Kheir MM, Tan TL, Gomez MM, Chen AF, Parvizi J. Patients with Failed Prior Two-Stage Exchange Have Poor Outcomes After Further Surgical Intervention. J Arthroplasty 2017; 32:1262–1265.

45. George J, Miller EM, Curtis GL, et al. Success of Two-Stage Reimplantation in Patients Requiring an Interim Spacer Exchange. J Arthroplasty 2018; 33:S228–S232.

46. Kuo F, Goswami K, Shohat N, et al. Two-Stage Exchange Arthroplasty is a Favorable Treatment Option Upon Diagnosis of a Fungal Periprosthetic Joint Infection. J Arthroplasty 2018; 33:3555–3560.

47. Nogler MM, Thaler MR. The Direct Anterior Approach for Hip Revision: Accessing the Entire Femoral Diaphysis Without Endangering the Nerve Supply. J Arthroplasty 2017; 32:510–514.

48. Spanyer JM, Beaumont CM, Yerasimides JG. The Extended Direct Anterior Approach in the Deficient Pelvis: A Novel Surgical Technique, and Case Series Report. J Arthroplasty 2017; 32:515–519.
49. Horsthemke MD, Koenig C, Gosheger G, Hardes J, Hoell S. The Minimal invasive Direct Anterior Approach in Aseptic Cup Revision Hip Arthroplasty: a Mid-term Follow-up. Archives of Orthopaedic and Trauma Surgery 2019; 139:121–126.
50. Sadhu A, Nam D, Coobs BR, et al. Acetabular Component Position and the Risk of Dislocation Following Primary and Revision Total hip Arthroplasty: A Matched Cohort Analysis. J Arthroplasty 2017; 32:987–991.
51. Abdel MP. Dual-Mobility Constructs in Revision Total Hip Arthroplasties. J Arthroplasty 2018; 331329–1330.
52. Harwin SF, Sultan AA, Khlopas A, et al. Mid-term Outcomes of Dual Mobility Acetabular Cups for Revision Total Hip Arthroplasty. J Arthroplasty 2018; 33:1494–1500.
53. Sutter EG, McClellan TR, Attarian DE, et al. Outcomes of Modular Dual Mobility Acetabular Components in Revision Total hip Arthroplasty. J Arthroplasty 2017; 32:S220–S224.
54. Scott TP, Weitzler MS, Salvatore A, Wright TM, Westrich GH. A Retrieval Analysis of Impingement in Dual-Mobility Liners. J Arthroplasty 2018; 33:2660–2665.
55. Levin JM, Sultan AA, O'Donnell JA, et al. Modern Dual-Mobility Cups in Revision Total Hip Arthroplasty: A Systematic Review and Meta-Analysis. J Arthroplasty 2018; 33:3793–3800.
56. Lange JK, Spiro SK, Westrich GH. Utilizing Dual Mobility Components for First-Time Revision Total Hip Arthroplasty for Instability. J Arthroplasty 2018; 33:505–509.
57. Hartzler MA, Abdel MP, Sculco PK, et al. Otto Aufranc Award: Dual-mobility Constructs in Revision THA Reduced Dislocations, Rerevision, and Reoperation Compared With Large Femoral Heads. Clin Orthop Relat Res 2018; 476:293–301.
58. Abdel MP, Miller LE, Hanssen AD, Pagnano MW. Cost Analysis of Dual-Mobility Versus Large Femoral Head Constructs in Revision Total Hip Arthroplasty. J Arthroplasty 2019; 34:260–264.
59. Huang RC, Malkani AL, Harwin SF, et al. Multicenter Evaluation of a Modular Dual Mobility Construct for Revision Total Hip Arthroplasty. J Arthroplasty 2019; 34:S287–S291.
60. Chalmers BP, Pallante GD, Taunton MJ, Sierra RJ, Trousdale RJ. Can Dislocation of a Constrained Liner be Salvaged With Dual-mobility Constructs in Revision THA? Clin Orthop Relat Res 2018; 476:305–312.
61. Blevins JL, Shen TS, Morgenstern R, DeNova TA, Su EP. Conversion of Hip Resurfacing With Retention of Monoblock Acetabular Shell Using Dual-Mobility Components. J Arthroplasty 2019; 34:2037–2044.
62. Gascoyne TC, Lanting BA, Derksen KJ, Teeter MG, Turgeon TR. Damage Assessment of Retrieved Birmingham Monoblock Cups: Is Conversion to Dual-Mobility Head a Viable Revision Option? J Arthroplasty 2018; 33:1242–1246.
63. Chalmers BP, Perry KI, Hanssen AD, Pagnano MW, Abdel MP. Conversion of Hip Hemiarthroplasty to Total Hip Arthroplasty Utilizing a Dual-Mobility Construct Compared to Large Femoral Heads. J Arthroplasty 2017; 32:3071–3075.
64. Chalmers BP, Mangold DG, Hanssen AD, et al. Uniformly Low Serum Cobalt Levels After Modular Dual-Mobility Total hip Arthroplasties With Ceramic Heads: A Prospective Study in High-Risk Patients. Bone Joint J 2019; 101-B:57–61.
65. Marie-Hardy L, O'Laughlin P, Bonnin M, Selmi T. Are Dual Mobility Cups Associated With Increased Metal ions in the Blood? Clinical Study of Nickel and Chromium Levels With 29 Months' Follow-up. Orthop Traumatol Surg Res 2018; 104:1179–1182.
66. Bruggemann A, Mallmin H, Hailer NP. Do Dual-mobility Cups Cemented into Porous Tantalum Shells Reduce the Risk of Dislocation After Revision Surgery? Acta Orthopaedica 2018; 89:156–162.
67. Chalmers BP, Ledford CK, Taunton MJ, et al. Cementation of a Dual Mobility Construct in Recurrently Dislocating and High Risk Patients Undergoing Revision Total Arthroplasty. J Arthroplasty 2018; 33:1501–1506.
68. Reina N, Pareek A, Krych AJ, et al. Dual-Mobility Constructs in Primary and Revision Total Hip Arthroplasty: A Systematic Review of Comparative Studies. J Arthroplasty 2019; 34:594–603.
69. Sultan AA, Cantrell WA, Khlopas A, et al. Evidence-Based Management of Trunionosis in Metal-on-Polyethylene Total Hip Arthroplasty: A Systematic Review. J Arthroplasty 2018; 33:3343–3353.
70. Weiser MC, Lavernia CJ. Trunionosis in Total Hip Arthoplasty. J Bone Joint Surg Am 2017; 99:1489–1501.
71. Persson A, Eisler T, Boden H, et al. Revision for Symptomatice Pseudotumor After Primary Metal-on-Polyethylene Total Hip Arthroplasty With a Standard Femoral Stem. J Bone Joint Surg Am 2018; 100: 942–949.
72. Taunton MJ. How to Interpret Metal Ions in THA. J Arthroplasty 2020; 35:S60–S62.
73. McGrory BJ, Payson AM, MacKenzie JA. Elevated Intra-articular Cobalt and Chromium Levels in Mechanically Assisted Crevice Corrosion in Metal-on-Polyethylene Total hip Arthroplasty. J Arthroplasty 2017; 32:1654–1658.

74. Morozov PP, Sana M, McGrory BJ, Farraher SW, Abrahams TG. Comparison of Pre-Revision Magnetic Resonance Imaging and Operative Findings in Mechanically Assisted Crevice Corrosion in Symptomatic Metal-on-Polyethylene Total Hip Arthroplasties. J Arthroplasty 2017; 32:2535–2545.

75. MacDonald DW, Chen AF, Lee G, et al. Fretting and Corrosion Damage in Taper Adapter Sleeves for Ceramic Heads: A Retrieval Study. J Arthroplasty 2017; 32:2887–2891.

76. Dickinson EC, Sellenschloh K, Morlock MM. Impact of Stem Taper Damage on the Fracture Strength of Ceramic heads With Adapter Sleeves. Clin Biomech 2019; 63:193–200.

77. McGrory BJ, Jorgensen AH. High Early Major Complication Rate After Revision for Mechanically Assisted Crevice Corrosion in Metal-on-Polyethylene Total Hip Arthroplasty. J Arthroplasty 2017; 32:3704–3710.

78. Kwon Y, Rossi D, MacAuliffe J, Peng Y, Arauz P. Risk Factors Associated With early Complications of Revision Surgery for head-neck Taper Corrosion in Metal-on-Polyethylene Total Hip Arthroplasty. J Arthroplasty 2018; 33:3231–3237.

79. Waterson HB, Whitehouse MR, Greidanus NV, et al. Revision for Adverse Local Tissue Reaction Following Metal-on-Polyethylene Total hip Arthroplasty is Associated With a High Risk of Early Major Complications. Bone Joint J 2018; 100-B:720–724.

80. Kwon Y, MacAuliffe J, Peng Y, Arauz P. The Fate of Elevated Metal Ion Levels After Revision Surgery for head-Neck Taper Corrosion in Patients With Metal-on-Polyethylene Total Hip Arthroplasty. J Arthroplasty 2018; 33:2631–2635.

81. Matharu GS, Berryman F, Dunlop DJ, et al. Has the threshold for Revision Surgery for Adverse Reactions to Metal Debris Changed in Metal-on-Metal Hip Arthroplasty Patients? A Cohort Study of 239 Patients Using an Adapted Risk-Stratification Algorithm. Acta Orthop 2019; 90:530–536.

82. Lainiala OS, Reito AP, Nieminen JJ, Eskelinen AP. Declining Revision Burden of Metal-on-Metal Hip Arthroplasties. J Arthroplasty 2019; 34:2058–2064.

83. Mata-Fink A, Philipson DJ, Keeney BJ, et al. Patient-Reported Outcomes After Revision of Metal-on-Metal Total Bearings in Total Hip Arthroplasty. J Arthroplasty 2017; 32:1241–1244.

84. Matharu GS, Eskelinen A, Judge A, Pandit HG, Murray DW. Revision Surgery of Metal-on-Metal Hip Arthroplasties for Adverse Reactions to Metal Debris. Acta Orthop 2018; 89:278–288.

85. Mathary GS, Judge A, Murray DW, Pandit HG. Outcomes After Metal-on-Metal Hip Revision Surgery Depend on the Reason for Failure: A Propensity Score-matched Study. Clin Orthop Relat Res 2018; 476:245–258.

86. Hug KT, Amanatullah DF, Huddleston JI, Maloney WJ, Goodman SB. Protocol-Driven Revision for Stiffness After Total Knee Arthroplasty Imporves Motion and Clinical Outcomes. J Arthroplasty 2018; 33:2952–2955.

87. Van Rensch PJH, Hannink G, Heesterbeek PJC, Wymenga AB, van Hellemondt GG. Long-Term Outcome Following Revision Total Knee Arthroplasty is Associated With Indication for Revision. J Arthroplasty 2020; 35:1671–1677.

88. Cohen JS, Gu A, Lopez NS, et al. Efficacy of Revision Surgery for the Treatment of Stiffness After Total Knee Arthroplasty: A Systematic Review. J Arthroplasty 2018; 33:3049–3055.

89. Rutherford RW, Jennings JM, Levy DL, et al. Revision Total Knee Arthroplasty for Arthrofibrosis. J Arthroplasty 2018; 33:S177–S181.

90. Hermans K, Vandenneucker H, Truijen J, Oosterbosch J, Bellemans J. Hinged versus CCK Revision Arthroplasty for the Stiff Total Knee. The Knee 2019; 26:222–227.

91. Maslaris A, Layher F, Bungartz M, et al. Saggital Profile has a Significant Impact on the Explantability of Well-fixed Cemented Stems in Revision Knee Arthroplasty: a Biomechanical Comparison Study of Five Established Knee Implant Models. Archives of Orthopaedic and Trauma Surgery 2019; 139:991–998.

92. Fleischman AN, Azboy I, Fuery M, et al. Effect of Stem Size and Fixation Method on Mechanical Failure After Revision Total Knee Arthroplasty. J Arthroplasty 2017; 32:S202–S208.

93. Ettinger M, Savov P, Balubaid O, Windhagen H, Calliess T. Influence of Stem Length on Component Flexion and Posterior Condylar Offset in Revision Total Knee Arthroplasty. The Knee 2018; 25:480–484.

94. Gomez-Vallejo J, Albareda-Albareda J, Seral Garcia B, Blanco-Rubio N, Ezquerra-Herrando L. Revision Total Knee Arthroplasty: Hybrid vs Standard Cemented Fixation. J Orthop Traumatol 2018; 19: 9.

95. Fleischman AN, Azboy I, Restrepo C, Maltenfort MG, Parvizi J. Optimizing Mechanical Alignment With Modular Stems in Revision TKA. J Arthroplasty 2017; 32:S209–S213.

96. Lei P, Hu R, Hu Y. Bone Defects in Revision Total Knee Arthroplasty and Management. Orthopaedic Surgery 2019; 11:15–24.

97. Angerame MR, Jennings JM, Holst DC, Dennis DA. Management of Bone Defects in Revision Total Knee Arthroplasty With Use of Stepped, Porous-Coated Metaphyseal Sleeve. J Bone Joint Surg Essential Surgical Techniques 2019; 9:e14.

98. Zanirato A, Formica M, Cavagnaro L, et al. Metaphyseal Cones and Sleeves in Revision Total Knee Arthroplasty: Two Sides of the Same Coin? Complications, Clinical and Radiological Results – a Systematic Review of the Literature. Muscoloskeletal Surgery 2020; 104:25–35.

99. Ihekweazu UN, Weitzler L, Wright TM, Padgett DE. Distribution of Bone Ongrowth in Metaphyseal Sleeves for Revision Total Knee Arthroplasty: A Retrieval Analysis. J Arthroplasty 2019; 34:760–765.

100. Fedorka CJ, Chen AF, Pagnotto MR, Crossett LS, Klatt BA. Revision Total Knee Arthroplasty With Porous-Coated Metaphyseal Sleeves Provides Radiographic Ingrowth and Stable Fixation. Knee Surg Sports Traumatol Arthrosc 2018; 26:1500–1505.

101. Bonanzinga T, Akkawi I, Zahar A, et al. Are Metaphyseal Sleeves a Viable Option to Treat bone Defect During Revision Total Knee Arthroplasty? A Systematic Review. Joints 2019; 7:19–24.

102. Wirries N, Winnecken HJ, von Lewinski G, Windhagen W, Skutek M. Osteointegrative Sleeves for Metaphyseal Defect Augmentation in Revision Total Knee Arthroplasty: Clinical and Radiological 5-year Follow-up. J Arthroplasty 2019; 34:2022–2029.

103. Burastero G, Cavagnaro L, Chiarlone F, et al. The Use of tantalum metaphyseal Cones for the Management of Severe Bone Defects in Septic Knee Revision. J Arhtroplasty 2018; 33:3739–3745.

104. Klim SM, Amerstorfer F, Bernhardt GA, et al. Septic Revision Total Knee Arthroplasty: Treatment of Metaphyseal Bone Defects Using Metaphyseal Sleeves. J Arthroplasty 2018; 33:3734–3738.

105. Fink B, Mittelstadt A. Treatment of Periprosthetic Fractures of the Knee Using Trabecular Metal Cones for Stabilization. Arthroplasty Today 2019; 5:159–163.

Chapter 8

What is new in sports medicine? Orthobiologics: An evidence-based review of the literature

Rocco Bassora

INTRODUCTION

The use of biological therapy dates back to the late 1980s, where it was implemented during cardiac surgery to help minimise post-operative blood loss. During this time, it was also used by maxillofacial surgeons as a method of minimising inflammation and increasing cell proliferation for wound healing [1,2]. In the ensuing decades, there has been an expansion of its role, namely, to aid in the restoration of musculoskeletal tissue. More recently, the use of platelet-rich plasma (PRP) to treat tendinopathy and ligament damage has increased significantly, and we are beginning to have a better understanding of how stem cells may potentially be utilised in the same realm. In this chapter, we will focus on PRP, and the potential role it plays in musculoskeletal healing, utilising an evidence-based review of the current literature.

PLATELET-RICH PLASMA

Platelet-rich plasma is defined as a sample of autologous blood with a high concentration of platelets, much higher than that observed at baseline levels. In order to achieve this high level of concentration, autologous blood is spun in a centrifuge at a rate between 1,500 and 7,000 RPM. This is often done in a two-stage process, allowing for the separation of platelets from red blood cells and leucocytes (**Figure 8.1**) [3]. Two types of preparations exist – leucocyte-rich PRP (Lr-PRP) and leucocyte-poor PRP (Lp-PRP), depending on whether the leucocyte count is above or below baseline levels, respectively. It is thought that the increased neutrophil content in Lr-PRP creates catabolic cytokines such as tumour necrosis factor-α (TNF-α) and interleukin-1β (IL-1β) that counteract the anabolic cytokines produced by platelets. Lr-PRP is thought to incite a higher inflammatory response when compared to the Lp-PRP, often causing increased pain at the site of injection, and the clinical and biological implications of this higher leucocyte concentration is a focus of many ongoing studies [4].

Rocco Bassora MD, Department of Sports Medicine, Rothman Orthopaedic Institute, Montvale, NJ
Email: rocco.bassora@rothmanortho.com

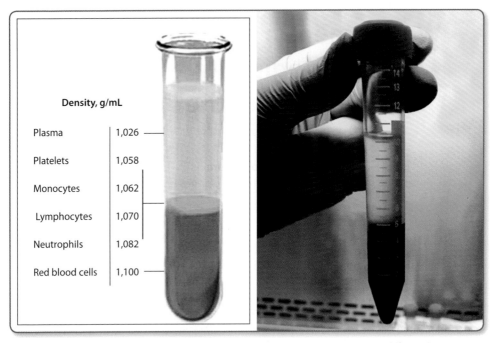

Density, g/mL	
Plasma	1,026
Platelets	1,058
Monocytes	1,062
Lymphocytes	1,070
Neutrophils	1,082
Red blood cells	1,100

Figure 8.1 After centrifugation, blood components are separated from plasma due to their different densities. Platelets have the lowest density. With permission from Alves et al. (2018) and Kolber et al. (2018) [1,39].

BASIC SCIENCE

Platelets are discoid, anucleated haematopoietic cells that play an important role in modulating haemostasis. They are involved in the host response to infection, inflammation, and malignancy. Platelets originate from megakaryocytes, and there are roughly 150,000–400,000 platelets per microliter of blood. They are directly involved in the process of healing, which is composed of three phases: inflammation, proliferation, and remodelling [5].

Platelets contain a myriad of growth factors within their granules that are essential for the healing response (**Figure 8.2**). These include transforming growth factor-β (TGF-β), platelet-derived growth factor (PDGF), vascular endothelial growth factor (VEGF), fibroblast growth factor (FGF), insulin-like growth factor (IGF), and epidermal growth factor (EGF) (**Table 8.1**). It is these growth factors that promote healing in tissue with otherwise poor, or limited blood supply by way of angiogenesis and chemotaxis [6].

In vitro studies have evaluated the effect of PRP on tendons and ligaments. PRP has been shown to increase tenocyte number and vascularity in culture. In addition, there appears to be an increased expression of VEGF as well as an increased production of collagen once they have been exposed to PRP [7]. Jo et al showed that cultured tenocytes from degenerated rotator cuff tendons had enhanced gene expression, as well as enhanced synthesis, and proliferation of the tendon matrix when exposed to PRP [8]; Cross et al showed promotion of collagen matrix synthesis along with decreased production of degradative cytokines associated with matrix degeneration [9].

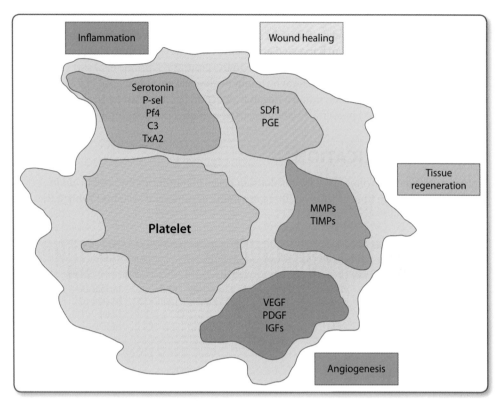

Figure 8.2 Platelets contain many cytokines that play significant roles in regulatory function [40]. IGF, insulin-like growth factor; MMP, matrix metalloproteinase; PDGF, platelet-derived growth factor; VEGF, vascular endothelial growth factor; TIMP, tissue inhibitors of metalloproteinase.

Table 8.1 Growth factors found in platelet alpha granules and their function [39]	
Growth factors in platelet alpha granules	
Growth factor (GF)	**Function**
Insulin-like GF-1 (IGF-I)	Cell growth, proliferation, and differentiation. Stimulates collagen synthesis. Proliferation and differentiation of mesenchymal cells [connective tissue (e.g. muscle, cartilage, and bone) and blood vessels]
Platelet-derived GF (PDGF)	Enhances collagen synthesis, macrophage activation, proliferation of bone cells, fibroblast chemotaxis, and mitosis. Stimulates angiogenesis and vasculogenesis
Vascular endothelial GF (VEGF)	Stimulates angiogenesis and vasculogenesis, migration and proliferation of endothelial cells, and stimulates chemotaxis of macrophages and neutrophils
Epidermal GF (EGF)	Accelerates reepithelialisation and influences cell proliferation
Transforming GF-β (TGF-β)	Proliferation and differentiation of mesenchymal cells. Stimulates synthesis of collagen, angiogenesis, reepithelialisation, and synthesis of protease inhibitors (prevent collagen breakdown). Inhibits osteoclast formation and bone resorption. Key regulator in balance between muscle fibrosis and myocyte regeneration. Some concerns exist over profibrotic effects in muscle
Fibroblastic GF (FGF) numerous subtypes exist	Proliferation of mesenchymal stem cells, chondrocytes, and osteoblasts. Growth and differentiation of chondrocytes, fibroblasts, and osteoblasts. Inhibits osteoclastic actions
Hepatocyte GF	Angiogenesis, mitogen for endothelial cells, and antifibrotic. Extracellular matrix synthesis. Anti-inflammatory effects
Source: With permission from Kolber M, et al. (2018) [39]	

Few basic science studies have evaluated the effects of PRP on ligaments, and their results have been mixed. Fallouh et al performed a study on cultured fresh cells from anterior cruciate ligaments, which were harvested at the time of surgery, and noted increased viability of the cells when exposed to PRP [10]. On the contrary, LaPrade et al showed no improvement in rabbit medial collateral ligament healing after a single dose of PRP when compared to controls, and even noted a negative effect on ligament strength and histological characteristics at 6 weeks post-injury when exposed to higher concentrations [11].

CLINICAL APPLICATION

Platelet-rich plasma is often used for recalcitrant cases of tendinopathy, and to aid in tendon healing at the time of surgery. There are many commercial systems (**Table 8.2**)

System	Company	Blood volume required (mL)	Concentrated volume produced (mL)	Processing time (min)	PPP produced?	Increase in (Platelets), times baseline	Platelet capture efficiency, % yield
Table 8.2 Characteristics of PRP preparations from different commercially available systems [12]							
Leucocyte-rich PRP:							
Angel	Arthrex (Florida, USA)	52	1–20	17	+	10	56–75%
Genesis CS	EmCyte (Florida, USA)	54	6	10	+	4–7	61% ± 12%
GPS III	Biomet (now known as Zimmer Biomet, Indiana, USA)	54	6	15	+	3–10	70% ± 30%
Magellan	Isto Biologics/ Arteriocyte (now known as Isto Biologics, Massachusetts, USA)	52	3.5–7	17	+	3–15	86% ± 41%
SmartPReP 2	Harvest (now known as Terumo BCT, Colorado, USA)	54	7	14	+	5–9	94% ± 12%
Leucocyte-poor PRP:							
Autologous conditioned plasma (ACP)	Arthrex	11	4	5	–	1.3	48% ± 7%
Cascade	MTF (New Jersey, USA)	18	7.5	6	–	1.6	68% ± 4%
Clear PRP	Harvest	54	6.5	18	+	3–6	62% ± 5%
Pure PRP	EmCyte	50	6.5	8.5	+	4–7	76% ± 4%

PPP, platelet-poor plasma; PRP, platelet-rich plasma.
Note: Plus–Minus sign signifies reported variance of platelet capture efficiency.
Source: With permission from Le ADK, et al. (2019) [12]

that have been developed to attain whole blood and isolate it into its various components. Once collected, whole blood is mixed with an anticoagulant and subsequently spun in a centrifuge. Red blood cells and platelet-poor plasma are then discarded, and the platelets are then injected directly into the tendon substance. Cytokines emitted by platelets help to facilitate the stages of healing mentioned above. It is these cytokines that are responsible for promoting neovascularisation, increasing blood supply to damaged cells, and attracting other reparative cells to the site of damage [12]. There are many studies that have evaluated the efficacy of PRP on various tendinopathies. In this chapter, we will evaluate these studies and attempt to draw up a conclusion on whether PRP injections are effective in treating several of the most common forms of tendinopathy.

Patellar tendinopathy

Patellar tendinopathy, also known as 'jumper's knee,' is a common cause of knee pain in the young athlete. Treatment often consists of extensive physical therapy and nonsteroidal anti-inflammatory drugs (NSAIDs), yet approximately one-third of athletes do not return to sport at 6 months, with 50% of patients often experiencing anterior knee pain for many years after the initial diagnoses [13]. PRP has become a common mode of treatment for patellar tendinopathy, despite the literature yielding mixed results with respect to its efficacy.

Abate et al compared outcomes of 54 patients receiving two ultrasound-guided injections (2 weeks apart), consisting of either PRP, saline, or a solution containing both. The Victorian Institute of Sport Assessment-Patella (VISA-P) and Visual Analogue Scale (VAS) scores were assessed at 3 and 6 months. The results revealed comparable results in the short term among the three groups, whereas in the long term, PRP alone, or in combination with saline, showed greater efficacy when compared to saline injection alone. They concluded that PRP injections, either alone or in combination with saline, improved symptoms related to patella tendinopathy [14].

In contrast to the above study, Scott et al performed a small, level-1 randomised controlled study evaluating whether a single ultrasound-guided PRP injection, either Lr-PRP or Lp-PRP, was superior to saline injection for the treatment of patellar tendinopathy. The VISA-P, pain during activity, and global rating of change were assessed at 6 and 12 weeks and 6 and 12 months. The results revealed no difference in outcomes among the three treatment arms and they concluded that PRP injections did not offer superior results when compared to saline injections alone [15].

Andriolo et al performed a systematic review and meta-analysis, analysing the outcomes of greater than 2,500 PRP injections for the treatment of patellar tendinopathy. They concluded that multiple injections yielded lower pain scores and better clinical outcomes 6 months after injections, with good results lasting up to 3 years. Unfortunately, based on the Coleman score, many of the PRP studies were of poor quality, consisting of case series analysis and retrospective reviews on a small number of patients [16].

Author's conclusion

Despite the dearth of high-quality studies evaluating the efficacy of PRP injections for patellar tendinopathy, smaller studies, and systematic reviews of the literature have yielded good results, and PRP injections should be considered as a treatment option for patellar tendonitis.

Lateral epicondylitis

Lateral epicondylitis (LE) is a common cause of elbow pain, affecting 1–3% of the general population, and up to 10% of heavy laborers. The extensor carpi radialis brevis (ECRB) is the most common tendon affected, with degeneration evident at the time of surgery (**Figure 8.3**). Histological studies typically reveal a process which involves angiofibroblastic hyperplasia, characterised by high cell counts, blood vessel hyperplasia, and collagen fibre breakdown. It is this tendinous degeneration, with the absence of local inflammation that points more towards a tendinosis, as opposed to a tendinitis [17].

Conservative treatment for LE is successful in >85% of cases, and often involves the use of a counter-force strap, NSAIDs and a regimented home exercise program. For patients who fail these conservative measures, cortisone injections have been proven to help alleviate symptoms. Unfortunately, steroid injections impart catabolic, degradative effects on tissue, and their use in the treatment of LE should remain limited [18].

Given the deleterious effects cortisone has on tissue, the use of PRP for LE has gained popularity in recent years and has become a more favourable alternative with good long-term results. Ben-nafa et al performed a systematic review comparing the use of corticosteroids versus PRP and concluded that corticosteroids were more effective than the latter in reducing symptoms in the short term (<2 months); however, PRP injections appeared to have longer lasting effects, alleviating pain for up to 2 years status post-injection. In addition, they also noted reduced tendon thickness and increased cortical erosion in the corticosteroid group when compared to the PRP group, indicating less atrophy in the latter. The authors concluded that despite the rapid therapeutic response corticosteroids provide after injection, their effects are short lived when compared to their PRP counterpart, and patients have a higher rate of recurrence in the long term [19].

These findings are consistent with a systematic review performed by Li et al, where they evaluated the short- and long-term effects of corticosteroids versus PRP. They noted that the corticosteroid group had significantly higher Disabilities of the Arm, Shoulder, and Hand (DASH) score at 4 and 8 weeks follow-up when compared to the PRP group, but lower DASH and VAS scores at 24 weeks. They concluded that PRP provided longer acting pain relief and improved function in the long term when compared to corticosteroid injections [20].

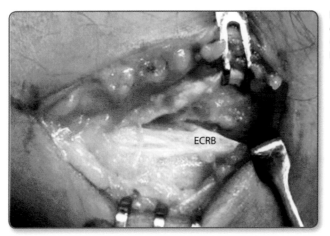

Figure 8.3 Tendinous degeneration of extensor carpi radialis brevis (ECRB). With permission from Inagaki K, et al. (2013) [41].

Leucocyte concentration also plays a role in clinical outcomes. One of the largest studies to date was performed by Mishra et al, where they evaluated 230 patients who failed conservative therapy for LE. After 24 weeks of treatment with Lr-PRP, patients experienced a significant improvement in pain (71.5% vs. 56.1%, $p = 0.019$) when compared with patients who received local anaesthetic [21].

Author's conclusion

High-quality systematic reviews of Level-I and Level-II randomised controlled studies have shown that PRP is an effective short- and long-term treatment regimen for LE, and that Lr-PRP is more effective than Lp-PRP, making it the concentration of choice.

Rotator cuff tendinopathy

Rotator cuff disease is a leading cause of shoulder disability, with a 19% and 32% prevalence of full thickness and partial thickness rotator cuff tears, respectively [22]. Approximately, 30% of patients over the age of 60 years and 62% over the age of 80 years have tears, and many are asymptomatic [23]. The aetiology of rotator cuff tendinopathy is unclear, and it appears that there are intrinsic and extrinsic contributory factors. One theory describes tendinopathy as a result of excessive force applied to the tendon, which exceeds the healing potential of tenocytes, hindering the tendon's ability to heal properly [24].

The use of PRP in patients with rotator cuff pathology has yielded mixed results, either as primary treatment for tendinopathy, or when used as an augment for rotator cuff tendon repair. Pauly et al studied the effects of PRP on human rotator cuff tenocytes by collecting tissue samples from 24 patients at the time of surgery, culturing the procured cells, and preserving them for 2 years. At the 2-year mark, the cultured tenocytes were exposed to PRP preparations obtained from the same patients, and the following were analysed – cell proliferation, collagen I synthesis, and expression of collagen I and III. They found that cell proliferation and collagen I synthesis were increased when compared to controls, and that PRP contained high levels of IGF-1 growth factor. The authors concluded that PRP had an anabolic effect on rotator cuff tenocytes [25].

Sari et al compared PRP, prolotherapy, and corticosteroid injections in patients with partial thickness rotator cuff tears and found lower short term (3 weeks) VAS and Western Ontario Rotator Cuff Index (WORC) scores in the corticosteroid group and lower long term (>24 weeks) scores in the PRP group [26]. A recent prospective randomised control study performed by Shams et al compared the effects of subacromial PRP versus corticosteroid injections in patients with partial thickness rotator cuff tears. They found statistically significant improvement in VAS and American Shoulder and Elbow Surgeons (ASES) scores in the PRP group at 12 weeks when compared with the corticosteroid group, but no difference at 6 months [27].

Recent studies have also evaluated the potential augmenting effects of PRP on rotator cuff tendon healing post-operatively. Malavolta et al performed a randomised control study on 54 patients – half of which received PRP at the time of surgery, and half who did not. Clinical and structural outcomes were assessed at 6, 12, 24, and 60 months. The authors found no difference in VAS scores between the PRP and control groups, and no structural differences in tendon quality throughout the aforementioned time period, and concluded that PRP did not provide added healing potential after single row rotator cuff tendon repair [28]. On the contrary, Hurley et al reviewed 18 randomised controlled trials (RCTs) comparing PRP or platelet-rich fibrin (PRF) to arthroscopic rotator cuff tendon repair alone and found significantly decreased rates of incomplete healing in small–medium and medium–complete tears in the PRP group when compared with controls. In addition, they found a significant decrease in VAS score in the PRP group 1 month after surgery [29]. Likewise, Wang and colleagues analysed eight RCTs comparing rotator cuff repair outcomes with and without PRP and found a significantly decreased short-term retear rate in the PRP group, but no significant difference in the long-term retear rate; VAS scores were significantly lower, while both Constant and University of California at Los Angeles (UCLA) scores were higher in the PRP group [30].

Author's conclusion

In vitro and RCT studies have shown positive effects of PRP on rotator cuff tendon healing and improvement in non-operative clinical outcomes, respectively. There appear to be some short-term benefits with subacromial PRP injections, negating the deleterious effects of cortisone on local tissue. With respect to the augmentation of rotator cuff tendon repairs, many studies have yielded mixed results, and there does not appear to be a clear-cut advantage supporting their use at the time of surgery.

Achilles tendinopathy

The Achilles tendon is the strongest and largest tendon in the body, with the ability to resist up to 12 times body weight during activity. It is a conjoined tendon which is comprised of the gastrocnemius and the soleus muscles, with little contribution from the plantaris muscle [31,32]. Achilles tendinopathy is a common disorder, affecting approximately 6% of the general population, and up to 9% of top-level runners. Anatomic studies have revealed a water-shed region of the tendon, predisposing it to ischaemic injury approximately 4–6 cm from its insertion onto the calcaneus [31,33]. There has been recent interest in determining whether PRP can help to alleviate symptoms secondary to Achilles tendinopathy, and perhaps aid in tendon healing.

Yan et al performed an in vivo study comparing the effects of intra-tendinous PRP injections using a rabbit chronic tendinopathy model. 4 weeks after tendons were injected with collagenase; they were either injected with Lp-PRP, Lr-PRP, or saline. Healing outcomes were measured 4 weeks after therapy with the use of MRI, histological analysis, transmission electron microscopy, and polymerase chain reaction analysis of gene expression. The results revealed an increased healing response with Lp-PRP when compared to Lr-PRP or saline, and the authors concluded that Lp-PRP injections should be considered when treating chronic tendinopathy [34].

Three meta-analysis studies evaluating the efficacy of PRP injections for Achilles tendinopathy were recently performed. Lin et al evaluated seven RCTs comparing PRP injections versus placebo and the results revealed equal effectiveness in Victorian Institute of Sports Assessment-Achilles (VISA-A) score at 6 weeks, 12 weeks, and 24 weeks [35]. The authors concluded that PRP injections were no more effective than placebo in treating Achilles tendinopathy. Likewise, Wang et al reviewed four level 1 RCTs where they evaluated VISA-A score, Doppler ultrasound index, and recovery time to normal sport and found no difference in outcomes between the PRP groups and control groups [36]. Finally, Liu et al reviewed five RCTs comparing PRP to placebo injections and found that despite better efficacy in the PRP group at 6 weeks, there was no difference in VISA-A score at 12 weeks and 1 year. They concluded that PRP injections remain an option in treating chronic Achilles tendinopathy and that further studies should be conducted to support their conclusion [37].

More recently, Boesen et al performed a randomised double-blinded prospective study comparing PRP, high-volume methylprednisolone injection (HVI), and sham injections in 60 males with Achilles tendinopathy >3 months. In addition to receiving injections, the participants also performed eccentric training exercises through a focussed rehabilitation program. The results revealed statistically significant improvement in pain and function in the PRP and HVI groups when compared with the sham group [38].

Author's conclusion

Despite positive results yielded by small in vivo studies as well as a recent randomised controlled study, the overall review of the literature points to decreased efficacy of PRP injections for Achilles tendinopathy and further high-quality studies are required to support their use.

CONCLUSION

The use of orthobiologics has been around for several decades, and its implementation in musculoskeletal tissue healing has gained interest in the field of regenerative medicine. PRP is derived from autologous blood and is composed of a high concentration of platelet-derived cytokines, which play an important role in tissue healing and reducing inflammation. Many studies assessing the efficacy of PRP have yielded mixed results, and more research is warranted to support its use for various tendinopathies. At this time, according to the most recent data available, it appears that PRP is safe and effective in treating LE and patellar tendinopathy, and less effective for Achilles tendinopathy. With respect to rotator cuff tendinopathy, there appear to be some short-term benefits with subacromial injections, and less benefit when used as an augment for rotator cuff tendon repair.

REFERENCES

1. Alves R, Grimalt R. A Review of Platelet-Rich Plasma: History, Biology, Mechanism of Action, and Classification. SAD 2018; 4:18–24.
2. DelRossi AJ, Cernaianu AC, Vertrees RA, et al. Platelet-rich plasma reduces postoperative blood loss after cardiopulmonary bypass. J Thorac Cardiovasc Surg 1990; 100:281–286.
3. Hsu WK, Mishra A, Rodeo SR, et al. Platelet-rich plasma in orthopaedic applications: evidence-based recommendations for treatment. J Am Acad Orthop Surg 2013; 21:739–748.
4. Dragoo JL, Braun HJ, Durham JL, et al. Comparison of the acute inflammatory response of two commercial platelet-rich plasma systems in healthy rabbit tendons. Am J Sports Med 2012; 40:1274–1281.
5. Elsevier Enhanced Reader. Role of platelets in immune system and inflammation https://reader.elsevier.com/reader/sd/pii/S2444866417300107?token=518B9DF3DE25D60D4FB53442AC3DBAE0A7D8770CF0B5965D1B78E22683D0170C7254C77B9BF72D11DC5919EDC815E9DE. [Last accessed 6 May 2022.]
6. Barrientos S, Stojadinovic O, Golinko MS, Brem H, Tomic-Canic M. Growth factors and cytokines in wound healing. Wound Repair Regen 2008; 16:585–601.
7. Geaney LE, Arciero RA, DeBerardino TM, Mazzocca AD. The effects of platelet-rich plasma on tendon and ligament: basic science and clinical application. Operat Tech Sports Med 2011; 19:160–164.
8. Jo CH, Kim JE, Yoon KS, Shin S. Platelet-rich plasma stimulates cell proliferation and enhances matrix gene expression and synthesis in tenocytes from human rotator cuff tendons with degenerative tears. Am J Sports Med 2012; 40:1035–1045.
9. Cross JA, Cole BJ, Spatny KP, et al. Leukocyte-reduced platelet-rich plasma normalizes matrix metabolism in torn human rotator cuff tendons. Am J Sports Med 2015; 43:2898–2906.
10. Fallouh L, Nakagawa K, Sasho T, et al. Effects of autologous platelet-rich plasma on cell viability and collagen synthesis in injured human anterior cruciate ligament. J Bone Joint Surg Am 2010; 92:2909–2916.

11. LaPrade RF, Goodrich LR, Phillips J, et al. Use of platelet-rich plasma immediately after an injury did not improve ligament healing, and increasing platelet concentrations was detrimental in an in vivo animal model. Am J Sports Med 2018; 46:702–712.

12. Le ADK, Enweze L, DeBaun MR, Dragoo JL. Platelet-Rich Plasma. Clin Sports Med 2019; 38:17–44.

13. Rosso F, Bonasia DE, Cottino U, et al. Patellar tendon: From tendinopathy to rupture. Asia Pac J Sports Med Arthrosc Rehabil Technol 2015; 2:99–107.

14. Abate M, Di Carlo L, Verna S, et al. Synergistic activity of platelet rich plasma and high-volume image guided injection for patellar tendinopathy. Knee Surg Sports Traumatol Arthrosc 2018; 26:3645–3651.

15. Scott A, LaPrade RF, Harmon KG, et al. Platelet-rich plasma for patellar tendinopathy: a randomized controlled trial of leukocyte-rich PRP or leukocyte-poor PRP versus saline. Am J Sports Med 2019; 47:1654–1661.

16. Andriolo L, Altamura SA, Reale D, et al. Nonsurgical treatments of patellar tendinopathy: multiple injections of platelet-rich plasma are a suitable option: a systematic review and meta-analysis. Am J Sports Med 2019; 47:1001–1018.

17. Lenoir H, Mares O, Carlier Y. Management of lateral epicondylitis. Orthop Traumatol Surg Res 2019; 105:S241–S246.

18. Calandruccio JH, Steiner MM. Autologous Blood and Platelet-Rich Plasma Injections for Treatment of Lateral Epicondylitis. Orthop Clin. 2017; 48:351–357.

19. Ben-Nafa W, Munro W. The effect of corticosteroid versus platelet-rich plasma injection therapies for the management of lateral epicondylitis: A systematic review. SICOT J 2018; 4:11.

20. Li A, Wang H, Yu Z, et al. Platelet-rich plasma vs corticosteroids for elbow epicondylitis: A systematic review and meta-analysis. Medicine (Baltimore) 2019; 98:e18358.

21. Mishra AK, Skrepnik NV, Edwards SG, et al. Efficacy of platelet-rich plasma for chronic tennis elbow: a double-blind, prospective, multicenter, randomized controlled trial of 230 patients. Am J Sports Med 2014; 42:463–471.

22. Weber S, Chahal J. Management of Rotator Cuff Injuries. JAAOS 2020; 28:e193.

23. May T, Garmel GM. Rotator Cuff Injury. In: StatPearls [Internet]. Treasure Island (FL): StatPearls Publishing; 2020. http://www.ncbi.nlm.nih.gov/books/NBK547664/. [Last accessed 6 May 2022.]

24. Spargoli G. Treatment of rotator cuff tendinopathy as a contractile dysfunction. A clinical commentary. Int J Sports Phys Ther 2019; 14:148–158.

25. Pauly S, Klatte-Schulz F, Stahnke K, Scheibel M, Wildemann B. The effect of autologous platelet rich plasma on tenocytes of the human rotator cuff. BMC Musculoskelet Disord 2018; 19:422.

26. Sari A, Eroglu A. Comparison of ultrasound-guided platelet rich plasma, prolotherapy, and corticosteroid injections in rotator cuff lesions. J Back Musculoskelet Rehabil 2019; 33:387–396.

27. Shams A, El-Sayed M, Gamal O, Ewes W. Subacromial injection of autologous platelet-rich plasma versus corticosteroid for the treatment of symptomatic partial rotator cuff tears. Eur J Orthop Surg Traumatol 2016; 26:837–842.

28. Malavolta EA, Gracitelli MEC, Assunção JH, et al. Clinical and structural evaluations of rotator cuff repair with and without added platelet-rich plasma at 5-year follow-up: A prospective randomized study. Am J Sports Med 2018; 46:3134–3141.

29. Hurley ET, Lim Fat D, Moran CJ, Mullett H. The efficacy of platelet-rich plasma and platelet-rich fibrin in arthroscopic rotator cuff repair: A meta-analysis of randomized controlled trials. Am J Sports Med 2019; 47:753–761.

30. Wang C, Xu M, Guo W, et al. Clinical efficacy and safety of platelet-rich plasma in arthroscopic full-thickness rotator cuff repair: A meta-analysis. PLoS One 2019; 14:e0220392.

31. Dayton P. Anatomic, vascular, and mechanical overview of the Achilles tendon. Clin Podiatr Med Surg 2017; 34:107–113.

32. Benjamin M, Toumi H, Ralphs JR, et al. Where tendons and ligaments meet bone: attachment sites ('entheses') in relation to exercise and/or mechanical load. J Anat 2006; 208:471–490.

33. Paoloni J. Current Strategy in the Treatment of Achilles Tendinopathy. Achilles Tendon [Internet]. 2012. https://www.intechopen.com/books/achilles-tendon/achilles-tendon-injury-management. [Last accessed 6 May 2022.]

34. Yan R, Gu Y, Ran J, et al. Intratendon delivery of leukocyte-poor platelet-rich plasma improves healing compared with leukocyte-rich platelet-rich plasma in a rabbit Achilles tendinopathy model. Am J Sports Med 2017; 45:1909–1920.

35. Lin MT, Chiang CF, Wu CH, Hsu HH, Tu YK. Meta-analysis comparing autologous blood-derived products (including platelet-rich plasma) injection versus placebo in patients with Achilles tendinopathy. Arthroscopy 2018; 34:1966–1975.e5.
36. Wang Y, Han C, Hao J, Ren Y, Wang J. Efficacy of platelet-rich plasma injections for treating Achilles tendonitis: Systematic review of high-quality randomized controlled trials. Orthopade 2019; 48:784–791.
37. Liu CJ, Yu KL, Bai JB, Tian DH, Liu GL. Platelet-rich plasma injection for the treatment of chronic Achilles tendinopathy: A meta-analysis. Medicine (Baltimore) 2019; 98:e15278.
38. Boesen AP, Hansen R, Boesen MI, Malliaras P, Langberg H. Effect of high-volume injection, platelet-rich plasma, and sham treatment in chronic midportion Achilles tendinopathy: A randomized double-blinded prospective study. Am J Sports Med 2017; 45:2034–2043.
39. Kolber M, Purita J, Paulus C, Carreno J, Hanney W. Platelet-rich plasma: basic science and biological effects. Strength Cond J 2018; 40:77–94.
40. Margraf A, Zarbock A. Platelets in inflammation and resolution. J Immunol 2019; 203:2357–2367.
41. Inagaki K. Current concepts of elbow-joint disorders and their treatment. J Orthop Sci 2013; 18:1–7.

Chapter 9

What is new in shoulder and elbow surgery?

Frank G Alberta, Christopher L Antonacci, Jeffrey D Tompson

ROTATOR CUFF

Non-arthroplasty options to address massive irreparable rotator cuff tear (MIRCT) continue to be the focus of much study. Partial repair with augmentation or inter-positional grafting has a role in the treatment of MIRCT. Inter-positional grafts have been used for some time to bridge irreparable defects in the rotator cuff [1,2], but clinical outcomes studies have been lacking. A recent large clinical study showed that pain scores, forward flexion and external rotation could be significantly improved with partial repair of the posterior portion of a MIRCT combined with xenograft patching of the remaining anterior defect. At >50 months follow-up, 92% of grafts remained fully intact and 3% were partially intact on ultrasound as well. Furthermore, Gupta et al observed 76% graft integrity by ultrasound when using human dermal allograft for interposition [3]. Pain scores and clinical parameters improved at 3 years follow-up.

The introduction of arthroscopic superior capsule reconstruction (ASCR) by Mihata gave many surgeons a new minimally invasive tool that could improve the functional losses seen following this difficult problem [4,5]. ASCR has been shown to improve function through two separate mechanisms. The graft acts both as a checkrein to limit the superior translation of the humeral head and as a sub-acromial 'spacer' that restores the acromiohumeral interval (AHI) and helps to re-centre the superiorly migrated humeral head. Reconstruction of the superior capsule as a static restraint protecting against superior translation of the humeral head was first described by Mihata et al [4] and has quickly gained momentum as an excellent option in these difficult problems. Attempts to reproduce the performance of autograft ASCR with dermal allograft tissue have mixed

Frank G Alberta MD, Associate Professor of Orthopaedic Surgery, Hackensack Meridian School of Medicine, Hackensack, Rothman Orthopaedics, Paramus, New Jersey
Email: Frank.Alberta@rothmanortho.com

Christopher L Antonacci MD MPH, Orthopaedic Surgery Resident at UConn Health, Farmington, Connecticut, United States
Email: antonacci@uchc.edu

Jeffrey D Tompson MD, Resident Physician, Department of Orthopaedic Surgery, Rutgers New Jersey Medical School, Newark, NJ
Email: Jdtompson@gmail.com

results. In a multi-centre short-term follow-up study, significant improvements were noted in forward flexion, external rotation, visual analogue scale (VAS) and ASES scores. However, early improvements in the AHI were not maintained at final follow-up and 11 patients underwent additional surgery including 7 (12%) who required arthroplasty. However, Pennington et al reported similar results in 88 patients undergoing ASCR with dermal allograft, with improvements in VAS, ASES scores and range of motion. In contrast, the improvements in AHI were maintained through the 1-year follow-up [6].

Differences in clinical results and rates of graft integrity have raised questions about graft material, source and thickness [4,7,8]. Scheiderer et al [7] showed that graft thickness was critically important. In a cadaveric model of MIRCT, 3 mm grafts could not restore superior translation or sub-acromial peak contact pressures. Thicker grafts (6 mm) restored translation and contact pressures and were significantly better than the thinner grafts and the torn conditions.

An inflatable balloon spacer has been proposed as an option to achieve the same effect [9–13]. This biodegradable balloon (InSpace Balloon, Orthospace, Caesarea, and Israel) is inserted through an enlarged arthroscopic portal and is then inflated in-situ (**Figure 9.1**). Of note, this implant has not been approved for use in the United States as of this writing, but its use in Europe has resulted in published clinical studies with 3 years of follow-up [12]. Biomechanical studies have shown that the balloon spacer can restore AHI, sub-acromial contact pressures and deltoid load but not sub-acromial contact areas [9,10]. Volume of inflation has also been studied and over-inflation was found to result in subluxation of the humerus [14]. Additional cadaveric studies comparing balloon

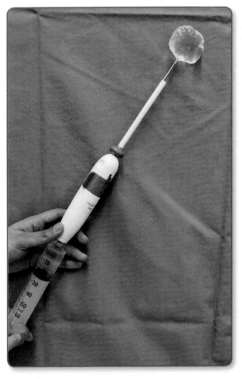

Figure 9.1 Inspace balloon spacer.
Source: Retrieved from http://orthospace.co.il/professionals/clinicians/inspace-benefits/#.

arthroplasty and ASCR showed that both techniques restored required abduction force to restore elevation but ASCR worked as a tether and the balloon directly depressed the humeral head [10].

Clinical outcomes of subacromial balloon spacers however, are limited to short- and mid-term case series. Twelve clinical studies included in a systematic review [11] netted pooled data in 291 shoulders treated with sub-acromial balloon spacers followed for a mean of 22.9 months. Improvements in mean constant scores and patient satisfaction rates varied but infrequent complications were noted (6 patients). Direct results have been reported as well [12]. Pain and functional outcomes were evaluated prospectively in 44 patients. Significant pain reduction and functional improvement was observed post-operatively and maintained at nearly 3 years with 82% patient satisfaction.

Castagna et al [13] attempted to define the cost benefits following balloon insertion, reverse total shoulder arthroplasty, partial MIRCT repair, or non-operative treatment. Arthroscopic balloon implantation resulted in a 0.05-increase in Quality Adjusted Life Years (QALYs) compared to non-operative care and 0.10 increase in QALY over reverse total shoulder arthroplasty. Furthermore, the sub-acromial balloon increased costs by only 522 Euro, resulting in an ICER which was significantly less than the threshold set for cost effectiveness. The authors concluded that the sub-acromial spacer is a safe, effective and cost-efficient option for patients with MIRCT.

There has also been a recent resurgence in the use of tendon transfers to address the functional limitations in younger patients with MIRCTs. Latissimus dorsi (LD) and, more recently, lower trapezius (LT) transfers for posterior superior, irreparable RCTs have gained momentum as a successful treatment option and are another tool in the armamentarium against this difficult problem. The LD was historically the most common tendon transfer for postero-superior rotator cuff tears. Multiple authors have reported on arthroscopically assisted LD transfer for MIRCT. In two recent trials [15,16], improved range of motion and functional scores have been reported following the procedure at >2-year follow-up. VAS decreased to 1–2 points and range of motion was significantly improved. Radiographs also confirmed improvement in AHI at final follow-up.

More recently, the lower portion of the trapezius muscle has been described as a potentially better alternative to LD transfer owing to its line of pull and in-phase firing pattern. Omid et al [15] demonstrated that the LT transfer is superior to the LD transfer in restoring glenohumeral kinematics and joint reaction forces. In a separate biomechanical study, Reddy et al [16] created a computer model to compare the LD and LT transfers using native insertion sites and force vectors. The authors noted the LT was able to recreate more efficient abduction and external rotation moment arms when transferred to the infraspinatus insertion site. Additionally, the LD performed better with transfer to the supraspinatus insertion site. Finally, the authors noted that transfer of the LT to the supraspinatus insertion placed increased muscle strain, necessitating an allograft to prevent over tensioning.

Elhassan et al [17] reported on the clinical outcomes of an arthroscopic LT transfer in 33 patients with an average follow-up of 47 months. Shoulder range of motion increased post-operatively in forward flexion to 120°, abduction to 90°, and external rotation to 50°. Subjective shoulder value (SSV) significantly increased from 54 to 78%. The authors concluded that the LT transfer was beneficial for patients with pseudo-paralytic shoulders at medium-term follow-up.

OPIOID USE IN SHOULDER AND ELBOW SURGERY

Risk factors for prolonged opioid use following shoulder surgery have been studied by multiple authors with somewhat consistent results reported [18–22]. History of alcohol abuse, history of psychiatric illness (depressive or anxiety disorders), female sex, obesity and higher Charlson Comorbidity Index scores were associated with an increased risk for prolonged opioid use after shoulder surgery. Patients undergoing open rotator cuff repair were also at higher risk. Pre-operative and peri-operative opioid use was consistently the most predictive risk factor for prolonged use with odds ratios as high as 11. Leroux et al [18] showed that 15% of opioid naïve patients were still using opioid pain medications 6 months after elective shoulder surgery. A clinical risk calculator to predict opioid dependence has been developed as well (**Figure 9.2**) [22]. Predictive accuracy reached 76% using 10 factors including pre-operative opioid use, insurance type (e.g. Medicare or Medicaid), smoking, body mass index and a history of psychiatric diagnosis.

Recent studies have shown that reducing opioid use through patient education is an achievable goal. In one study of shoulder arthroplasty patients treated with a multimodal regimen for pain control [23], only 3 out of 35 patients required a rescue dose of narcotic pain medicine in the post-operative period and 97% of patients reported being satisfied with their pain control. In a Neer Award-winning study on the effect of pre-operative education on opioid use following rotator-cuff repair, patients in the education group were 2.2 times more likely to discontinue opioid use and consumed up to 42% fewer narcotic dosages by 3 months post-operatively [24].

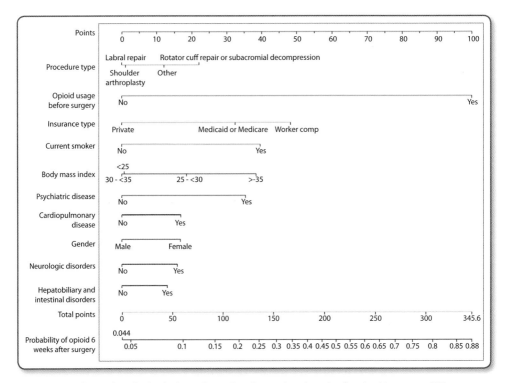

Figure 9.2 Predictive clinical risk calculator of opioid use longer than 6 weeks after shoulder surgery [22].

SHOULDER ARTHROPLASTY

The growth of shoulder arthroplasty continues to outpace all other joint replacement procedures. In 2019, there were 1,53,800 shoulder replacement procedures performed in the US, an increase of 8.2% over the previous year [25]. By comparison, hip and knee replacement grew by just over 4% in the same period. This growth has led to an equally rapid and impressive cycle of innovation and technological advancement. One such advancement is the introduction of shorter humeral components. Many authors have published clinical outcome studies of short-stem and stemless humeral components [26–30]. Concerns have remained over early radiographic signs of loosening, however. 2-year outcome data in two separate studies [26,28] were consistent in showing excellent clinical outcome scores and objective range of motion data comparable to historical outcomes in standard length stems. Patient satisfaction was reported as high as 95%. Up to 9% of stems showed radiographic lucencies or lucent lines around the stem and were considered at risk of loosening. First generation short stems without proximal porous coating were at higher risk and are no longer recommended. Other factors that may lead to increased radiographic changes or risk of loosening include larger stems with higher filling ratios and cortical contact of the stem [30]. The influence of these radiographic changes on clinical outcomes was not significantly different between patients with low or high degree of changes [29]. Clinical outcomes were worse, however, in women and patients over 65 years old if they had higher levels of changes.

Stemless arthroplasty, while in use for more than a decade in Europe, has recently achieved Federal Drug Administration approval in the USs. Short- and mid-term results are now available for these prostheses. Multiple authors have recently reported clinical outcomes at up to 6 years. Constant and ASES scores significantly improved [27,31]. At 2 years, no stemless implant showed migration or loosening. In a review of the Nordic Arthroplasty Register, adjusted cumulative survival rates were comparable for stemmed and stemless arthroplasties at 6 years, with rates >95% for both groups and revision for loosening occurring in 0.7% of stemless arthroplasties compared to 0.4% of stemmed procedures [31].

AUGMENTED GLENOID COMPONENTS

A more pervasive problem than humeral fixation has historically been the ability and means to address glenoid deficiency in shoulder arthroplasty. Bone grafting of contained defects has been shown to be technically demanding with mixed clinical results [32]. Recently, implant manufacturers have provided augmented glenoid components for both anatomic and reverse arthroplasty indications. The effect of implant design on biomechanical stresses in augmented components was studied in a simulated model [19]. The authors concluded that their model showed a wedge design provides better fixation and stress profiles with less micromotion when compared to step-shaped implants.

Recent clinical data has been encouraging as well. In Walch B2 or B3 glenoid deformities in patients with osteoarthritis implanted with a step-type component for correction of retroversion, clinical outcomes showed significant improvement over pre-operative evaluation with consistent improvement in humeral head centering and correction of retroversion assessed by radiographs. Higher amounts of pre-operative posterior subluxation were associated with worse outcomes and persistent posterior subluxation at follow-up was associated with worse pre-operative fatty infiltration of the teres minor and greater component retroversion [32].

Wedge-type components have achieved similar results [33–35]. In a case-control series comparing wedge-type components to non-augmented glenoid components in anatomic TSA, improvements in clinical outcomes scores, range of motion and VAS scores were no different between the groups. While there was no difference in glenoid component loosening, higher grade lucencies were more common in the augmented group and increased with the size of the augment. The authors recommended against using the largest wedge-type components due to these findings [33]. In another report of wedge-type augments used in Walch B type glenoids, 98% of patients were 'better' or 'much better' and >90% exceeded the MCID for all outcomes measures. Radiolucent lines were seen in 36.8% but were not significantly different between glenoid subtypes [34].

Augmented glenoid components have been used in reverse TSA as well. Approximately 90% of patients implanted with an 8° augmented baseplate for a Walch B2, B3 or C type glenoid achieved the MCID for clinical outcome measures and range of motion with no signs of loosening and a low complication rate. There were no differences noted in clinical outcomes when stratified by Walch type [35].

PERI-PROSTHETHIC SHOULDER JOINT INFECTION

Cutibacterium acnes (formerly *propionibacterium*) remains a challenge from preventative, diagnostic and treatment perspectives. While overall infection rates are generally low following shoulder arthroplasty (approximately 1%) [36], it can be a devastating complication. A majority of these infections are caused by *C. acnes* (39%), a slow growing, low virulence organism that fails to induce a strong inflammatory response [37]. These characteristics make typical diagnostic testing less predictive, and newer modalities borrowed from the hip and knee experience have been investigated [38]. Historical treatments for acne vulgaris, caused by *C. acnes*, have also been studied as a means of reducing surgical field contamination and have been somewhat successful [39–41]. Others have evaluated the effectiveness of different treatment strategies once the peri-prosthetic joint infection (PJI) has been confirmed [42].

Many authors have shown that skin preparation at the time of surgery does not necessarily remove all *C. acnes* prior to surgery. Sixty-five percent of patients had at least one positive culture at the time of elective arthroscopy and the rate of positive cultures increased until the end of the procedure [43]. In deep tissue culture, nearly 19% are positive for *C. acnes* with nearly double occurring after prosthetic implantation [44]. More concerning, skin preparation with typical agents had no effect on the rate of positive cultures.

Study of the microbiome of shoulder tissues with advanced DNA sequencing techniques failed to produce *C. acnes* DNA in any deep tissue, however, indicating that *C. acnes* infections are most likely the result of contamination of deep tissues from the skin and not from an expansion of resident colonies within the joint [45].

New skin preparation protocols have been introduced following the findings of positive *C. acnes* cultures from the skin following standard techniques. Benzoyl peroxide (BPO), clindamycin and hydrogen peroxide have all been investigated with variable results [39–41]. A small study on 12 volunteers showed no significant difference in the rate of positive cultures following BPO and clindamycin application to the skin while BPO significantly outperformed chlorhexidine gluconate standard skin prep in 80 patients undergoing shoulder surgery. These authors showed a nearly 10-fold decrease in *C. acnes* burden in patients treated with BPO [40].

Some patients report skin sensitivity, cost difficulties, and non-compliance with home application of BPO. Hydrogen peroxide, the active agent and breakdown product of BPO, has been studied in isolation for its effectiveness in limiting *C. acnes* positive cultures. No patients in a study cohort treated with pre-operative HPO skin preparation developed triple positive cultures (skin, dermis, and joint) compared to 19% of the control group with a significantly lower percentage of peroxide treated patients having positive joint cultures (10% vs. 35%) [41].

Unfortunately, diagnosis of *C. acnes* infections remains challenging. Advanced synovial fluid and serum assays have not performed as well in shoulder PJI as they have in the lower extremities. Synovial alpha-defensin enzyme linked immuno-sorbent assay and leucocyte esterase and serum C-reactive protein levels have been compared to establish sensitivities and specificities in diagnosing shoulder PJI [38]. The overall accuracy for alpha-defensin was 91% with 75% sensitivity and 96% specificity whereas leucocyte esterase had accuracy of 76%, sensitivity of 50% and specificity of 87%. One potential explanation is the lower amounts and quality of synovial fluid typically obtained in shoulder PJI compared to that in the hip and knee.

Consensus best practices for treatment of prosthetic shoulder PJI is lacking. In a systematic review of the literature, 34 studies were identified that specifically addressed the outcomes of revision shoulder arthroplasty following PJI [42]. In 754 pooled cases, *C. acnes* was the most common infecting organism (33%) with male gender, hemi-arthroplasty and anatomic TSA being relative risk factors. Irrigation and debridement alone performed the worst in terms of both functional outcome and eradication of infections leading. Functional outcomes were not different between two-stage and one-stage revision protocols and both were significantly higher than resection arthroplasty, irrigation and debridement or permanent spacer placement. One-stage revision procedures achieved eradication of infection in 96% compared to 86% of two-stage with a lower complications rate leading the authors to conclude that one-stage revision for PJI is recommended in most cases.

ELBOW ARTHROPLASTY

Post-traumatic and inflammatory arthritic conditions of the elbow remain a challenging problem. Due to the relatively smaller size of the humerus and ulna, the component size, and the high loads placed across the elbow, fixation and longevity of the prosthetic components typically utilised do not parallel those in the other major joints. Patients with post-traumatic arthritis are usually higher demand patients and find it difficult to comply with lifting restrictions following total elbow arthroplasty (TEA). As a result, arthroscopic and open osteocapsular arthroplasty (OCA) techniques have been used, but only recently have outcomes been described [46]. TEA for the treatment of acute fracture has become a very successful option for treating these sometimes difficult fractures in the elderly population. Long-term results are now being reported and are encouraging [47]. Our understanding of risks and complications has also been expanded recently [48–50], as has the role for revision elbow arthroplasty [51]. Elbow arthroplasty has not escaped the trend towards out-patient surgery either [52].

As with other joint replacements, obesity has a negative effect on TEA outcomes [50]. Morrey et al reviewed their database as well as current literature on the subject and found that all major complications were increased in patients with obesity including intra-operative fracture, heterotopic ossification (HO), extensor mechanism failure, vascular compromise and loosening, but not infection. Most importantly, survivorship decreased to only 35% at 8 years (vs. 75% at 14 years) in patients with BMI over 40. In a systematic review of the occurrence of HO that included over 2,200 patients, 10% of patients undergoing TEA developed HO, and only 3% were symptomatic [49]. Less than 1% of patients pursued surgical treatment. Risk factors for HO development included TEA performed for ankylosis, primary arthritis and distal humerus fractures. Based on these findings, routine prophylaxis is no longer recommended.

Long-term clinical outcome studies have recently been reported and have the potential to change practice habits in relation to distal humerus fracture and rheumatoid arthritis. In a study performed in combination with the Canadian Orthopaedic Trauma Society, Dehgnan et al [47] reported the 12.5-year follow-up of 42 patients treated for distal humerus fracture. Of the 25 patients treated with TEA, 7 were living with the original arthroplasty, 15 died with a well-functioning arthroplasty during the follow-up period, and only 1 underwent a revision arthroplasty. 4 of the 15 patients in the open reduction group had undergone at least 1 re-operation. These results led the authors to conclude that TEA for distal humerus fracture was a reliable operation that was likely to be the last elbow procedure needed. Furthermore, Federer et al [53] showed in a recent cost-analysis that TEA was slightly more cost-effective. The incremental cost-effectiveness ration (ICER) for TEA was $2375/QALY versus $2677/QALY for ORIF.

In rheumatoid arthritis patients, 85% of prostheses were in and well-functioning at 10 years. Clinical outcomes scores were excellent but complications (26%) and revisions (13%) are common. Triceps weakness, ulnar paresthesias, and infection were the most common complications noted [47]. Bushing wear was common but no patient needed bushing exchange. The trend towards out-patient arthroplasty spilled over into TEA recently as well. Ninety-day complication and re-admission rates were reviewed major complications within 90 days occurred in 7.1% and minor wound complications, correlated with smoking, occurred in 39.2%. As with all ambulatory joint replacement procedures, patient selection is key but is even more critical in avoiding soft-tissue complications in elbow arthroplasty.

Complication rates in elbow arthroplasty have remained high and therefore, revision surgery is not uncommon. A systematic review of the outcomes following revision TEA was performed by Guerts et al [51]. Results in over 500 combined cases confirmed the difficulties associated with these procedures as a full 44% of patients experienced at least one complication the most common of which are aseptic loosening (22%), transient ulnar or radial symptoms (21%) and peri-prosthetic fractures (15%). Importantly, functional outcomes were significantly better when a linked prosthesis was used but patients with linked prostheses underwent significantly more re-operations.

Young and high-demand patients who sustain complex trauma to the elbow continue to be a treatment challenge. Both acute treatment options and their sequelae (i.e. post-traumatic arthritis) are difficult problems to adequately address in this population. OCA has been a useful tool for these patients and arthroscopic options have been described and utilised for years. Results of minimally invasive, arthroscopic OCA have recently been reported to outperform the open alternative in flexion improvement only, with no other significant differences noted between the procedures. The most important finding in this study, however, was that patients with 2 mm of joint space remaining had worse function and more pain at final follow-up [54].

While significant functional loss is not unexpected following elbow trauma, it is especially debilitating in young patients. In 57 such patients treated with radial head replacement for Mason type 3 fractures, only 53% could return to sports and those that were able to, did so at lower rates, frequency and demands [55]. Regression analysis showed that a MEPS < 85 points and a replacement performed secondarily were independent risk factors for inability to return to sports.

ELBOW TRAUMA: INTERNAL JOINT STABILISER

'Terrible triad' injuries – the combination of elbow dislocation, radial head fracture and coronoid fracture – almost always result in recurrent instability as both the bony and soft-tissue restraints are compromised. Historically, lengthy periods of immobilisation, external fixation, or both have sometimes been required to achieve and maintain stability in these injuries. The potential complications as well as the discomfort and cumbersome nature of external fixation lead to the development of other options. Treatment for this challenging problem continues to evolve.

In an effort to predict the causes of failure of treatment in terrible triad injuries, Jung et al [56] found that recurrent instability was more likely in those patients with high-energy trauma, increased time between injury and surgery, Mason type III radial head fractures, medial collateral ligament injuries and those patients who did not undergo coronoid fracture repair. The rate of post-traumatic arthritis was significantly higher in the group of patients with recurrent instability.

Multiple authors have evaluated the optimal treatment for the radial head fracture component of these injuries [57,58]. Two clinical studies failed to discern a difference between treatment options, however. No difference in outcomes scores or range of motion was noted in a meta-analysis comparing replacement to reconstruction. High complication rates were noted in both (65%) with 18% re-operation rates. When replacement was compared to resection alone, no differences were identified either [57]. VAS, range of motion and clinical outcomes were similar as were the rates of post-traumatic arthritis.

The internal joint stabiliser (IJS-E, Skeletal Dynamics) has been developed and used as a temporary stabilising device to maintain concentric reduction of the elbow joint. The concept was validated in 24 patients and all but one remained concentrically reduced (**Figure 9.3**) [59]. Good or excellent results were observed in the 23 patients who remained stable. However, other authors have not been able to achieve the same level of clinical success [60]. In 10 patients with terrible triad injuries treated with the IJS-E, mean

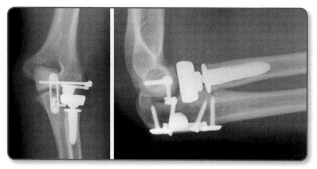

Figure 9.3 Anteroposterior and lateral radiograph of the patient after stabilisation surgery with the internal joint stabiliser of the elbow [59].

Broberg–Morrey scores of 68.7 at 14 months were reported. Range of motion was similar to the proof-of-concept study but 4 out of the 10 patients required subsequent procedures in addition to device removal.

INTERNAL BRACING OF ELBOW LIGAMENT INJURIES

Ulnar collateral ligament injuries are a common problem in the elbow in both trauma and sports medicine injuries. Traumatic injuries to these ligaments have historically been treated acutely with repair, while chronic, attritional overuse injuries usually seen in athletes have been addressed with reconstruction of the medial ulnar collateral ligament (MUCL). In both cases, internal bracing (IB) or load sharing on repaired tissues has been used to accelerate rehabilitation and improve outcomes. Biomechanical studies have shown the additional benefits of IB augmentation with woven polyester tapes [61–63]. The addition of an IB to docking constructs restored stiffness, ultimate failure torque, gapping and valgus opening back to the native ligament levels [61,62]. In lateral ulnar collateral ligament (LUCL) studies, IB repair was as effective as reconstruction in restoring the elbow to native state in terms of ultimate load and cyclic loading [63]. Additionally, when LUCL repair was augmented with an IB in a cadaveric model of LUCL insufficiency, fewer suture anchors were necessary to achieve stability. These studies taken in combination confirm the biomechanical validity of IB augmented repairs and support the use of this exciting new technique for both acute traumatic injuries and throwing injuries.

CONCLUSION

Shoulder arthroplasty is one of the fastest growing segments in orthopaedics today. This coincides with the more active lifestyles now common in the ageing population and has fueled the major increase in interest in shoulder and elbow surgery in general. Advances in surgical techniques have played a large role in this growth which has been accelerated by the technological feats categorised above. In turn, interest from residents and fellows has steadily increased as well. This continues to have a positive effect on the volume and quality of shoulder and elbow research. The application of these technical advancements and the lessons learned via the latest scientific endeavours will continue to improve shoulder and elbow care in the future.

REFERENCES

1. Bond JL, Dopirak RM, Higgins J, Burns J, Snyder SJ. Arthroscopic replacement of massive, irreparable rotator cuff tears using a Graft- Jacket allograft: technique and preliminary results. Arthroscopy 2008; 24:403–409.
2. Neumann, JA, Zgonis MH, Rickert KD. Interposition dermal matrix xenografts: a successful alternative to traditional treatment of massive rotator cuff tears. Am J Sports Med 2017; 45:1261–1268.
3. Gupta AK, Hug K, Berkoff DJ. Dermal tissue allograft for the repair of massive irreparable rotator cuff tears. Am J Sports Med 2012; 40:141–147.
4. Mihata T, McGarry MH, Pirolo JM, Kinoshita M, Lee TQ. Superior capsule reconstruction to restore superior stability in irreparable rotator cuff tears: a biomechanical cadaveric study. Am J Sports Med 2012; 40(10):2248–2255.
5. Mihata T. Editorial commentary: superior capsule reconstruction: grafts for superior capsular reconstruction must be thick and stiff. Arthroscopy 2019; 35:2535–2536.

6. Pennington WT, Bartz BA, Pauli JM, Walker CE, Schmidt W. Arthroscopic superior capsular reconstruction with acellular dermal allograft for the treatment of massive irreparable rotator cuff tears: short-term clinical outcomes and the radiographic parameter of superior capsular distance. Arthroscopy 2018; 34:1764–1773.
7. Scheiderer B, Kia C, Obopilwe E, et al. Biomechanical Effect of Superior Capsule Reconstruction Using a 3-mm and 6-mm Thick Acellular Dermal Allograft in a Dynamic Shoulder Model. Arthroscopy 2020; 36:355–364.
8. Zastrow RK, London DA, Parsons BO, Cagle PJ. Superior capsule reconstruction for irreparable rotator cuff tears: a systematic review. Arthroscopy 2019; 35:2525–2534.
9. Lobao MH, Canham RB, Melvani RT, et al. Biomechanics of biodegradable subacromial balloon spacer for irreparable superior rotator cuff tears: study of a cadaveric model. J Bone Joint Surg Am 2019; 101:e49.
10. Singh S, Reeves J, Langohr GDG, Johnson JA, Athwal GS. The subacromial balloon spacer versus superior capsular reconstruction in the treatment of irreparable rotator cuff tears: a biomechanical assessment. Arthroscopy 2019; 35:382–389.
11. Stewart RK, Kaplin L, Parada SA, et al. Outcomes of subacromial balloon spacer implantation for massive and irreparable rotator cuff tears: a systematic review. Orthop J Sports Med 2019; 7(10):2325967119875717.
12. Piekaar RSM, Bouman ICE, van Kampen PM, van Eijk F, Huijsmans PE. The subacromial balloon spacer for massive irreparable rotator cuff tears: approximately 3 years of prospective follow-up. Musculoskelet Surg 2019.
13. Castagna A, Garofalo R, Maman E, Gray AC, Brooks EA. Comparative cost-effectiveness analysis of the subacromial spacer for irreparable and massive rotator cuff tears. Int Orthop. 2019; 43:395–403.
14. Singh S, Reeves J, Langohr GDG, Johnson JA, Athwal GS. The effect of the subacromial balloon spacer on humeral head translation in the treatment of massive, irreparable rotator cuff tears: a biomechanical assessment. J Shoulder Elbow Surg. 2019; 28:1841–1847.
15. Omid R, Heckmann N, Wang L, et al. Biomechanical comparison between the trapezius transfer and latissimus transfer irreparable posterosuperior rotator cuff tears. J Shoulder Elbow Surg 2015; 24:1635–1643.
16. Reddy A, Gulotta LV, Chen X, et al. Biomechanics of lower trapezius and latissimus dorsi transfers in rotator cuff-deficient shoulders. J Shoulder Elbow Surg 2019; 28:1257–1264.
17. Elhassan BT, Wagner ER, Werthel JD. Outcome of flower trapezius transfer to reconstruct massive irreparable posterior-superior rotator cuff tear. J Shoulder Elbow Surg 2016; 25:1346–1353.
18. Leroux TS, Saltzman BM, Sumner SA, et al. Elective shoulder surgery in the opioid naïve: rates of and risk factors for long-term postoperative opioid use. Am J Sports Med 2019; 47:1051–1056.
19. Sabesan VJ, Meiyappan A, Montgomery T, et al. Diagnosis can predict opioid usage and dependence in reverse shoulder arthroplasty. JSES Open Access. 2019; 3:316–319.
20. Gil JA, Gunaseelan V, DeFroda SF, et al. Risk of prolonged opioid use among opioid-naïve patients after common shoulder arthroscopy procedures. Am J Sports Med 2019; 47:1043–1050.
21. Khazi ZM, Lu Y, Shamrock AG, et al. Opioid use following shoulder stabilization surgery: risk factors for prolonged use. J Shoulder Elbow Surg 2019; 28:1928–1935.
22. Nicholson AD, Kassam HF, Steele JL, et al. Development of a clinical risk calculator for prolonged opioid use after shoulder surgery. J Shoulder Elbow Surg 2019; 28:2225–2231.
23. Leas DP, Connor PM, Schiffern SC, et al. Opioid-free shoulder arthroplasty: a prospective study of a novel clinical care pathway. J Shoulder Elbow Surg 2019; 28:1716–1722.
24. Syed UAM, Aleem AW, Wowkanech C, et al. Neer Award 2018: the effect of preoperative education on opioid consumption in patients undergoing arthroscopic rotator cuff repair: a prospective, randomized clinical trial. J Shoulder Elbow Surg 2018; 27:962–967.
25. Killeen K. A 2020 Extremity Update. Orthopedic Network News. 2020; 31:1–2.
26. Romeo AA, Thorsness RJ, Sumner SAet al. Short-term clinical outcome of an anatomic short-stem humeral component in total shoulder arthroplasty. J Shoulder Elbow Surg 2018; 27:70–74.
27. Krukenberg A, McBirnie J, Bartsch S, et al. Sidus stem-free shoulder system for primary osteoarthritis: short-term results of a multicenter study. J Shoulder Elbow Surg 2018; 27:1483–1490.
28. Szerlip BW, Morris BJ, Laughlin MS, Kilian CM, Edwards TB. Clinical and radiographic outcomes after total shoulder arthroplasty with an anatomic press-fit short stem. J Shoulder Elbow Surg 2018; 27:10–16.
29. Schnetzke M, Wittmann T, Raiss P, Walch G. Short-term results of a second generation anatomic short-stem shoulder prosthesis in primary osteoarthritis. Arch Orthop Trauma Surg 2019; 139:149–154.
30. Raiss P, Schnetzke M, Wittmann T, et al. Postoperative radiographic findings of an uncemented convertible short stem for anatomic and reverse shoulder arthroplasty. J Shoulder Elbow Surg 2019; 28:715–723.

31.   Rasmussen JV, Harjula J, Arverud ED, et al. The short-term survival of total stemless shoulder arthroplasty for osteoarthritis is comparable to that of total stemmed shoulder arthroplasty: a Nordic Arthroplasty Register Association study. J Shoulder Elbow Surg 2019; 28:1578–1586.

32.   Ho JC, Thakar O, Chan WW, et al. Early radiographic failure of reverse total shoulder arthroplasty with structural bone graft for glenoid bone loss. J Shoulder Elbow Surg 2020; 29:550–560.

33.   Priddy M, Zarezadeh A, Farmer KW, et al. Early results of augmented anatomic glenoid components. J Shoulder Elbow Surg 2019; 28:S138–S145.

34.   Grey SG, Wright TW, Flurin PH, et al. Clinical and radiographic outcomes with a posteriorly augmented glenoid for Walch B glenoids in anatomic total shoulder arthroplasty. J Shoulder Elbow Surg 2020; 29:e185–e195.

35.   Virk M, Yip M, Liuzza L, et al. Clinical and radiographic outcomes with a posteriorly augmented glenoid for Walch B2, B3, and C glenoids in reverse total shoulder arthroplasty. J Shoulder Elbow Surg 2020; 29:e196–e204.

36.   Padegimas EM, Maltenfort M, Ramsey ML, et al. Periprosthetic shoulder infection in the United States: incidence and economic burden. J Shoulder Elbow Surg 2015; 24:741–746.

37.   Nelson GN, Davis DE, Namdari S. Outcomes in the treatment of periprosthetic joint infection after shoulder arthroplasty: a systematic review. J Shoulder Elbow Surg 2016; 25:1337–1345.

38.   Unter Ecker N, Koniker A, Gehrke T, et al. What is the diagnostic accuracy of alpha-defensin and leukocyte esterase test in periprosthetic shoulder infection? Clin Orthop Relat Res 2019; 477:1712–1718.

39.   Heckmann N, Heidari KS, Jalali O, et al. Cutibacterium acnes persists despite topical clindamycin and benzoyl peroxide. J Shoulder Elbow Surg 2019; 28:2279–2283.

40.   Kolakowski L, Lai JK, Duvall GT, et al. Neer Award 2018: Benzoyl peroxide effectively decreases preoperative Cutibacterium acnes shoulder burden: a prospective randomized controlled trial. J Shoulder Elbow Surg 2018; 27:1539–1544.

41.   Chalmers PN, Beck L, Stertz I, Tashjian RZ. Hydrogen peroxide skin preparation reduces Cutibacterium acnes in shoulder arthroplasty: a prospective, blinded, controlled trial. J Shoulder Elbow Surg 2019; 28:1554–1561.

42.   Mercurio M, Castioni D, Iannò B, Gasparini G, Galasso O. Outcomes of revision surgery after periprosthetic shoulder infection: a systematic review. J Shoulder Elbow Surg 2019; 28:1193–1203.

43.   Pauzenberger L, Heller V, Ostermann RC, et al. Cutibacterium acnes (formerly Propionibacterium acnes) contamination of the surgical field during shoulder arthroscopy. Arthroscopy 2019; 35:1750–1757.

44.   Torrens C, Marí R, Alier A, et al. Cutibacterium acnes in primary reverse shoulder arthroplasty: from skin to deep layers. J Shoulder Elbow Surg. 2019; 28:839–846.

45.   Qiu B, Al K, Pena-Diaz AM, et al. Cutibacterium acnes and the shoulder microbiome. J Shoulder Elbow Surg 2018; 27:1734–1739.

46.   Kwak JM, Kholinne E, Sun Y, et al. Clinical outcome of osteocapsular arthroplasty for primary osteoarthritis of the elbow: comparison of arthroscopic and open procedure. Arthroscopy 2019; 35:1083–1089.

47.   Dehghan N, Furey M, Schemitsch L, et al. Long-term outcomes of total elbow arthroplasty for distal humeral fracture: results from a prior randomized clinical trial. J Shoulder Elbow Surg 2019; 28:2198–2204.

48.   Lee H, Vaichinger AM, O'Driscoll SW. Component fracture after total elbow arthroplasty. J Shoulder Elbow Surg 2019; 28:1449–1456.

49.   Liu EY, Hildebrand A, Horner NS, et al. Heterotopic ossification after total elbow arthroplasty: a systematic review. J Shoulder Elbow Surg 2019; 28:587–595.

50.   Morrey ME, Hevesi M. The influence of obesity on total elbow arthroplasty. Orthop Clin North Am 2018; 49:361–370.

51.   Geurts EJ, Viveen J, van Riet RP, Kodde IF, Eygendaal D. Outcomes after revision total elbow arthroplasty: a systematic review. J Shoulder Elbow Surg 2019; 28:381–386.

52.   Stone MA, Singh P, Rosario SL, Omid R. Outpatient total elbow arthroplasty: 90-day outcomes. J Shoulder Elbow Surg 2018; 27:1311–1316.

53.   Federer AE, Mather RC 3rd, Ramsey ML, Garrigues GE. Cost-effectiveness analysis of total elbow arthroplasty versus open reduction-internal fixation for distal humeral fractures. J Shoulder Elbow Surg 2019; 28:102–111.

54.   Kim DM, Han M, Jeon IH, Shin MJ, Koh KH. Range-of-motion improvement and complication rate in open and arthroscopic osteocapsular arthroplasty for primary osteoarthritis of the elbow: a systematic review. Int Orthop 2020; 44:329–339.

55.   Jung M, Groetzner-Schmidt C, Porschke F, et al. Low return-to-sports rate after elbow injury and treatment with radial head arthroplasty. J Shoulder Elbow Surg 2019; 28:1441–1448.

56. Jung SW, Kim DH, Kang SH, et al. Risk Factors That Influence Subsequent Recurrent Instability in Terrible Triad Injury of the Elbow. J Orthop Trauma 2019; 33:250–255.

57. Mazhar FN, Ebrahimi H, Jafari D, Mirzaei A. Radial head resection versus prosthetic arthroplasty in terrible triad injury: a retrospective comparative cohort study: a retrospective comparative cohort study. Bone Joint J 2018; 100-B:1499–1505.

58. Kyriacou S, Gupta Y, Bains HK, Singh HP. Radial head replacement versus reconstruction for the treatment of the terrible triad injury of the elbow: a systematic review and meta-analysis. Arch Orthop Trauma Surg 2019; 139:507–517.

59. Orbay JL, Ring D, Kachooei AR, et al. Multicenter trial of an internal joint stabilizer for the elbow. J Shoulder Elbow Surg 2017; 26:125–132.

60. Pasternack JB, Ciminero ML, Choueka J, Kang KK. Patient outcomes for the Internal Joint Stabilizer of the Elbow (IJS-E). J Shoulder Elbow Surg 2020; 29:e238–e244.

61. Bernholt DL, Lake SP, Castile RM, et al. Biomechanical comparison of docking ulnar collateral ligament reconstruction with and without an internal brace. J Shoulder Elbow Surg 2019; 28:2247–2252.

62. Bodendorfer BM, Looney AM, Lipkin SL, et al. Biomechanical comparison of ulnar collateral ligament reconstruction with the docking technique versus repair with internal bracing. Am J Sports Med 2018; 46:3495–3501.

63. Scheiderer B, Imhoff FB, Kia C, et al. LUCL internal bracing restores posterolateral rotatory stability of the elbow. Knee Surg Sports Traumatol Arthrosc 2020; 28:1195–1201.

Chapter 10

What is new in orthopaedic trauma?

Brianna R Fram, Taylor Paziuk, Gerard Chang, James C Krieg

INTRODUCTION

Orthopaedic trauma care continues to evolve, as clinicians optimise outcomes, while minimising complications. Published research over the past 2 years has not only impacted the current treatment of traumatic musculoskeletal injuries, but has also laid groundwork for future investigations. Various well-designed studies, from randomised controlled trials to meta-analyses, have clarified our understanding of injury patterns, fixation constructions, post-operative protocols, and outcomes. Further, the scope of study has included other aspects of trauma care from wound management, antibiotic usage and pain management to cost considerations and radiation exposure. Each year, the granularity of research seems to improve, as the field of orthopaedic trauma seeks to clarify the ideal treatment for a given individual.

By reviewing major orthopaedic journals over the past 2 years, this chapter aims to update the reader on research related to orthopaedic trauma. Sections include upper extremity, lower extremity, pelvis and acetabulum, and general orthopaedic trauma. While we have attempted to place articles into a larger context along with their strengths and limitations, we encourage readers to review articles of interest in full.

Brianna R Fram MD, Thomas Jefferson University, Department of Orthopaedic Surgery and the Rothman Orthopaedic Institute, Philadelphia, USA
Email: brfram@gmail.com

Taylor Paziuk MD, Thomas Jefferson University, Department of Orthopaedic Surgery and the Rothman Orthopaedic Institute, Philadelphia, USA
Email: taylor.paziuk@rothmanortho.com

Gerard Chang MD, University of Texas Health Science Center at Houston, Department of Orthopaedic Surgery, Houston, USA
Email: gerard.chang@gmail.com

James C Krieg MD, Thomas Jefferson University, Department of Orthopaedic Surgery and the Rothman Orthopaedic Institute, Philadelphia, USA
Email: james.krieg@rothmanortho.com

GENERAL ORTHOPAEDIC TRAUMA

Wound care

Negative pressure wound therapy (NPWT) has revolutionised wound care in many ways. However, its role in the care of open fractures remains unclear. A recent meta-analysis of 10 studies compared NPWT to conventional dressings in open fractures [1]. One of the included studies was the WOLFF randomised controlled trial of 460 patients in the United Kingdom [2]. They found that the deep infection rate with conventional dressings was 17.5%, compared to 9.0 % with NWPT. They also identified a significant decrease in the secondary outcome of flap failure with NPWT (3.3%) compared to conventional dressings (9.6%). There were not significant differences in rates of fracture nonunion, amputation, or hospital length of stay. The conclusions of this study contradict those of the WOLFF trial, which was the single largest study included in this meta-analysis. The WOLFF trial found no difference in functional scores or surgical site infections (SSIs) between NPWT and conventional dressings [2]. The evidence-guiding use of NPWT in open fractures following initial surgical debridement without ability to primarily close the wound therefore, remains unclear.

For those without affordable access to commercially available NPWT devices, Cocjin et al published a randomised controlled trial comparing a low-cost clinician-assembled vacuum-assisted closure apparatus (termed "AqauVac") to the vacuum-assisted closure advanced therapy system (VAC-ATS; KCI) [3]. Their system was constructed from an aquarium pump with a pressure gauge and regulator, and a dressing assembled from food plastic wrap, surgical gauze, nasogastric tubing, and IV bottles for effluent. Over 7 days of treatment, they did not find significant differences in time to apply the systems (AquaVAC 5.5 minutes vs. VAC-ATS 7.5 minutes, $p = 0.093$), amount of wound exudate, reduction in wound size, pain by VAS scores, deep infections or periwound complications, or rates of pump malfunction. Over 7 days, the AquaVac system was significantly less expensive at $63.75 USD per patient versus $491.38 USD per patient for the VAC-ATS. Though performed on a small number of patients, this study suggests equivalent outcomes between the setups and illustrates a system by which clinicians in practice settings without access to commercial NPWT devices can nevertheless provide the benefits of this wound care to their patients.

Antibiotics

We know that early administration of antibiotics is integral for prevention of infection in the setting of an open fracture [4]. But, the ideal duration of antibiotic treatment following surgical irrigation and debridement with wound closure is not known. Stennett et al performed an international multicentre retrospective cohort study (level III) looking at the duration of antibiotic therapy following definitive fracture wound closure and its association with deep infection [5]. Of 2,400 patients with open fractures, 42% received >72 hours antibiotics after closure. Deep SSI within 1 year of surgery was divided by level of wound contamination, with 5% of patients with mild wound contamination developing deep SSI, 8% with moderate contamination, and 23% with severe contamination. They found >72 hours of prophylactic antibiotics, when compared to a shorter duration, was associated with a trend towards increased deep SSI in mildly contaminated wounds [adjusted odds ratio (OR) 1.39, 95% confidence interval (CI) 0.92–2.11]. In severely contaminated wounds, >72 hours antibiotics was strongly protective against deep SSI (adjusted odds ratio 0.20, 95% CI 0.07–0.60). There was no association with antibiotic duration and deep SSI for those with moderately contaminated wounds. This suggests open fractures should be treated differently following thorough operative debridement and definitive closure, with severely contaminated wounds receiving longer durations of post-closure antibiotics and mildly contaminated wounds shorter durations.

While we study ways to avoid deep orthopaedic infections, there are also questions about the ideal treatment when infections occur. Many orthopaedists think of IV antibiotics as more efficacious than their PO counterparts. However, a multi-centre randomised controlled trial by Li et al, published in the New England Journal of Medicine in 2019, suggests that this is not the case [6]. The study, Oral versus Intravenous Antibiotics for Bone and Joint Infection (OVIVA), included 1,015 patients with acute or chronic infections of the axial skeleton or spine, including those without implants, and those with fracture-related infection with retained implants or peri-prosthetic joint infection. Patients were randomised to 6 weeks of IV or PO antibiotics with the specific medication chosen by infectious disease specialists. The primary endpoint was definite treatment failure within 1 year (defined by clinical, microbial, or histologic criteria for frank infection) with secondary endpoints of early discontinuation of the randomised treatment, IV catheter complications, *Clostridium difficile*-associated diarrhoea, serious adverse events, resource use, health status measured by EQ-5D-3L and Oxford Hip and Knee Scores, and adherence to treatment. Treatment failure occurred in 14.6% of the IV group and 13.2% of the PO group, with PO being non-inferior to IV on analysis. The IV group, as might be expected, had significantly higher rates of early treatment discontinuation and of IV catheter associated complications, and significantly longer hospital stays (18.9% vs. 12.8%, $p = 0.006$, 9.4% vs. 1.0%, $p < 0.001$, and 14 days vs. 11 days, $p < 0.001$, respectively). Cases of *C. difficile*-associated diarrhoea and serious adverse events did not differ significantly, nor did EQ-5D-3L or Oxford Hip Scores, though Oxford Knee Scores were significantly better in the PO group at 120 and 365 days. In all, this paper found PO antibiotics were non-inferior to IV during the first 6 weeks of treatment for a wide range of orthopaedic infections, and had lower rates of secondary complications. This could make appropriate medical treatment of deep infections more accessible for many patients.

Pain control and the opioid epidemic

As the opioid epidemic continues, Parzych et al reported retrospectively on 30 patients with a unique presentation of compartment syndrome of the buttocks/thigh, lower leg, or forearm after being "found down" following drug overdose [7]. Given that patients are frequently sedated on presentation, have baseline hyperalgesia and opioid tolerance, and often have an unclear time course, the question for surgeons is which patients will benefit from emergent fasciotomies. In the 25 managed with fasciotomies, there was a 20% infection rate, 12% amputation rate, and an average of 4.2 surgeries. Of those who were examinable with incomplete neurological deficits on presentation, 70% had some functional recovery after fasciotomy. Of six with complete neurological deficits on presentation, four underwent fasciotomy, with two resultant deep infections, and none had meaningful functional return. They did not find lactate, creatinine, or creatine phosphokinase levels predictive of limb outcomes. This limited experience suggests those presenting after being "found down" with concern for compartment syndrome and partial deficits may benefit from emergent fasciotomies, though with high expected complication rates, but those with complete deficits likely will not benefit and may experience harm.

Peri-operative pain control in geriatric patients is a balancing act between adequate analgesia to allow mobilisation and side effects related to polypharmacy, delirium, constipation, nephrotoxicity and GI injury. Thompson et al prospectively studied pre-operative fascia iliaca compartment blocks (FICBs) for geriatric hip fracture patients, with 23 randomised to receive blocks and 24 controls [8]. Single-shot blocks of 30 mL 0.25% ropivacaine were given under ultrasound guidance by an anaesthesiologist pre-operative, and patients had a standardised post-operative pain management protocol of acetaminophen, tramadol, and morphine for mild, moderate, or severe pain respectively. Primary outcome was total consumption of pain medication through post-operative day 3, with patient in the FICB group using a mean of 0.4 mg morphine versus 19.4 mg for controls ($p = 0.05$). The secondary outcome of distance ambulated on post-operative day 3 did not differ significantly (20.2 feet for FICB vs. 13.5 feet, $p = 0.23$), but patient satisfaction on post-operative day 3 was significantly (31%) higher in the FICB group ($p = 0.01$). While further study is needed on the effects of these blocks at later post-operative time points, this is compelling early data on a high-risk patient population.

Thromboprophylaxis

Another perennial question when treating trauma patients is how to best prevent venous thromboembolism (VTE) while balancing the risks of injury- and procedure-related bleeding. The most feared outcome of VTE is clinically significant pulmonary embolus (PE), reported to occur in 0.4–4.2% of trauma patients and account for 12% of deaths after major trauma. It is not uncommon for trauma patients to have contraindications to systemic anti-coagulation, such as intracranial haemorrhage. In these cases, inferior vena cava (IVC) filters are often placed, despite limited data supporting this practice.

Ho and colleagues from Australia randomised 240 adult polytrauma patients (injury severity scores >15, median 27) with contraindications to systemic prophylactic anti-coagulation into two groups: 122 patients received a retrievable IVC filter and 118 did not [9]. Most (57.5%) were contraindicated due to intracranial haemorrhage. Both groups had sequential compression devices on uninjured legs and began prophylactic anti-coagulation as early as deemed safe. Patients had screening ultrasonography of their legs 2 weeks after enrolment and CT pulmonary angiography only when symptomatic per study protocol. There was no significant difference between the groups in the primary end-points of symptomatic PE or death within 90 days (13.9% filter vs. 14.4% control, HR 0.99, 95% CI 0.51–1.94, $p = 0.98$). Only age and ISS correlated with these primary end-points. The IVC filter group did far better in the secondary outcome of symptomatic PE from day 8 to 90 among patients not receiving systemic anti-coagulation within 7 days of injury (0% filter vs. 14.7% control, HR 0, 95% CI 0–0.55). However, this result may have been confounded by clinician decision making, as only 29% of the controls versus 38% of the IVC filter group were included. Other secondary end-points of death, major and non-major bleeding, and lower limb DVT, did not differ significantly. Finally, as noted by the authors, IVC filters are not without complications such as filter adherence to vessel walls, difficulty with removal, and retained clots within the filter. This study suggests early prophylactic IVC filters do not reduce symptomatic PE or death at 90 days in polytrauma patients with early contraindications to prophylactic anti-coagulation.

Radiation exposure

Polytraumatised patients undergo a lot of medical imaging. Many centres now perform routine CT of the chest, abdomen and pelvis in all high-energy trauma patients, in addition to more focussed imaging, such as studies of head and extremities. In addition to screening imaging, many times there are studies ordered after intervention. Prior studies have evaluated the utility of routine post-operative CT in both pelvic ring and acetabular surgery [10,11]. For pelvic ring injuries, post-operative CT led to revision surgery in only 2/331 (0.6%) patients in a single-centre retrospective study, and in no patients without pelvic dysmorphism. This led the authors to recommend that routine post-operative CTs may not be warranted [10]. Regarding post-operative CTs after acetabular fixation, they led to revision surgery in 14/563 (2.5%) patients for reasons including intra-articular screw placement, malreduction, and residual retained osteochondral fragments, in another single-centre retrospective study. No analysed risk factors correlated significantly with risk for second procedure [11]. Post-operative imaging may provide data that is not reflected in revision rates, with regard to activity, prognosis, and treatment learning curve.

A group in the UK recently attempted to model lifetime risk of fatal carcinogenesis attributable to medical radiation exposure in the first year following injury. They followed a cohort of 2,394 patients, with mean injury severity score (ISS) of 28.66 [12]. After adding the radiation doses from radiographs and CTs (fluoroscopy was excluded) in the 12 months following injury, and converting these to millisieverts (mSv), the authors used patient age and sex to calculate attributable lifetime fatal cancer risk based on models developed by the International Commission on Radiological Protection. Mean and median radiation doses were 30.45 mSv and 18.46 mSv, respectively, with the majority of this coming from CTs (mean 5.26 studies/patient). The mean additional lifetime fatal cancer risk was 3.56% (median 3.43%), translating to 85 of the cohort patients developing cancer in their lifetime due to this radiation exposure. ISS correlated with higher radiation exposure up to score of 50, after which the data became less clear. This study is limited by its use of models, instead of clinical follow-up, to determine carcinogenesis risk. As the authors point out, there are many variables between patient lifestyles and exposures which could confound such a study. This study emphasises that polytrauma patients receive significant radiation exposure in ranges clearly correlated with increased cancer risk. It should prompt orthopaedists to question their CT practices, especially in scenarios with low demonstrated clinical impact.

Bone defects

In open fractures, the classical teaching is that bone fragments devoid of attached soft tissue should be discarded to prevent infection. This bone loss can contribute to osseous defects requiring multiple surgeries over extended periods. Al-Hourani and colleagues published on a single-centre consecutive cohort of 113 patients with type IIIB open diaphyseal tibia fractures who, when present, underwent retention of these devitalised fragments, coupled with early plastic reconstruction [13]. Median patient age was 44.3 years, median follow-up was 1.7 years, and 44/113 had "orthoplastic reconstruction using mechanically relevant devitalised bone" (ORDB). The protocol consisted of two stages: (1) initial thorough surgical debridement of the open fracture with provisional stabilisation using a 3.5 mm dynamic compression plate, application of a wound VAC, limb splinting, and antibiotics until stage two; (2) plate removal, re-debridement, application of fresh 3.5 mm plate, tibial intramedullary nailing, and definitive soft-tissue coverage with plastic surgery. When present, mechanically relevant devitalised bone was debrided and lavaged and re-incorporated into the fracture at stage 1, and again cleaned and reincorporated at stage 2. There was no significant difference in the primary outcomes of deep infection [ORDB 1/44 (2.3%), non-ORDB 7/69 (10.1%), $p = 0.119$] and number of operations (median two operations/patient, $p = 0.389$), or in secondary outcomes of overall complications [ORDB 3/44 (6.8%), non-ORDB 8/69 (11.6%)], non-union, or flap failure. A major caveat in this protocol is the presence of experienced plastic surgeons who were able to provide coverage at median 64 hours after presentation. They report only 5-flap failures (4.4%), 4 of which were associated with deep infection. As early soft-tissue coverage has been shown to decrease infection rate in open fracture, results using this algorithm may not be replicable at centres with less readily available coverage [14].

UPPER EXTREMITY

General

Outcomes of amputation versus limb salvage have been studied extensively for the lower extremities, but less so for the uppers. Mitchell et al evaluated 155 Global War on Terror veterans pulled from the Military Extremity Trauma Amputation/Limb Salvage (METALS) study who had sustained major upper-extremity injuries treated with amputation or limb salvage [15]. They compared social support, personal habits, and patient-reported outcomes limb salvage and amputation in the 137 patients with unilateral injuries, at a mean of 40 months follow-up. They found participants reported moderate to high levels of physical and psychosocial disability, with 19.4% screening positive for post-traumatic stress disorder (PTSD) and 12.3% screening positive for depression. However, 63.6% were either working, on active duty, or attending school, and 38.7% were involved in vigorous recreational activities. The limb salvage and amputation groups did not differ significantly.

Shoulder girdle

Treatment of clavicle fractures remains a controversial and much-studied topic. One thing that seems clear, despite questions about function benefits of treatment, is that operative fixation decreases the risk of non-union. In order to help to predict which non-operatively treated clavicle fractures might be going on to non-union, Nicholson et al compared the ability of two models, one based on information at the time of injury and the other on information at 6 weeks post-injury, to predict midshaft clavicle fracture nonunion at 6 months [16]. This was a prospective consecutive cohort study of 200 patients aged 16+ years who presented with a displaced midshaft clavicle fracture which was treated nonoperatively. At 6 months, 173 had healed and 27 (14%) had CT-confirmed nonunion. The time-of-injury model included smoking, fracture comminution and displacement. On analysis of multiple patient, injury, and outcome factors, quick disabilities of the arm, shoulder and hand (DASH) score, lack of callus on radiographs, and fracture movement on exam at 6 weeks were most predictive of progression to nonunion. If 0/3 were present, non-union risk as 3%, while if ≥2 were present (the case in 23.5% of the cohort), non-union risk was 60%. This model had superior characteristics to the predictive model at time of injury, with improved accuracy (area under curve 87.3% vs. 64.8%). As there is evidence that outcome score and complications do not increase when clavicle fractures are fixed sub-acutely (3–12 weeks post-injury), this model may allow surgeons to counsel patients who are at high-risk for non-union at their 6-week visit about crossing over to operative treatment [17,18].

We have long accepted that clavicle fractures have high rates of symptomatic hardware removal. A recent Level 3 meta-analysis comparing antero-inferior plating to superior plating for midshaft clavicle fractures found this may occur far less often following anteroinferior plating (OR 2.51 for symptomatic hardware, $p = 0.005$; OR 2.36 of implant removal with superior plating, $p = 0.008$) [19]. This study included 34 studies reporting on 390 patients with anteroinferior plating and 1,104 patients with superior plating. There were no significant differences between these groups on the secondary measures of DASH and constant scores, probability of union ($p = 0.41$), malunion ($p = 0.28$), nonunion ($p = 0.29$), or implant failure ($p = 0.39$). One caveat of this study is that hardware prominence and removal are subjective, and could have been susceptible to surgeon bias.

In recent years, the focus on midshaft clavicle fractures has shifted to include distal clavicle fractures and acromioclavicular (AC) joint dislocations. These injuries are often on a spectrum with certain morphologies of clavicle fracture variably affecting the AC joint and coracoclavicular (CC) ligaments. Robinson et al performed a retrospective study on medium-term outcomes in 67 patients with displaced lateral-end clavicle fractures who underwent open reduction and tunnelled suspensory device (ORTSD) fixation [20]. Patient-reported outcome scores (DASH) were assessed post-operative at 6 weeks, 3, 6, and 12 months, and for 55/64 surviving patients at mean 69 months for DASH and OSS, level of satisfaction, and complications. They found durable outcomes without significant changes in functional scores from 1 year post-operative (mean DASH: 2.4, mean OSS: 46.5) to latest follow-up (mean DASH: 2.2, mean OSS: 46.5). Two patients went on to symptomatic non-union warranting re-operation, and two went on to asymptomatic non-union without further intervention. Overall, they found 5-year survival without implant-related revision surgery to be 97%, and concluded that ORTSD is associated with durable medium-term outcomes and that routine implant removal is not necessary with this technique.

Proximal humerus

The question of which proximal humerus fractures benefit from surgical fixation remains. Two recent papers displaced on Neer 3- and 4-part proximal humerus fractures in the elderly (70–80+ years), one a randomised controlled trial and one a retrospective cohort, compared reverse total shoulder arthroplasty (rTSA) to non-operative treatment and found no clinically significant benefits to arthroplasty [21,22]. The danger of large-scale studies of this injury type is the heterogeneity in injury characteristics, patient demand levels, and surgical modalities. A recent meta-analysis of non-operative treatment (may any modality) in patients over 65 years did not find significant differences in functional scores at 1 year [23].

Certain types, such as head split fractures, are considered to necessitate surgery. Peters et al recently published on a retrospective cohort of 30 head-split proximal humerus fractures treated with open reduction internal fixation [(ORIF), 24/30, mean age 60 years], reverse total shoulder arthroplasty (rTSA, 4/30, mean age 76 years), or hemi-arthroplasty (2/30, mean age 74 years) at a minimum 12 months and mean follow-up of 49 months [24]. They evaluated functional outcomes with subjective shoulder value, simple shoulder test, and constant score, and used radiographs to assess fracture pattern and reduction quality. They found a whopping 83% complication rate [ORIF: 21/24 (88%), rTSA 3/4 (75%); hemi-arthroplasty 1/2 (50%)]. After ORIF, 42% had humeral head osteonecrosis, 33% has lesser tuberosity malunion, and 29% has screw protrusion, with 7/24 (29%) undergoing non-elective revision surgery (4 converted to rTSA, 3 penetrated screw removed). All arthroplasty-related problems had to do with tuberosity healing (3/5 with non-union of both tuberosities) and none underwent revision surgery. Clinical failure rate (constant score < 40) was 50% (ORIF: 12/24, rTSA: 1/4, hemi-arthroplasty: 2/2), with expectedly lower functional scores in those requiring revision surgery. Functional scores were higher in those undergoing ORIF and primary rTSA than those undergoing hemi-arthroplasty and secondary rTSA. They did not identify any pre-operative or clinical risk factors for treatment failure. Given the rTSA patients were less likely to need revision surgery than their ORIF counterparts, the authors suggest that rTSA may be the most reliable primary procedure for elderly patients presenting with head split proximal humerus fractures. However, any conclusions are limited by the small size and retrospective nature of this study.

Robinson et al of the Edinburgh Shoulder Clinic in the UK reported on long-term (mean 10.8 years) outcomes in 368 patients, mean age 55.3 years, who had undergone ORIF of a proximal humerus fracture [25]. In that period, 5,436/5,897 patients with proximal humerus fracture presenting to their clinic had been treated non-operatively. Patients who underwent surgery had presented with either unreduced glenohumeral fracture-dislocation, tuberosity involvement with >1 cm displacement in a 3- or 4-part pattern, disengagement of the head from the shaft, or angular deformity with head-shaft angle <90° or >160°. All had minimum 2 years clinical and radiographic follow-up, and 208 who were >5 years post-operative were successfully contacted to complete a questionnaire. Outcome scores included Oxford Shoulder Score (OSS), QuickDASH, subjective assessments of pain, stiffness, instability, satisfaction, and overall function. Complications included symptomatic stiffness (87/368, 23.6%, with 66 undergoing arthrolysis, subacromial decompression, and implant removal for this), mechanical failure/nonunion (25/368, 6.8%, with 12 undergoing revision ORIF, 5 conversion to arthroplasty, and 8 no further surgery), and osteonecrosis or post-traumatic arthritis (16/368, 4.3%, with 11 undergoing conversion to arthroplasty). With reoperation for any causes as the end-point, 5-year survivorship was 74.5% and 10-year survivorship 74.0%. Excluding reoperations for stiffness, survivorship without revision ORIF or conversion to arthroplasty was 90.4% at 5 years and 90.0% at 10 years. Survivorship with conversion to arthroplasty as the end-point was 95.2% at 5 years and 92.6% at 10 years. Patients reports median shoulder function of 90% compared to their other shoulder, and 82.7% reported high levels of satisfaction with their outcome. While this study is limited by its lack of a control group and loss to long-term follow-up of 43.5% of the cohort due to death, development of cognitive impairment, or loss of contact, it is valuable in both its stringent selection of the proximal humerus fracture morphologies that are likely most likely to warrant surgery, its introduction of a protocol for addressing post-operative stiffness, and its long-term follow-up.

Humeral shaft and elbow

Most humeral shaft fractures have historically been treated non-operatively with a functional brace. However, some patients cross over to surgical treatment. Serrano et al published a multi-centre retrospective series of 1,182 patients with closed humeral shaft fractures initially managed with functional bracing [26]. Their primary outcome was conversion to surgery. In all, 334 (29%) of fractures proceeded to surgery, with reported reasons as non-union (60%), malalignment beyond acceptable parameters (24%), inability to tolerate functional bracing (12%), and persistent radial nerve palsy warranting exploration (3.7%). In their analysis, females, whites, alcoholics, those with proximal shaft fractures, and those with comminuted, segmental, or butterfly fractures had increased rates of conversion to surgery. While retrospective in nature, these results may be helpful in counselling patients regarding functional bracing versus surgical fixation of humeral shaft fractures.

Conversely, iatrogenic nerve palsy is a known complication following operative fixation of humeral shaft fractures. Streufert et al retrospectively evaluated rates of iatrogenic injury with humeral plate fixation through posterior triceps-sparing, posterior triceps-splitting, and anterolateral approaches, and compared rates of recovery [27]. Of 261 humeral shaft fractures, 18.4% had pre-operative radial nerve palsies and 12.2% experienced iatrogenic radial nerve palsies. Broken down by approach, this consisted of 17.9% for posterior triceps-sparing, 11.7% for posterior triceps-splitting, and 7.1% for anterolateral, though these rates were not statistically significantly different. For the anterolateral approach, they found significantly higher rates of iatrogenic radial nerve palsy for middle shaft fractures (14.2%) than for proximal shaft fractures (0%) ($p = 0.0258$). Interestingly, they found higher rates of resolutions (95% vs. 74%, $p = 0.064$) in iatrogenic radial nerve palsies than for injury-associated palsies, along with shorter time to palsy resolution and lower likelihood of undergoing surgery for residual palsy (4.1 months vs. 5.5 months, $p = 0.91$; 6 patients vs. 0 patients, $p = 0.006$). Of note, their study was likely underpowered to detect clinically meaningful significance in palsy rate between the approaches. Their findings will assist surgeons in counselling patients both pre- and post-operatively about approaches, risks, and rates of recovery, and may steer surgeons away from using anterolateral approaches for distal shaft fractures.

For intra-articular distal humerus fractures in the elderly, total elbow arthroplasty (TEA) has gained acceptance as an option for acute treatment. However, given the lifting and weight-bearing restrictions following TEA and concern for bone loss or prosthesis loosening, many surgeons and patients remain cautious in choosing this option over attempted fixation. It was previously unknown how the results of primary TEA compare to those of delayed TEA following attempted open reduction internal fixation. Logli et al published a retrospective cohort study comparing 22 patients with distal humerus fractures who underwent primary TEA to 66 patients with distal humerus fractures who underwent salvage TEA for non-union, post-traumatic arthritis, hardware failure, stiffness, instability, or malunion at mean 7.3 years after initial fixation [28]. The majority of these were indicated for conversion due to non-union (36%) or post-traumatic arthritis (32%). The salvage group was younger (74 years acute vs. 60 years salvage, $p < 0.0001$) and more likely to use tobacco (0% acute vs. 23% salvage, $p = 0.02$). The authors compared Mayo Elbow Performance Scores (MEPS), range of motion (ROM), and complications between the groups. Outcomes did not differ significantly for primary or delayed TEA (MEPS mean 85 acute vs. 81 salvage, $p = 0.32$; flexion-extension arc/pronation/supination 95/82/75° acute vs. 112/81/72° salvage, $p = 0.07/0.85/0.65$; re-operation 36% acute vs. 39% salvage, $p = 1.00$). This was true even after excluding those who underwent delayed TEA for post-traumatic arthritis with 75% of patients classified as having good or excellent results. This suggests elderly patients with distal humerus fractures who fail initial attempted fixation may not compromise the outcome of an eventual TEA. Despite the limitations of its retrospective nature, this study provides helpful information for physicians and patients when deciding on acute treatment of these injuries.

LOWER EXTREMITY

Pelvic ring

Pelvic ring injuries occur as a result of both high and low energy mechanisms. Injuries resulting from low energy mechanisms often go undiagnosed. Natoli et al demonstrated that advanced imaging in the form of computed tomography (CT) or magnetic resonance imaging (MRI) was able to detect an additional 57.1% of posterior pelvic ring injuries relative to plain radiographs [29]. While this difference was significant, the clinical impact of these missed diagnoses was limited. There was no significant difference in the degree of post-mobilisation displacement after weight-bearing as tolerated mobilisation [29]. Pulley et al performed a study that also highlights the importance of advanced imaging in the geriatric population [30]. They found that spinopelvic dissociation in the form of "U-Type" sacral insufficiency fractures represents about 16.7% of all pelvic ring injuries in the elderly population. Without advanced imaging, these potentially debilitating injuries will often go undiagnosed [30]. They demonstrated that early surgical stabilisation of these injuries, in the form of posterior percutaneous fixation, allowed for early weight-bearing and rapid pain relief while decreasing the risk of progressive kyphotic deformity and potential malunion relative to delayed stabilisation. A prospective multi-centre observational assessment of minimally displaced lateral compression (LC) sacral fractures determined that operative stabilisation can result in a significant decrease in post-operative pain relative to non-operative management [31]. While these results were statistically significant at all time points, the clinical significance has been called into question, given that the absolute difference in VAS pain scores only ranged from 2.7 to 0.9 over 3-months [31]. Further evaluation of LC injuries was undertaken by Beckman et al as they attempted to validate a scoring system for the management of the specific LC subtypes [32]. They surveyed 111 OTA/OA members on 27 different cases of LC injuries to determine the operative tendencies associated with each injury. They subsequently compared those tendencies to scores that were assigned to each case based on their proposed scoring system [32]. This scoring system was validated via 33 separate cases and demonstrated an intra-class correlation coefficient of 0.77 [32]. These analyses determined that <10% of survey respondents would offer surgical stabilisation for a case with a score of <7 but over 90% of respondents would offer stabilisation for a case with a score of >9 [32]. Further comparative studies evaluating outcomes associated with this scoring system will hopefully provide insight into the optimal threshold for surgical stabilisation.

Hip

There is little debate about the benefits of surgical fixation of hip fractures. However, given the heterogeneity associated with these injuries, there has been significant investigation into the optimal timing and treatment modality for these fractures. Anthony et al performed a retrospective multi-centre database analysis of 4,215 patients on the temporal impact of hip fracture fixation and determined that there is an association between increased complications and those patients undergoing non-arthroplasty fixation of hip fractures beyond 48-hours (18.7% vs. 23.4%; $p < 0.01$) [33]. This temporal association was not seen in those patients undergoing arthroplasty for their hip fracture on multivariate analysis [33]. In an international randomised control trial (RCT) of almost 3,000 patients that was published in *The Lancet*, it was determined that fixation of hip fractures within 6-hours of admission, relative to within 24-hours of admission, had no impact on mortality or complication rates [34]. Therefore, although expeditious hip fracture fixation is optimal, they concluded that there is no benefit in rushing patients to the operating room as long as they have their fixation within 48 hours of admission. Lastly, a database analysis of nearly 90,000 hip fracture patients >60 years of age deemed that after-hours fixation of these fractures, including weekends, was not associated with increased rates of adverse outcomes [35].

Arthroplasty is standard of care for displaced femoral neck fractures in the elderly. The 12-year follow-up from a RCT conducted in the Netherlands that evaluated hemi-arthroplasty versus total hip arthroplasty for displaced femoral neck fractures in active patients >70 years old determined that there is no significant difference in complication rates, revision surgery rates, mortality rates, or functional outcome scores [36]. Unfortunately, only 20% of participating patients were alive for follow-up and patients with underlying osteoarthritis were excluded from their index cohorts which limits the impact of these results [36]. With that being said, another recently published international multi-centre RCT published in the *New England Journal of Medicine*, albeit with only 2-year follow-up, also demonstrated that there is largely no difference in functional scores between patients treated with total hip or hemi-arthroplasty for their displaced femoral neck fracture, despite a trend towards an increased incidence of serious adverse events (41.8% vs. 36.7%; $p = 0.13$) and dislocations (4.7% vs. 2.4%) in the total hip arthroplasty cohort [37]. To further evaluate the optimal treatment for displaced femoral neck fractures in the elderly, a meta-analysis of 21 studies looked at impact of the surgical approach on outcomes following hemi-arthroplasty and determined that the posterior approach, relative to the anterior (OR 2.61; $p = 0.01$) or lateral (OR 2.90; $p = 0.0003$) approach was associated with higher dislocation rates [38]. Furthermore, the posterior approach, compared with the lateral approach, was associated with a higher rate of reoperation (OR 1.25; 95% CI 1.12–1.41; $p < 0.0001$) [38]. Although the orthopaedic community often considers preinjury level of function in deciding total hip versus hemi-arthroplasty in the treatment of displaced femoral neck fractures, high level evidence suggests that hemi-arthroplasty, relative to total hip arthroplasty, may provide similar functional outcomes, especially if performed from a lateral or anterior approach, while minimising post-operative issues [36–38].

Hip fractures in the elderly are pathologic in nature and therefore many treating physicians apply oncologic principles for their subsequent treatment, i.e. protect the entire bone. However, in a RCT of 220 patients by Shannon et al, the use of a long cephalomedullary nail, relative to a short nail, was not associated with a decrease in post-operative peri-implant fracture rates, despite longer operative times, greater blood loss, and longer overall hospital stay for the treatment of pertrochanteric hip fractures [39]. The authors state that although the incidence of these peri-implant fractures was similar between the cohorts, operative fixation of subsequent fractures in the setting of a long cephalomedullary nail may be more challenging and thus warrants consideration when utilising these implants [39].

Femur

Intramedullary reaming is associated intravascular emboli. Tarride et al performed an RCT to evaluate whether the utilisation of a reamer-irrigator-aspirator (RIA) would decrease this embolic load relative to that of a standard reamer during the treatment of femoral shaft fractures [40]. Their investigation determined that while the RIA did modestly decrease the overall embolic load, as assessed via a continuous intra-operative transoesophageal echocardiogram, it offered no physiologic benefit in terms of arterial pressure, end-tidal carbon dioxide, oxygen saturation, pH, partial pressure of oxygen, or partial pressure of carbon dioxide [40]. Therefore, although the RIA did decrease the overall embolic load relative to a standard reamer, its clinical benefits may be limited but warrants further clinical investigation.

Tibia

Several approaches exist for the utilisation of intra-medullary nails to fix tibial shaft fractures. A retrospective review performed by Metcalf et al demonstrates that while there is no difference in functional scores, infection rates, or non-union, an infra-patellar approach, relative to a supra-patellar approach, is independently associated with an increased risk for malunion (adjusted OR 0.165, 95% CI 0.054–0.501, $p = 0.001$) and post-operative anterior knee pain (adjusted OR 0.272, 95% CI 0.083–0.891, $p = 0.032$) [41]. Further prospective evaluations are required to validate these findings.

Fractures of the tibia have a relatively high incidence of being open, due to the limited soft-tissue envelope and associated high energy mechanisms. Traditionally, devitalised bone fragments associated with these open fragments are disposed of due to the theoretical risk they pose for infection. However, in a retrospective review of Type 3B open tibia fractures out of the UK, there was no increased risk for infection when these devitalised fragments were retained in the setting of early-staged "orthoplastic" reconstruction, even after they were completely stripped of their associated soft-tissue [13]. The results of this study challenge orthopaedic dogma associated with thorough debridement of devitalised tissue in the setting of open fractures and thus warrant prospective clinical evaluation for validation.

Ankle

Syndesmotic injury is common in the setting of ankle fractures, but optimal reduction and fixation of these injuries has not been standardised. An RCT out of Norway compared single quadcortical screw fixation to suture button fixation for these injuries and determined that although there was no difference in initial syndesmotic reduction between the fixation strategies, the maintenance of that reduction was significantly better in the suture button cohort at 1 and 2 years post-operatively as assessed via CT scan [42]. Unfortunately, the single quadcortical screw cohort was subject to routine screw removal performed at an average of 86 days post-operatively and no sub-group analysis was conducted on those patients who had their screws maintained for longer periods of time. Similarly, functional scores were significantly higher in the suture button cohort relative to the screw cohort at all post-operative time points, but no sub-group analysis was conducted on those patients who had their screw fixation maintained for longer periods of time [42]. In another RCT evaluating the optimal reduction and fixation of syndesmotic injuries, the *Canadian Orthopaedic Trauma Society* determined that suture button fixation, relative to two screw syndesmotic fixation, had fewer malreductions at 3 months post-operatively (39% vs. 15%; $p = 0.03$) but was associated with a greater diastasis (4.1 ± 1.3 vs. 3.3 ± 1.4 mm; $p = 0.01$) relative to the screw cohort [43]. Therefore, the suture button functioned superiorly in its ability to aid in syndesmotic reduction but was unable to maintain said reduction relative to quad-cortical screw fixation. In addition, the screw fixation cohort required a greater number of re-operations relative to the suture button cohort, albeit this was primarily driven by removal of hardware (30% vs. 4%; $p = 0.02$) [43]. Unlike the previous RCT, the Canadian study demonstrated that there was no difference in functional outcome scores at any time point, up to 1 year post-operatively, between the screw and suture button fixation cohorts [43]. This contrast in functional outcomes between these two RCTs may represent the importance of longer hardware retention in the setting of syndesmotic fixation with screws. Further prospective evaluation with hopefully provides insight into this discrepancy.

REFERENCES

1. Grant-Freemantle MC, Lane O'Neill B, Clover AJP. The Effectiveness of Negative Pressure Wound Therapy Versus Conventional Dressing in the Treatment of Open Fractures: A Systematic Review and Meta-Analysis. J Orthop Trauma 2020; 34:223–230.
2. Costa ML, Achten J, Bruce J, et al. Negative-pressure wound therapy versus standard dressings for adults with an open lower limb fracture: the WOLLF RCT. Health Technol Assess Winch Engl 2018; 22:1–162.
3. Cocjin HGB, Jingco JKP, Tumaneng FDC, Coruña JMR. Wound-Healing Following Negative-Pressure Wound Therapy with Use of a Locally Developed AquaVac System as Compared with the Vacuum-Assisted Closure (VAC) System [published online ahead of print, 2019 Oct 9]. J Bone Joint Surg Am 2019; 10.2106/JBJS.19.00125.
4. Gosselin RA, Roberts I, Gillespie WJ. Antibiotics for preventing infection in open limb fractures. Cochrane Database Syst Rev 2004; 1:CD003764.
5. Stennett CA, O'Hara NN, Sprague S, et al. Effect of Extended Prophylactic Antibiotic Duration in the Treatment of Open Fracture Wounds Differs by Level of Contamination. J Orthop Trauma 2020; 34:113–120.
6. Li HK, Rombach I, Zambellas R, et al. Oral versus Intravenous Antibiotics for Bone and Joint Infection. N Engl J Med 2019; 380:425–436.
7. Parzych L, Jo J, Diwan A, Swart E. "Found Down" Compartment Syndrome: Experience from the Front Lines of the Opioid Epidemic. J Bone Joint Surg Am 2019; 101:1569–1574.
8. Thompson, Jeffrey, Long, Mitchell, Rogers, Eloise, et al. Fascia Iliaca Block Decreases Hip Fracture Postoperative Opioid Consumption: A Prospective Randomized Controlled Trial. J Orthop Trauma 2020; 34:49–54.
9. Ho KM, Rao S, Honeybul S, et al. A multicenter trial of vena cava filters in severely injured patients. N Engl J Med 2019; 381:328–337.
10. Cronin KJ, Hockensmith L, Hayes CB, et al. Are Routine Postoperative Computer Tomography Scans Warranted for All Patients After Operative Fixation of Pelvic Ring Injuries? J Orthop Trauma 2019; 33:e360–e365.
11. Archdeacon MT, Dailey SK. Efficacy of routine postoperative CT scan after open reduction and internal fixation of the acetabulum. J Orthop Trauma 2015; 29:354–358.
12. Howard A, West R, Iball G, et al. An Estimation of Lifetime Fatal Carcinogenesis Risk Attributable to Radiation Exposure in the First Year Following Polytrauma: A Major Trauma Center's Experience Over 10 Years. J Bone Joint Surg Am 2019; 101:1375–1380.
13. Al-Hourani K, Stoddart M, Khan U, Riddick A, Kelly M. Orthoplastic reconstruction of type IIIB open tibial fractures retaining debrided devitalized cortical segments: the Bristol experience 2014 to 2018. Bone Joint J 2019; 101-B:1002–1008.
14. Mathews J, Ward J, Chapman T, Khan U, Kelly M. Single-stage orthoplastic reconstruction of Gustilo–Anderson Grade III open tibial fractures greatly reduces infection rates. Injury 2015; 46:2263–2266.
15. Mitchell SL, Hayda R, Chen AT, et al. The Military Extremity Trauma Amputation/Limb Salvage (METALS) Study: Outcomes of Amputation Compared with Limb Salvage Following Major Upper-Extremity Trauma. J Bone Joint Surg Am 2019; 101:1470–1478.

16. Nicholson JA, Clement ND, Clelland AD, et al. Displaced Midshaft Clavicle Fracture Union Can Be Accurately Predicted with a Delayed Assessment at 6 Weeks Following Injury: A Prospective Cohort Study. J Bone Joint Surg Am 2020; 102:557–566.
17. Das A, Rollins KE, Elliott K, et al. Early versus delayed operative intervention in displaced clavicle fractures. J Orthop Trauma. 2014; 28:119–123.
18. Sawalha S, Guisasola I. Complications associated with plate fixation of acute midshaft clavicle fractures versus non-unions. Eur J Orthop Surg Traumatol 2018; 28:1059–1064.
19. Nourian A, Dhaliwal S, Vangala S, Vezeridis PS. Midshaft Fractures of the Clavicle: A Meta-analysis Comparing Surgical Fixation Using Anteroinferior Plating Versus Superior Plating. J Orthop Trauma 2017; 31:461–467.
20. Robinson CM, Bell KR, Murray IR. Open Reduction and Tunneled Suspensory Device Fixation of Displaced Lateral-End Clavicular Fractures: Medium-Term Outcomes and Complications After Treatment. J Bone Joint Surg Am 2019; 101:1335–1341.
21. Chivot M, Lami D, Bizzozero P, Galland A, Argenson JN. Three- and four part displaced proximal humeral fractures in patients older than 70 years: reverse shoulder arthroplasty or nonsurgical treatment? J Shoulder Elbow Surg 2019; 28:252–259.
22. Lopiz Y, Alcobía-Díaz B, Galán-Olleros M, et al. Reverse shoulder arthroplasty versus nonoperative treatment for 3- or 4-part proximal humeral fractures in elderly patients: a prospective randomized controlled trial. J Shoulder Elbow Surg 2019; 28:2259–2271.
23. Beks RB, Ochen Y, Frima H, et al. Operative versus nonoperative treatment of proximal humeral fractures: a systematic review, meta-analysis, and comparison of observational studies and randomized controlled trials. J Shoulder Elbow Surg 2018; 27:1526–1534.
24. Peters PM, Plachel F, Danzinger V, et al. Clinical and Radiographic Outcomes After Surgical Treatment of Proximal Humeral Fractures with Head-Split Component. J Bone Joint Surg Am 2020; 102:68–75.
25. Robinson CM, Stirling PHC, Goudie EB, MacDonald DJ, Strelzow JA. Complications and Long-Term Outcomes of Open Reduction and Plate Fixation of Proximal Humeral Fractures. J Bone Joint Surg Am 2019; 10.2106/JBJS.19.00595.
26. Serrano R, Mir HR, Sagi HC, et al. Modern Results of Functional Bracing of Humeral Shaft Fractures: A Multicenter Retrospective Analysis. J Orthop Trauma 2020; 34:206–209.
27. Streufert BD, Eaford I, Sellers TR, et al. Iatrogenic Nerve Palsy Occurs With Anterior and Posterior Approaches for Humeral Shaft Fixation. J Orthop Trauma 2020; 34:163–168.
28. Logli AL, Shannon SF, Boe CC, et al. Total Elbow Arthroplasty for Distal Humerus Fractures Provided Similar Outcomes When Performed as a Primary Procedure or After Failed Internal Fixation. J Orthop Trauma 2020; 34:95–101.
29. Natoli RM, Fogel HA, Holt D, et al. Advanced imaging lacks clinical utility in treating geriatric pelvic ring injuries caused by low-energy trauma. J Orthop Trauma 2017; 31:194–199.
30. Pulley BR, Cotman SB, Fowler TT. Surgical Fixation of Geriatric Sacral U-Type Insufficiency Fractures: A Retrospective Analysis. J Orthop Trauma 2018; 32:617–622.
31. Tornetta P 3rd, Lowe JA, Agel J, et al. Does Operative Intervention Provide Early Pain Relief for Patients With Unilateral Sacral Fractures and Minimal or No Displacement? J Orthop Trauma 2019; 33:614–618.
32. Beckmann J, Haller JM, Beebe M, et al. Validated Radiographic Scoring System for Lateral Compression Type 1 Pelvis Fractures. J Orthop Trauma 2020; 34:70–76.
33. Anthony CA, Duchman KR, Bedard NA, et al. Hip fractures: appropriate timing to operative intervention. J Arthroplasty 2017; 32:3314–3318.
34. HIP ATTACK Investigators. Accelerated surgery versus standard care in hip fracture (HIP ATTACK): an international, randomised, controlled trial. Lancet 2020; 395(10225):698–708.
35. Pincus D, Desai SJ, Wasserstein D, et al. Outcomes of after-hours hip fracture surgery. J Bone Joint Surg Am 2017; 99:914–922.
36. Tol MCJM, van den Bekerom MPJ, Sierevelt IN, et al. Hemiarthroplasty or total hip arthroplasty for the treatment of a displaced intracapsular fracture in active elderly patients: 12-year follow-up of randomised trial. Bone Joint J 2017; 99-B:250–254.
37. Bhandari M, Einhorn TA, Guyatt G, et al. Total hip arthroplasty or hemiarthroplasty for hip fracture. N Engl J Med 2019; 381:2199–2208.
38. van der Sijp MPL, van Delft D, Krijnen P, Niggebrugge AHP, Schipper IB. Surgical approaches and hemiarthroplasty outcomes for femoral neck fractures: a meta-analysis. J Arthroplasty 2018; 33:1617–1627.
39. Shannon SF, Yuan BJ, Cross WW 3rd, et al. Short Versus Long Cephalomedullary Nails for Pertrochanteric Hip Fractures: A Randomized Prospective Study. J Orthop Trauma 2019; 33:480–486.

40. Hall JA, McKee MD, Vicente MR, et al. Prospective randomized clinical trial investigating the effect of the Reamer-Irrigator-Aspirator on the volume of embolic load and respiratory function during intramedullary nailing of femoral shaft fractures. J Orthop Trauma 2017; 31:200–204.

41. Metcalf KB, Du JY, Lapite IO, et al. Comparison of Infrapatellar and Suprapatellar Approaches for Intramedullary Nail Fixation of Tibia Fractures [published online ahead of print, 2020 Jul 8]. J Orthop Trauma 2020; 10:1097.

42. Andersen MR, Frihagen F, Hellund JC, Madsen JE, Figved W. Randomized trial comparing suture button with single syndesmotic screw for syndesmosis injury. J Bone Joint Surg Am. 2018; 100:2–12.

43. Sanders D, Schneider P, Taylor M, et al. Improved reduction of the tibiofibular syndesmosis with Tight Rope compared with screw fixation: results of a randomized controlled study. J Orthop Trauma 2019; 33:531–537.

Chapter 11

What is new in hand surgery?

Kevin Lutsky, Michael Nakashian, Samir Sodha,
Jonas Matzon, Pedro Beredjiklian

TENDON INJURY AND REPAIR

Flexor tendon injury

Management of flexor tendon injuries remains challenging for hand surgeons and is an area of continued active research. The technical challenges of primary flexor tendon repair were investigated by Irwin et al. They compared repair strength and speed between a tendon coupler and a standard core suture repair, and found that the coupler repair had better residual load to failure and was faster to perform [1]. Surgical technique including wide-awake hand surgery has been found to be valuable in flexor tendon repair [2] and rehabilitation techniques such as early active motion have been shown to be beneficial [3,4]. Predicting outcomes after flexor tendon repair is difficult, but Rigo et al [5] demonstrated multiple factors including age, smoking, injury between sub-zones 1C and 2C, injury to the little finger, soft tissue and bony damage, and technical repair factors that are associated with poor outcomes.

Repair of zone 1 flexor digitorum profundus (FDP) injuries has historically required use of a pull out suture tied over a button. Several recent studies have described techniques which do not require an external repair. Putnam et al compared biomechanical strength

Kevin Lutsky MD, Department of Orthopaedic Surgery, University of Vermont Medical Center, Burlington, VT
Email: kevin.lutsky@uvmhealth.org

Michael Nakashian MD, Department of Orthopaedic Surgery, Thomas Jefferson University, Division of Hand Surgery, Rothman Institute, Philadelphia, PA
Email: mikenakashian@gmail.com

Samir Sodha MD, Department of Orthopaedic Surgery, Thomas Jefferson University, Division of Hand Surgery, Rothman Institute, Philadelphia, PA
Email: samir.sodha@rothmanortho.com

Jonas Matzon MD, Department of Orthopaedic Surgery, Thomas Jefferson University, Division of Hand Surgery, Rothman Institute, Philadelphia, PA
Email: Jonas.Matzon@jefferson.edu

Pedro Beredjiklian MD, Department of Orthopaedic Surgery, Thomas Jefferson University, Division of Hand Surgery, Rothman Institute, Philadelphia, PA
Email: Pedro.Beredjiklian@rothmaninstitute.com

of a fully threaded titanium suture anchor with standard mini-anchor or suture button techniques for zone 1 repairs [6]. They found the fully threaded anchor had a higher load to failure than the other techniques. Polfer et al [7] described a technique for all-inside repair of zone 1 FDP avulsions using a combination of a suture anchor and buried backup suture tied dorsally over the distal phalanx, but buried beneath the skin.

Extensor tendon

Recent studies on extensor tendon repair have been focussed on advancing rehabilitation techniques, in particular the use of relative motion splints. Merritt et al [8] and Hirth et al [9] have investigated the use of relative motion splints for extensor tendon rehabilitation and noted increasing popularity of this technique.

Closed sagittal band injury can be treated non-operatively with good outcomes. Roh et al [10] described outcomes after 5 weeks of finger extension orthosis use followed by 2 weeks of intermittent use and found 71% had resolution of tendon subluxation. Manual labourers, those with longer duration of symptoms or grade III injury were less likely to have a good outcome.

Central slip injuries are challenging, particularly in the chronic setting. Patel et al [11] described a reconstruction technique using a slip of the flexor digitorum superficialis through a bone tunnel for this difficult problem.

Extensor tendon injuries are typically traumatic in nature. However, attenuation can occur due to hardware or bony prominence or inflammatory arthropathy. Tobimatsu et al [12] described a case of index finger extensor tendon rupture from multiple gouty tophi.

WRIST, CARPUS AND HAND

Scaphoid injury

Obtaining healing of scaphoid fractures is paramount to avoid sequelae of non-union and/ or avascular necrosis. Screw fixation is the mainstay of treatment for operative management of scaphoid fractures. Ilyas et al [13] evaluated the compressive force obtained with three headless compression screws. They found equal compression among all screws tested unless the fracture gap increased to 4 mm, in which case the Acutrak 2 screw had less compression. Yildirim et al [14] reported excellent healing rates for both acute fractures and non-unions using two-screw fixation of scaphoid fractures. For waist fractures, fixation can be performed either through a volar or dorsal approach. The technical objective of screw placement is to obtain central positioning in the scaphoid. Lucenti et al [15] found that this objective was more often reached through the dorsal, ante-grade approach. **Figures 11.1** and **11.2** demonstrate a minimally displaced scaphoid fracture treated with a headless compression screw via a dorsal approach.

Pre-operative considerations that can predispose an acute scaphoid fracture for non-union were pointed out by Prabhakar et al [16]. The authors noted that delayed ORIF beyond 31 days from injury and smaller proximal pole volumes <38% of size of the scaphoid are associated with a higher risk of nonunion. Guidance on post-operative clearance to normal activity after scaphoid fracture repair was clarified by a recent biomechanical study [17]. This cadaveric study determined that a 50% intact scaphoid with a centrally placed screw behaved similarly to an intact scaphoid with biomechanical loading. This finding suggests that the threshold of 50% scaphoid fracture healing after surgical treatment is warranted to safely allow patients to return to unrestricted activity.

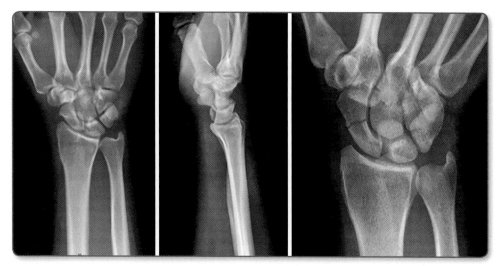

Figure 11.1 Posteroanterior (PA), lateral, and scaphoid X-ray view of a patient with minimally displaced scaphoid waist fracture.

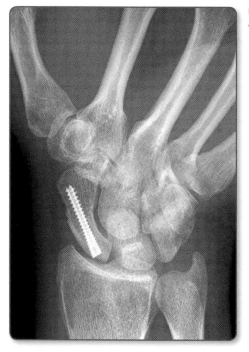

Figure 11.2 Post-operative radiograph after headless compression screw fixation through a dorsal approach.

Several contemporary approaches to management of scaphoid non-unions have been reported. Vascularised grafting has been described to have favourable healing rates using free vascularised medial femoral condyle (MFC) grafts [18]. Other authors have utilised local vascularised bone graft based on the palmar radiocarpal artery [19]. Volar plate fixation of scaphoid non-union has been suggested and shown to have excellent union rates and favourable functional outcomes [20,21].

A single institution's retrospective review of managing scaphoid non-unions compared iliac crest bone graft (ICBG), 1,2 inter-compartmental supra-retinacular artery (1,2-ICSRA) flap and a free vascularised MFC flap [22]. The results are summarised in **Table 11.1**. Each treatment group had differing non-union characteristics. The ICBG group consisted of non-unions with some carpal collapse but without prior surgery and intact vascularity of the proximal pole. The 1,2-ICSRA group had osteonecrosis of the proximal pole with half of them having some carpal collapse and up to a one-third had prior surgery. The MFC group consisted of those with osteonecrosis, almost all had carpal collapse and two-thirds of them had prior surgery. Studies reporting on non-vascularised grafts are also summarised in **Table 11.1** for comparison [20,23]. Locking plate fixation is an alternative method to address scaphoid non-unions with encouraging results as reported by Putnam et al. Just over 40% of their patient cohort had failed prior surgery and all had osteonecrosis [20]. Rancy et al reported their results using non-vascularised bone grafting with cannulated screw fixation in their series of patients of which 9 of the 23 patients had ischaemia on MRI [23]. Once again, the disparate groups in each of these studies make comparisons difficult, but the newly available data does help the surgeon on patient education on which of these available strategies are best applicable.

Distal radius fracture

Distal radius fractures are the most common upper extremity fracture. While many can be treated non-operatively, surgical fixation is often necessary for fractures that are unstable or with malalignment. While generally considered to be a safe procedure, surgical fixation has been reported to have relatively high rate of complications. The most common, transient paresthesia, can occur in almost 10% of patients [24].

Complications referable to the fracture hardware or loss of reduction can occur as well. Minimising prominence of the distal locking screws is necessary to avoid risk of extensor tendon issues. Care should be taken to drill and measure appropriately. The dorsal tangential view can help intra-operatively to identify screws that are too long [25]. Stabilisation of small volar rim fragments can be challenging. The loop-wiring technique can be used to support these small fragments that are otherwise not amenable to plate stabilisation [26].

Table 11.1 Healing rates of scaphoid nonunion by graft type.				
	Number of patients	Union rate	Time to union	Complications
Aibinder et al				
ICBG	31	71%	19 weeks	23%
1,2 ICSRA	33	79%	26 weeks	12%
MFC	45	89%	16 weeks	16%
Putnam et al				
BG+ volar plate	13	100%	18 weeks	8%
Rancy et al				
BG+ screw	35	94%	12 weeks	–

Several studies have evaluated the treatment of distal ulna fractures in conjunction with operatively treated fractures of the distal radius. While one study described use of an intra-medullary screw for stabilisation of these injuries [27], another demonstrated that fractures of the distal ulna do not need to be routinely stabilised after fixation of the radius [28].

Vitamin C has been suggested as a method for decreasing the risk of complex regional pain syndrome after distal radius fracture. However, Özkan et al did not find that the use of vitamin C improved recovery after distal radius fracture [29].

INFECTION

Animal bites remain a common source of morbidity in the general population. Seegmueller and co-authors examined if differences between the treatment of animal bite injuries within the first 24 hours after injury compared to >24 hours after injury [30]. A total of 69 patients with cat and dog bite injuries were treated in the emergency room, with 45 patients treated within 24 hours after the injury and 24 patients were treated >24 hours after injury. An operation was performed in 22 patients, and two were treated conservatively. In five patients, a second surgery was necessary in the late group. Based on this study, it appears that early treatment of cat and dog bite injuries leads to less second-look operations and a shorter hospitalisation.

Open hand fractures have historically been reported to have lower infection rates than open long bone fractures. Reasoner et al retrospectively reviewed 67 patients with 107 open hand fractures [31]. The overall rate of infection was 9% (6 out of 67 patients). No Gustilo–Anderson type 1 or type 2 fractures developed infection in contrast to 12.2% of type 3 fractures, an association which was significant. Patients who received antibiotics in <3 hours and underwent debridement in <6 hours did not have lower infection or nonunion rates than those who did not. Fracture type as defined by a modified Gustilo–Anderson classification was the factor most strongly related to the development of infection or non-union in these fractures.

Ovalle et al evaluated the epidemiology of the intravenous drug use (IDU) in a patient population presenting to a Midwestern academic medical centre emergency room [32]. A retrospective review of 1,482 patients with 1,754 emergency room visits was performed, including 308 patients with IDU-acquired infections (396 visits) and 1,174 patients with non-IDU infections (1,358 visits). Psychiatric co-morbidities and hepatitis C were common in the IDU group (51% and 39%, respectively). Heroin use was identified in 96% of visits. The IDU infections were more likely to have surgical intervention than those in non-IDU patients (16% vs. 6%), and a longer mean length hospital stay (2.4 vs. 0.9 days). In multi-variable analysis, IDU, psychiatric comorbidity, and insurance status were independent predictors ($p < 0.05$) for leaving the hospital against medical advice.

KIENBOCK'S DISEASE

Several long-term outcome studies have reported the results of treatment of this complex problem. DeCarli and colleagues, in an analysis of patients with Stage IIIA disease who underwent distal radius metaphyseal core decompression followed for at least 10 years, favourable results were demonstrated [33]. In a similar study, Viljakka et al in a clinical outcome study of titanium lunate arthroplasty found range of motion 70% compared to the contralateral wrist, and 81% strength at a mean of 11 years after surgery [34]. However, 20% of these patients had a dorsally dislocated implant. In a retrospective study by Hegazi et al comparing distal capitate shortening and arthrodesis to the third metacarpal base, results in patients with either stage II or stage IIIA disease showed pain level and range of motion was improved only in stage II patients, and was unable to prevent carpal collapse in stage IIIA patients [35]. Preliminary results of medial femoral trochlea osteochondral free flap for stage IIIA and IIIB disease showed a cessation of radiocarpal collapse, without improvement on range of motion but acceptable levels of pain and function [36].

In a systematic review of patients treated with vascularised bone grafts, Tsantes et al found that 13% of cases had progression of disease, with strength increasing from 52 to 84%, and ROM increasing from 66 to 77% of normal [37]. In an evaluation of inter-observer agreement on diagnosing early stage Kienbock's disease on radiographs and MRI, there was fair agreement with hand surgeons evaluating radiographs alone, and moderate agreement when MRI was evaluated in combination with radiographs [38]. A retrospective long-term analysis of radial shortening osteotomy for stage IIIA disease found that motion and grip strength were significantly improved, mean DASH score was 12, and patient's satisfaction was high although radiographic progression of disease was not prevented [39]. In 27 patients undergoing pronator quadratus pedicled bone graft from treatment of stage II, IIIA and IIIB disease, satisfactory pain relief was achieved in two-thirds of patients [40]. **Figures 11.3** and **11.4** demonstrate a patient with Kienbock's disease treated with radial shortening osteotomy.

CUBITAL TUNNEL SYNDROME

Cubital tunnel syndrome (CuTS) is the second most commonly treated compressive neuropathy of the upper extremity.

In an estimation of the incidence of CuTS in the United States (US) population, a commercial insurance database study was performed [41]. The authors estimated an adjusted incidence rate of 30 per 100,000 person-years, of which 53,401 cases were

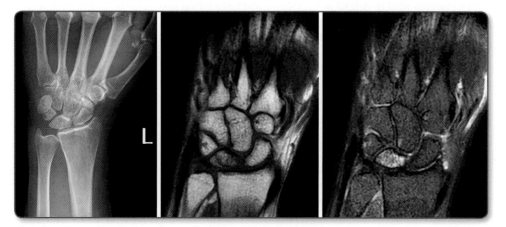

Figure 11.3 X-ray and MRI appearance of a patient with Kienbock's disease.

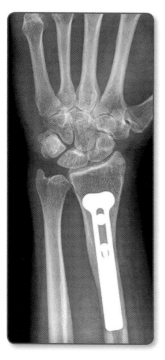

Figure 11.4 Post-operative appearance after radial shortening osteotomy for Kienbock's disease.

identified over the 6-year study period. In addition to finding that incident cases are more common with increasing age, the percentage of cases treated surgically also increases with age (surgery in 34.4% of cases in 18–30 age group vs. 48.8% in 60–65 years age group), with an overall 41.3% of cases treated surgically across all cases.

When performing cubital tunnel release (CuTR) surgery, the surgeon must decide between performing an in situ decompression or nerve transposition. In a meta-analysis comparing in situ decompression to transposition published in 2019, the authors found that there was no statistically significant difference between clinical outcomes or revision rates between groups. However, the study did identify significantly more complications within the transposition group, with the top three complications being scar sensitivity, infection and wound complications [42].

Regarding in situ decompression technique, a systematic review published in 2017 by Fowler et al looking at endoscopic versus open decompression found that the pooled rate of excellent/good outcomes was 92% for endoscopic and 82.7% for open surgery. Further looking at complication rates, they found a pooled odds ratio of 0.280 favouring endoscopic surgery [43]. This study suggests that endoscopic CuTR may be superior when considering complication rates and patient satisfaction. A similar study performed in 2019 by Byvalstev et al found that there was no statistically significant difference between techniques based on the Bishop score, visual analogue scale, post-operative satisfaction rate or secondary procedures [4]. They did find, however, a significant improvement in scar tenderness/elbow pain in the endoscopic group compared to open surgery [44].

Medial epicondylectomy as a surgical treatment for CuTS is a well-known alternative technique. In a systematic review of this technique published in 2017, O'Grady et al found an improvement of one or more McGowan grades in 79% of patients, with the mean percentage of good/excellent results of 83% [45]. With the existing literature regarding this technique found to be of limited methodological quality, definitive conclusions regarding comparison of medial epicondylectomy to other surgical techniques are unable to be made, and this topic requires further study.

Recurrence of CuTS is a complex problem and often requires revision surgery. Long-term revision rates were evaluated, comparing subcutaneous transposition versus in situ decompression in a retrospective multi-centre cohort study, comparing patients at minimum 5 years follow-up. The study found a higher re-operation rate for in situ decompression (25% vs. 12%), with 78% of revisions being performed within the first 3 years after surgery. Independent factors predicting need for revision were younger age and female sex [46].

CARPAL TUNNEL SYNDROME

Carpal tunnel syndrome (CTS) is the most common compressive neuropathy of the upper extremity and carpal tunnel release (CTR) is one of the most common procedures performed by hand surgeons.

For non-operative treatment of CTS, cortisone injection is one option that may be considered. In a comparison of ultrasound-guided versus landmark-based injection, a 2019 prospective randomised trial was conducted on 102 patients. Evaluating patients 6 months after injection, the authors found that, based on grip strength and Boston Carpal Tunnel Questionnaire (BCTQ), pain level and functional results were similar in both groups, although symptoms of median nerve irritation were more likely to occur in landmark-based injections (14% vs. 2%) [47]. In another study, 756 simulated carpal tunnel injections were performed in patients prior to open CTR, and the position of the needle was evaluated during the surgery. In 75.7% of patients, the needle was found to be appropriately located within the carpal tunnel; however, the needle was found to have either pierced the median nerve or missed the carpal tunnel in 8.7% and 15.6% of patients respectively [48].

Jansen et al evaluated 1,049 patients over a 4-year period and looked at symptoms relief on the BCTQ. They found that clinical severity of CTS at intake was the most important factor contributing to symptoms improvement [49].

Electromyography and nerve conduction studies are commonly performed prior to CTR surgery. In a prospective study evaluating CTR outcomes in relation to electrodiagnostic (EDX) testing, Rivlin et al found that CTR leads to significant improvement in outcomes at 2 weeks and 3 months post-operative time points, regardless of EDX severity grade. In addition, they found that the extent of improvement was not statistically different between groups with mild, moderate or severe disease [50].

The ability of diagnostic testing to accurately confirm CTS diagnosis and severity a controversial topic. In a prospective comparison of diagnostic tools, NCS, CTS-6, Wainner, Kamath and Lo tests were compared, using clinical diagnosis as the reference standard. They found that while NCS had the highest sensitivity (94%), it also had the lowest specificity (50%), whereas the CTS-6 had the highest specificity (99%) [51].

In 2018, a prospective randomised, double-blinded study comparing acetaminophen, ibuprofen and oxycodone as pain management after CTR surgery, the authors found that patients were content with the pain medicine prescribed with equal pain scores across all groups. This was regardless of which pain medicine they received, hence their recommendation to prescribe only non-opioid pain medication [52].

Surgical treatment with open versus endoscopic CTR has been evaluated extensively. In 2020, a prospective randomised trial comparing open and endoscopic CTR within the same patient undergoing surgery for bilateral CTS. While there were no statistically significant objectively evaluated differences between either group at any time point the authors note that, subjectively, 24 out of 30 patients preferred the endoscopic technique [53].

TRAPEZIOMETACARPAL ARTHRITIS

Arthritis of the trapeziometacarpal or basilar joint of the thumb is a very common source of morbidity in the general population, preferentially affecting middle aged female patients. Currently, there is a myriad of surgical procedures addressing basal thumb arthritis. Given that there is limited evidence on which technique is optimal, the choice regarding technique is predominantly based on surgeon preference. This was recently illustrated by a study which found that one quarter of surveyed hand surgeons had changed their surgical procedure for basal thumb arthritis within the past 5 years [54]. While there is considerable variation in surgical technique, a retrospective study conducted by Wilkens et al [55] demonstrated a low overall re-operation rate with trapeziometcarpal arthroplasty regardless of the technique employed. The authors reviewed 458 basal thumb arthroplasties performed over a 9-year span and found only a 4% re-operation rate. Of these, 16 of the 19 re-operations were performed within the 1st year after the initial surgery. Risk factors correlating with unplanned re-operation were younger patient age, surgeon inexperience, and surgeries performed without using ligament reconstruction or suspension arthroplasty.

Non-traditional arthroplasty techniques have been gaining popularity. Yao and Cheah [56] demonstrated favourable outcomes using suture button arthroplasty in 14 patients with a mean follow-up of >5 years. Moreover, a biomechanical cadaveric study evaluated 2-strand versus 4-strand suture button fixation for trapeziometacarpal arthroplasty and found that pinch pressure and load to failure results were equivalent in both groups [57]. The authors concluded that utilising the 2-strand construct with a 1.1-mm bone tunnel versus a 4-strand suture button arthroplasty (using a 2.7-mm bone tunnel) would produce similar mechanical stability and decrease the risk of index metacarpal fracture. Another similar technique that is gaining popularity is suture suspension arthroplasty. Weiss et al [58] retrospectively reviewed 320 patients who underwent trapezial excision and metacarpal suspension using #2 high-strength suture weaved between the abductor pollicis longus and flexor carpi radialis. At an average of 5.4 years, the patients had an average VAS score of 0.6. The authors cite the advantages of this technique as shortened operative time, inherent stability, and no necessity for K-wire fixation, tendon transfers, or implants.

Some recent studies have provided insight regarding the use of allograft material in trapeziometacarpal arthroplasty in order to avoid donor site morbidity. Marks et al [59] investigated two groups of patients in a prospective randomised study, comparing trapeziectomy and suspension arthroplasty using either half of the flexor carpi radialis or allograft tendon. Both groups had similar 12-month clinical results, but there was a higher complication rate in the allograft tendon group. There were 10 complications in allograft tendon cohort of 31 patients, and 5 complications out of the 29 patients in the flexor carpi radialis tendon group. The findings of this study led the authors to recommend against routine use tendon allograft for suspension arthroplasty.

In another study, Logli et al [60] reported their 5-year results of 24 patients who underwent an arthroscopic partial trapeziectomy with dermal matrix allograft interposition. All patients reported improvements in their pre-operative status, but one patient had painful instability. None of the 24 patients at the 5-year follow-up had undergone revision surgery.

Traditionally, all of the arthroplasty procedures have been met with consternation in younger patients; however, Rhee et al [61] demonstrated excellent outcomes for suspension-plasty and ligament reconstruction with tendon interposition in patients under the age of 55 years. A total of 57 wrists were evaluated at 10 years and none warranted revision surgery with all reporting improved grip strength and less pain. While radiographic studies did show progressive metacarpal subsidence, this finding did not correlate with clinical outcome.

In contrast to the various arthroplasty options, CMC joint denervation is a technique that preserves the joint anatomy, and therefore it may have particular appeal for younger patients. In a cadaveric and clinical study, Tuffaha et al [62] found that nerve branches to the CMC joint arise from the lateral cutaneous nerve (10/10 specimens), the palmar cutaneous branch of the median nerve (710 specimens), and the radial sensory nerve (4/10 specimens). In the same study, 11 out of 12 patients who underwent denervation demonstrated complete or near complete pain relief at an average of 15 months follow-up. In a prospective study of 31 patients undergoing denervation, Giesen et al [63] found that all of their patients reported less pain and improved key pinch strength at 1-year follow-up. However, the authors noted that 6 patients were unsatisfied with the procedure, and 4 of these 6 had stage IV CMC arthritis.

Finally, pre-operative hyper-extension deformity of the thumb metacarpophalangeal (MCP) joint and its impact on basal thumb arthroplasty outcomes is controversial. In a retrospective comparative study of 203 patients, Brogan et al [64] divided patients into those without pre-operative thumb MCP joint deformity and those with hyperextension <30°. Both groups demonstrated equivalent outcomes at an average 27.3 months, and therefore, the authors concluded that intervention for thumb MCP extension <30° is not warranted.

DUPUYTREN'S DISEASE

Dupuytren's disease continues to be a vexing problem for hand surgeons. Recently, less invasive alternatives to the standard fasciectomy have been introduced and have been gaining popularity. These include needle aponeurotomy (NA) and injection of collagenase *Clostridium histolyticum* (CCH) into the diseased cords. In a randomised controlled trial of 152 patients comparing NA and CCH, Stromberg et al [65] found no advantage of CCH compared to NA in terms of clinical outcomes at any time during 2-year follow-up. Similarly, in a prospective randomised controlled trial of 50 patients with isolated proximal inter-phalangeal joint Dupuytren's contracture, Skov et al [66] demonstrated no superiority of CCH to NA at 2 years follow-up. However, CCH was associated with a higher complication rate (93% to 24%). Fortunately, these complications were mainly transient. Long-term research is ultimately necessary to determine if either option is superior to the other.

Surgical fasciectomy continues to be a reasonable option for Dupuytren's contracture. Post-operatively, patients have historically been recommended to use a night-time splint for several months to maintain the surgical correction. In a systematic review,

Samargandi et al [67] set out to determine the role of a night orthosis. Seven studies met the standard for inclusion, which allowed 659 patients to be studied. There was no significant improvement in range of motion of hand joints or patient reported functional status for patients who received a static night orthosis after Dupuytren's surgery compared to patient without an orthosis. This study brings to question whether night-time splinting following surgery is necessary.

FRACTURES OF HAND

The type of fixation utilised for many phalangeal fractures is predominantly at the surgeon's discretion. However, some findings in recent studies could influence this decision-making process. A multi-centre retrospective study looked at 159 proximal phalangeal fractures treated by Kirschner wire (K-wire), lag screw, or plate fixation [68]. There was no advantage of any fixation method over the other when comparing outcome measures; however, the plate fixation group had a significantly higher unplanned re-operation rate and overall complication rate. Similarly, another study looking at 181 fractures of the middle and proximal phalanges also concluded open reduction with plate fixation resulted in higher re-operation rates than the other operative fixation techniques [69]. Furthermore, if K-wire fixation is the selected mode of treatment, Terndup et al found that keeping the wires exposed may avoid unnecessary trips to the operating room for incarcerated buried K-wires [70]. They also determined no difference in the rate of infections between buried and exposed K-wires for hand fracture fixation. With regard to metacarpal fracture fixation, Jones et al analysed three mechanical repair constructs and found the 2.0-mm locking plate fixation superior in its ability to resist displacement with cyclical loading [71]. The locking plate outperformed both the 3.0-mm intramedullary headless screw and a two 1.2-mm K-wire fixation construct.

REFERENCES

1. Irwin CS, Parks BG, Means KR. Biomechanical Analysis of Zone 2 Flexor Tendon Repair With a Coupler Device Versus Locking Cruciate Core Suture. J Hand Surg Am 2020.
2. Prasetyono TOH, Tunjung N. Long-Term Follow-up of Full-Awake Hand Surgery in Major Flexor Tendon Injury of the Hand and Forearm. Ann Plast Surg 2019; 83:163–168.
3. Pan ZJ, Pan L, Fei Xu Y. Infrequent need for tenolysis after flexor tendon repair in zone 2 and true active motion: a four-year experience. J Hand Surg Eur Vol 2019; 44:865–866.
4. Moriya K, Yoshizu T, Tsubokawa N, et al. Outcomes of flexor tendon repairs in zone 2 subzones with early active mobilization. J Hand Surg Eur Vol 2017; 42:896–902.
5. Rigo IZ, Røkkum M. Predictors of outcome after primary flexor tendon repair in zone 1, 2 and 3. J Hand Surg Eur Vol 2016; 41:793–801.
6. Putnam JG, Adamany D. Biomechanical Comparison of Flexor Digitorum Profundus Avulsion Repair. J Wrist Surg 2019; 8:312–316.
7. Polfer EM, Sabino JM, Katz RD. Zone I Flexor Digitorum Profundus Repair: A Surgical Technique. J Hand Surg Am 2019; 44:164.e1–164.e5.
8. Merritt WH, Wong AL, Lalonde DH. Recent Developments Are Changing Extensor Tendon Management. Plast Reconstr Surg 2020; 145:617e–628e.
9. Hirth MJ, Howell JW, Feehan LM, Brown T, O'Brien L. Postoperative hand therapy management of zones V and VI extensor tendon repairs of the fingers: An international inquiry of current practice. J Hand Ther 2020.
10. Roh YH, Hong SW, Gong HS, Baek GH. Prognostic Factors for Nonsurgically Treated Sagittal Band Injuries of the Metacarpophalangeal Joint. J Hand Surg Am 2019; 44:897.e1–897.e5.

11. Patel SS, Singh N, Clark C, Stone J, Nydick J. Reconstruction of Traumatic Central Slip Injuries: Technique Using a Slip of Flexor Digitorum Superficialis. Tech Hand Up Extrem Surg 2018; 22:150–155.
12. Tobimatsu H, Nakayama M, Sakuma Y, et al. Multiple Tophaceous Gout of Hand with Extensor Tendon Rupture. Case Rep Orthop 2017; 2017:7201312.
13. Ilyas AM, Mahoney JM, Bucklen BS. A Mechanical Comparison of the Compressive Force Generated by Various Headless Compression Screws and the Impact of Fracture Gap Size. Hand (N Y) 2019; 1558944719877890.
14. Yildirim B, Deal DN, Chhabra AB. Two-Screw Fixation of Scaphoid Waist Fractures. J Hand Surg Am 2020.
15. Lucenti L, Lutsky KF, Jones C, et al. Antegrade Versus Retrograde Technique for Fixation of Scaphoid Waist Fractures: A Comparison of Screw Placement. J Wrist Surg 2020; 9:34–38.
16. Prabhakar P, Wessel L, Nguyen J, et al. Factors Associated with Scaphoid Nonunion following Early Open Reduction and Internal Fixation. J Wrist Surg 2020; 9:141–149.
17. Guss MS, Mitgang JT, Sapienza A. Scaphoid Healing Required for Unrestricted Activity: A Biomechanical Cadaver Model. J Hand Surg Am 2018; 43:134–138.
18. Pulos N, Kollitz KM, Bishop AT, Shin AY. Free Vascularized Medial Femoral Condyle Bone Graft After Failed Scaphoid Nonunion Surgery. J Bone Joint Surg Am 2018; 100:1379–1386.
19. Sommerkamp TG, Hastings H, Greenberg JA. Palmar Radiocarpal Artery Vascularized Bone Graft for the Unstable Humpbacked Scaphoid Nonunion With an Avascular Proximal Pole. J Hand Surg Am 2020; 45:298–309.
20. Putnam JG, DiGiovanni RM, Mitchell SM, Castañeda P, Edwards SG. Plate Fixation With Cancellous Graft for Scaphoid Nonunion With Avascular Necrosis. J Hand Surg Am 2019; 44:339.e1–339.e7.
21. Esteban-Feliu I, Barrera-Ochoa S, Vidal-Tarrason N, et al. Volar Plate Fixation to Treat Scaphoid Nonunion: A Case Series With Minimum 3 Years of Follow-Up. J Hand Surg Am 2018; 43:569.e1–569.e8.
22. Aibinder WR, Wagner ER, Bishop AT, Shin AY. Bone Grafting for Scaphoid Nonunions: Is Free Vascularized Bone Grafting Superior for Scaphoid Nonunion? Hand (N Y) 2019; 14:217–222.
23. Rancy SK, Swanstrom MM, DiCarlo EF, et al. Success of scaphoid nonunion surgery is independent of proximal pole vascularity. J Hand Surg Eur Vol 2018; 43:32–40.
24. DeGeorge BR, Brogan DM, Becker HA, Shin AY. Incidence of Complications following Volar Locking Plate Fixation of Distal Radius Fractures: An Analysis of 647 Cases. Plast Reconstr Surg 2020; 145:969–976.
25. Bergsma M, Bulstra A-E, Morris D, et al. Accuracy of Dorsal Tangential Views to Avoid Screw Penetration with Volar Plating of Distal Radius Fractures. J Orthop Trauma 2020.
26. Minato K, Yasuda M, Shibata S. A Loop-Wiring Technique for Volarly Displaced Distal Radius Fractures With Small Thin Volar Marginal Fragments. J Hand Surg Am 2020; 45:261.e1–261.e7.
27. Oh JR, Park J. Intramedullary Stabilization Technique Using Headless Compression Screws for Distal Ulnar Fractures. Clin Orthop Surg 2020; 12:130–134.
28. Lutsky KF, Lucenti L, Beredjiklian PK. Outcomes of Distal Ulna Fractures Associated With Operatively Treated Distal Radius Fractures. Hand (N Y) 2020; 15:418–421.
29. Özkan S, Teunis T, Ring DC, Chen NC. What Is the Effect of Vitamin C on Finger Stiffness After Distal Radius Fracture? A Double-blind, Placebo-controlled Randomized Trial. Clin Orthop Relat Res 2019; 477:2278–2286.
30. Seegmueller J, Arsalan-Werner A, Koehler S, Sauerbier M, Mehling I. Cat and dog bite injuries of the hand: early versus late treatment. Arch Orthop Trauma Surg 2020.
31. Reasoner K, Desai MJ, Lee DH. Factors Influencing Infection Rates after Open Hand Fractures. J Hand Microsurg 2020; 12:56–61.
32. Ovalle F, Dembinski D, Yalamanchili S, Minkara A, Stern PJ. Hand and Upper Extremity Infections in Intravenous Drug Users: Epidemiology and Predictors of Outcomes. J Hand Surg Am 2020.
33. De Carli P, Zaidenberg EE, Alfie V, et al. Radius Core Decompression for Kienböck Disease Stage IIIA: Outcomes at 13 Years Follow-Up. J Hand Surg Am 2017; 42:752.e1–752.e6.
34. Viljakka T, Tallroth K, Vastamäki M. Long-Term Clinical Outcome After Titanium Lunate Arthroplasty for Kienböck Disease. J Hand Surg Am 2018; 43:945.e1–945.e10.
35. Hegazy G, Akar A, Abd-Elghany T, et al. Treatment of Kienböck's Disease With Neutral Ulnar Variance by Distal Capitate Shortening and Arthrodesis to the Base of the Third Metacarpal Bone. J Hand Surg Am 2019; 44:518.e1–518.e9.
36. Pet MA, Assi PE, Giladi AM, Higgins JP. Preliminary Clinical, Radiographic, and Patient-Reported Outcomes of the Medial Femoral Trochlea Osteochondral Free Flap for Lunate Reconstruction in Advanced Kienböck Disease. J Hand Surg Am 2020.
37. Tsantes AG, Papadopoulos DV, Gelalis ID, et al. The Efficacy of Vascularized Bone Grafts in the Treatment of Scaphoid Nonunions and Kienbock Disease: A Systematic Review in 917 Patients. J Hand Microsurg 2019; 11:6–13.

38. van Leeuwen WF, Janssen SJ, Guitton TG, Chen N, Ring D. Interobserver Agreement in Diagnosing Early-Stage Kienböck Disease on Radiographs and Magnetic Resonance Imaging. Hand (N Y) 2017; 12:573–578.

39. Luegmair M, Goehtz F, Kalb K, Cip J, van Schoonhoven J. Radial shortening osteotomy for treatment of Lichtman Stage IIIA Kienböck disease. J Hand Surg Eur Vol 2017; 42:253–259.

40. Ho Shin Y, Yoon JO, Ryu JJ, et al. Pronator quadratus pedicled bone graft in the treatment of Kienböck disease: follow-up 2 to 12 years. J Hand Surg Eur Vol 2020; 45:396–402.

41. Osei DA, Groves AP, Bommarito K, Ray WZ. Cubital Tunnel Syndrome: Incidence and Demographics in a National Administrative Database. Neurosurgery 2017; 80:417–420.

42. Said J, Van Nest D, Foltz C, Ilyas AM. Ulnar Nerve In Situ Decompression versus Transposition for Idiopathic Cubital Tunnel Syndrome: An Updated Meta-Analysis. J Hand Microsurg 2019; 11:18–27.

43. Toirac A, Giugale JM, Fowler JR. Open Versus Endoscopic Cubital Tunnel In Situ Decompression: A Systematic Review of Outcomes and Complications. Hand (N Y) 2017; 12:229–235.

44. Byvaltsev VA, Stepanov IA, Kerimbayev TT. A systematic review and meta-analysis comparing open versus endoscopic in situ decompression for the treatment of cubital tunnel syndrome. Acta Neurol Belg 2020; 120:1–8.

45. O'Grady EE, Vanat Q, Power DM, Tan S. A systematic review of medial epicondylectomy as a surgical treatment for cubital tunnel syndrome. J Hand Surg Eur Vol 2017; 42:941–945.

46. Hutchinson DT, Sullivan R, Sinclair MK. Long-term Reoperation Rate for Cubital Tunnel Syndrome: Subcutaneous Transposition Versus In Situ Decompression. Hand (N Y) 2019:1558944719873153.

47. Roh YH, Hwangbo K, Gong HS, Baek GH. Comparison of Ultrasound-Guided Versus Landmark-Based Corticosteroid Injection for Carpal Tunnel Syndrome: A Prospective Randomized Trial. J Hand Surg Am 2019; 44:304–310.

48. Green DP, MacKay BJ, Seiler SJ, Fry MT. Accuracy of Carpal Tunnel Injection: A Prospective Evaluation of 756 Patients. Hand (N Y) 2020; 15:54–58.

49. Jansen MC, Evers S, Slijper HP, et al. Predicting Clinical Outcome After Surgical Treatment in Patients With Carpal Tunnel Syndrome. J Hand Surg Am 2018; 43:1098–1106.e1.

50. Rivlin M, Kachooei AR, Wang ML, Ilyas AM. Electrodiagnostic Grade and Carpal Tunnel Release Outcomes: A Prospective Analysis. J Hand Surg Am 2018; 43:425–431.

51. Wang WL, Buterbaugh K, Kadow TR, Goitz RJ, Fowler JR. A Prospective Comparison of Diagnostic Tools for the Diagnosis of Carpal Tunnel Syndrome. J Hand Surg Am 2018; 43:833–836.e2.

52. Ilyas AM, Miller AJ, Graham JG, Matzon JL. Pain Management After Carpal Tunnel Release Surgery: A Prospective Randomized Double-Blinded Trial Comparing Acetaminophen, Ibuprofen, and Oxycodone. J Hand Surg Am 2018; 43:913–919.

53. Michelotti BM, Vakharia KT, Romanowsky D, Hauck RM. A Prospective, Randomized Trial Comparing Open and Endoscopic Carpal Tunnel Release Within the Same Patient. Hand (N Y) 2020; 15:322–326.

54. Deutch Z, Niedermeier SR, Awan HM. Surgeon Preference, Influence, and Treatment of Thumb Carpometacarpal Arthritis. Hand (N Y) 2018; 13:403–411.

55. Wilkens SC, Xue Z, Mellema JJ, Ring D, Chen N. Unplanned Reoperation After Trapeziometacarpal Arthroplasty: Rate, Reasons, and Risk Factors. Hand (N Y) 2017; 12:446–452.

56. Yao J, Cheah AE-J. Mean 5-Year Follow-up for Suture Button Suspensionplasty in the Treatment of Thumb Carpometacarpal Joint Osteoarthritis. J Hand Surg Am 2017; 42:569.e1-569.e11.

57. Grasu BL, Trontis AJ, Parks BG, Wittstadt RA. Four-Strand Versus 2-Strand Suture-Button Constructs in First Carpometacarpal Arthroplasty: A Biomechanical Study. Hand (N Y) 2019; 14:626–631.

58. Weiss A-PC, Kamal RN, Paci GM, Weiss BA, Shah KN. Suture Suspension Arthroplasty for the Treatment of Thumb Carpometacarpal Arthritis. J Hand Surg Am 2019; 44:296–303.

59. Marks M, Hensler S, Wehrli M, et al. Trapeziectomy With Suspension-Interposition Arthroplasty for Thumb Carpometacarpal Osteoarthritis: A Randomized Controlled Trial Comparing the Use of Allograft Versus Flexor Carpi Radialis Tendon. J Hand Surg Am 2017; 42:978–986.

60. Logli AL, Twu J, Bear BJ, et al. Arthroscopic Partial Trapeziectomy With Soft Tissue Interposition for Symptomatic Trapeziometacarpal Arthritis: 6-Month and 5-Year Minimum Follow-Up. J Hand Surg Am 2018; 43:384.e1-384.e7.

61. Rhee PC, Paul A, Carlsen B, Shin AY. Outcomes of Surgical Management for Thumb Basilar Arthritis in Patients 55 Years of Age and Younger. Hand (N Y) 2019; 14:641–645.

62. Tuffaha SH, Quan A, Hashemi S, et al. Selective Thumb Carpometacarpal Joint Denervation for Painful Arthritis: Clinical Outcomes and Cadaveric Study. J Hand Surg Am 2019; 44:64.e1–64.e8.

63. Giesen T, Klein HJ, Franchi A, Medina JA, Elliot D. Thumb carpometacarpal joint denervation for primary osteoarthritis: A prospective study of 31 thumbs. Hand Surg Rehabil 2017; 36:192–197.

64. Brogan DM, van Hogezand RM, Babovic N, Carlsen B, Kakar S. The Effect of Metacarpophalangeal Joint Hyperextension on Outcomes in the Surgical Treatment of Carpometacarpal Joint Arthritis. J Wrist Surg 2017; 6:188–193.

65. Strömberg J, Ibsen Sörensen A, Fridén J. Percutaneous Needle Fasciotomy Versus Collagenase Treatment for Dupuytren Contracture: A Randomized Controlled Trial with a Two-Year Follow-up. J Bone Joint Surg Am 2018; 100:1079–1086.

66. Skov ST, Bisgaard T, Søndergaard P, Lange J. Injectable Collagenase Versus Percutaneous Needle Fasciotomy for Dupuytren Contracture in Proximal Interphalangeal Joints: A Randomized Controlled Trial. J Hand Surg Am 2017; 42:321–328.e3.

67. Samargandi OA, Alyouha S, Larouche P, et al. Night Orthosis After Surgical Correction of Dupuytren Contractures: A Systematic Review. J Hand Surg Am 2017; 42:839.e1–839.e10.

68. Kootstra TJM, Keizer J, Bhashyam A, et al. Patient-Reported Outcomes and Complications After Surgical Fixation of 143 Proximal Phalanx Fractures. J Hand Surg Am 2020; 45:327–334.

69. von Kieseritzky J, Nordström J, Arner M. Reoperations and postoperative complications after osteosynthesis of phalangeal fractures: a retrospective cohort study. J Plast Surg Hand Surg 2017; 51:458–462.

70. Terndrup M, Jensen T, Kring S, Lindberg-Larsen M. Should we bury K-wires after metacarpal and phalangeal fracture osteosynthesis? Injury 2018; 49:1126–1130.

71. Jones CM, Padegimas EM, Weikert N, et al. Headless Screw Fixation of Metacarpal Neck Fractures: A Mechanical Comparative Analysis. Hand (N Y) 2019; 14:187–192.

Chapter 12

What's new in foot and ankle surgery?

Tara Gaston Moncman, Joseph Daniel, Rachel Shakked

INTRODUCTION

This chapter provides a summary of the most recent orthopaedic foot and ankle literature. Most studies were published between January 2017 and May 2020. The following journals were included, *The Journal of Bone and Joint Surgery, Foot and Ankle International,* and *The American Journal of Sports Medicine.* The chapter includes evidence about Achilles tendon disorders in the active population and how functional rehabilitation affects various outcomes and parameters, such as tendon elongation, calf size, and muscle strength. In addition, there is an abundance of literature being published on operative treatment of osteochondral lesions of the talus, including micro-fracture, allograft versus autograft transplantation, as well as a series of consensus statements on the clinical management of cartilage repair. Minimally invasive surgery (MIS) is also of recent interest with the goal of reduced pain, scar formation, and post-operative wound complications. In particular, MIS is being utilised in the forefoot for hallux rigidus and hallux valgus correction, but also for operative treatment of Lisfranc injuries, calcaneal osteotomies, and Achilles tendon rupture repairs. While ankle arthrodesis (AA) has been the historical gold standard for operative treatment of end-stage ankle arthritis, there are now more intermediate to long-term studies that report good to excellent outcomes and adequate survivorship of various total ankle arthroplasty (TAA) implants. These studies provide a comparison of fixed and mobile bearing implants, report on risk factors for revision surgery, highlight an algorithm for the treatment of periprosthetic fractures, and guide treatment of periprosthetic joint infections. How depression is correlated to outcomes after bunion correction, as well as the time to return to safe driving after first metatarsal osteotomy has been recently studied, as well. Furthermore, a few studies have suggested that the stages of hallux rigidus do not always correlate with the operative treatment and outcomes. Likewise, hydrogel hemi-arthroplasty implants for hallux rigidus continue to demonstrate variability of success. Higher level

Tara Gaston Moncman DO, The Rothman Institute, Thomas Jefferson University, Philadelphia, USA
Email: tara.moncman@rothmanortho.com

Joseph Daniel DO, The Rothman Institute, Thomas Jefferson University, Philadelphia, USA
Email: joe.daniel@rothmanortho.com

Rachel Shakked MD, The Rothman Institute, Thomas Jefferson University, Philadelphia, USA
Email: rachel.shakked@rothmanortho.com

studies are also proving the syndesmotic suture button to be a safe, reliable, and effective option to improve pain and function after syndesmosis injury. Lisfranc injuries in the active population may also be better treated with open reduction internal fixation instead of primary arthrodesis. For the difficult problem of Charcot arthropathy, various implants that provide a more stable, robust construct have been reported, including intramedullary beam fixation and tibiotalocalcaneal (TTC) intra-medullary nails with external fixation. Orthobiologics, such as platelet rich plasma (PRP) and recombinant human platelet-derived growth factor BB homodimer (rhPDGF-BB) are also being utilised to provide augmentation in surgery and perhaps allow for a quicker return to work or sport. Lastly, the opioid epidemic has fueled surgeons to be more judicious with narcotic prescriptions. Especially since studies are showing that patients may not need as many narcotics as they are being prescribed, and alternative analgesics such as ketorolac and acetaminophen can be just as effective.

SPORTS AND BIOLOGICS

Achilles tendinitis/rupture

Achilles tendon injuries are some of the most commonly treated orthopaedic injuries in the active population. It is unclear why this occurs in certain individuals and not others, despite participating in the same level of physical activity. In a large, level-II prospective study by Wezenbeek et al [1] 250 young, active individuals were followed for two consecutive years while participating in an identical recreational sports programme as part of their school education. Twenty seven (11%) developed Achilles tendinopathy, with notably decreased blood flow after running being the major risk factor. Female sex was also found to be a risk factor [1]. In professional athletes, acute Achilles tendon ruptures can decrease performance. In a level-III retrospective cohort study by Trofa et al [2] evaluating all National Football League (NFL), National Basketball Association (NBA), National Hockey League (NHL), and Major League Baseball (MLB) players who sustained an acute Achilles tendon rupture during the 1988–1989 and 2012–2013 seasons with subsequent operative repair, 19 of the 62 (30.6%) players did not return to play. At 1 year and 2 years post-operative, NBA players had the greatest reduction in playing time, while NFL players had the greatest decrease in performance overall, when compared to matched non-injured players, those who sustained acute Achilles tendon ruptures played significantly fewer games, had significantly reduced playing time, and performed worse at 1 year post-operative (**Figure 12.1**). However, at 2 years post-operative, there was no difference, suggesting professional athletes may be able to return to play and compete at their pre-injury level by 2 years [2]. With one of the longest follow-up periods of 8 years, Schipper et al [3] compared a cohort of general patients and elite athletes after repair of acute Achilles tendon avulsions. After trans-osseous bone tunnels or bone suture anchor fixation, all patients reported high satisfaction with good to excellent clinical outcomes. The average return to play in elite athletes was 13.4 months [3].

According to the 2010 American Academy of Orthopaedic Surgeons (AAOS) Clinical Practice Guidelines (CPG) for the diagnosis and treatment of acute Achilles tendon ruptures (**Table 12.1**), both non-operative and operative management are acceptable options for treatment [4]. In addition, both open and percutaneous techniques can be used for repair with good outcomes. The greatest theoretical advantage of percutaneous repair is reduced wound complications. An updated meta-analysis of eight randomised controlled

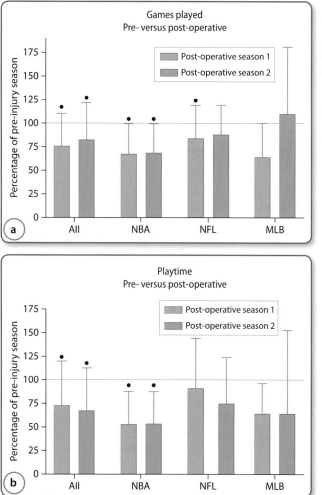

Figure 12.1 Playing time and games played after Achilles tendon repair. Pre-operative versus post-operative comparison of playing time (a) and games played (b) after operative repair of Achilles tendon ruptures in professional athletes. Post-operative data was collected after 1 and 2 seasons from surgery [2]. With permission from Trofa DP, , et al. (2017)

trials (RCT) was performed by Grassi et al [5] to evaluate MIS versus open Achilles tendon rupture repair. On risk reduction analysis, the authors found that one wound complication could be avoided with every 10 MIS procedures performed. Additionally, one post-operative complication could be avoided with every four MIS procedure performed. However, a recent retrospective, level-III study by Stavenuiter et al [6] including 615 patients reported no difference in post-operative complications between MIS and open repair. With open repair, the incidence of post-operative complications was 11.6% (65/562). The most common complications for open repair included surgical wound healing problems (5%), symptomatic venous thromboembolism (3.4%), and sural nerve injury (2%). For those treated with MIS, post-operative complications occurred in 13.2% (7/53) of patients. The most common complications for MIS repair included surgical wound healing problems (7.6%), symptomatic venous thromboembolism (5.7%), and sural nerve injury (1.9%). However, no significant difference was found for overall complications and wound healing problems between the two groups. Advanced age and active tobacco use were risk factors for complications [6].

Table 12.1 Selected 2010 the American Academy of Orthopaedic Surgeons (AAOS) clinical practice guidelines (CPG) for acute Achilles tendon rupture [4]

Work-up	Recommendation	Recommendation grade (Level of evidence)*
Physical examination	The physical examination should include two or more of the following tests to establish the diagnosis: Thompson test, palpable gap, decreased plantar-flexion, increased passive dorsiflexion	Consensus (opinion)
Imaging	Unable to recommend for or against the routine use of MRI, ultrasonography, and radiography to confirm the diagnosis	Inconclusive (insufficient)
Nonsurgical, treatment	Non-surgical treatment is an option	Weak (Level-II, conflicting)
Surgical, treatment	Surgical treatment is an option	Weak (Level-IV)
Surgical, risk factors	Surgical treatment should be approached more cautiously in patients with diabetes or neuropathy, those in immuno-compromised states or aged >65 years, those who use tobacco or have a sedentary lifestyle, those who are obese (body mass index > 30), and those with peripheral vascular disease, or local/systemic dermatologic disorders	Consensus (opinion)
Surgical, technique	Open, limited open, and percutaneous techniques are options for surgical treatment	Weak (Level-II, III; insufficient)
Post-operative, DVT prophylaxis	Unable to recommend for or against the use of anti-thrombotic therapy	Inconclusive (insufficient)
Post-operative, weight bearing	Suggest early (≥2 weeks) post-operative protected weight bearing (including limiting dorsiflexion)	Moderate (Level-II)

*Recommendations are based on the following [4]:
- We recommend: Recommendation grade, Strong. Level of evidence: Level-I evidence from more than one study with consistent findings for recommending for or against the intervention or diagnostic
- We suggest: Recommendation grade, Moderate. Level of evidence: Level-II or III evidence from more than one study with consistent findings, or Level-I evidence from a single study for recommending for or against the intervention or diagnostic
- Option: Recommendation grade, Weak. Level of evidence: Level IV or V evidence from more than one study with consistent findings, or Level II or III evidence from a single study for recommending for or against the intervention or diagnostic
- We are unable to recommend for or against: Recommendation grade, Inconclusive. Level of evidence: There is insufficient or conflicting evidence not allowing a recommendation for or against intervention
- In the absence of reliable evidence, it is the opinion of the work group: Recommendation grade, Consensus. Level of evidence: There is no supporting evidence. In the absence of reliable evidence, the work group is making a recommendation based on their clinical opinion, considering the known harms and benefits associated with the treatment

Interestingly, the American Academy of Orthopaedic Surgeons (AAOS) Clinical Practice Guidelines (CPG) do not indicate the optimal time to repair for acute Achilles tendon ruptures. In a retrospective study by Svedman et al [7], the authors found that at 1 year post-operative, reduced time to surgery reduced complications and improved patient reported outcomes. In particular, patients who had surgery <48 hours from their injury had significantly better functional outcomes and fewer adverse events at final follow-up. Whereas, significantly worse functional outcomes and pain were reported when surgery was performed between 72 hours and 10 days post-injury [7].

With the advent of accelerated functional rehabilitation, there has been increased support for non-operative management. Two recent prospective studies compared non-operative to operative treatment in which all patients received identical post-operative immobilisation and functional rehabilitation protocols [8,9]. Lim et al [8] found that at

2–6.5 years post-operative, there was no significant difference in outcomes comparing non-operative and operative treatment. On the other hand, in a level-I RCT, Heikkinen et al [9] found that those treated non-operatively experienced increased soleus muscle atrophy, reduced plantar-flexion strength, and increased fatty degeneration. In the non-operative group, the Achilles tendon lengthened by 19 mm within the first 3 months. Other studies have also reported on how tendon elongation affects outcomes. A follow-up prospective study evaluating operative and non-operative treatment of Achilles rupture found that at 18 months after injury greater muscle atrophy of the soleus muscle occurred with non-operative management [10]. In addition, the Achilles tendon was a mean 19 mm longer after non-operative treatment and this tendon elongation was proposed as being responsible for the soleus atrophy. Furthermore, the increased muscle atrophy seen with non-operative treatment was significantly associated with reduced peak plantar-flexion torque. Both operative and non-operative management results in compensatory deep flexor muscle hypertrophy[10]. An RCT by Eliasson et al [11] evaluated Achilles tendon elongation in 75 patients up to 1 year after operative repair comparing three different 8-week post-operative protocols (late weight-bearing-immobilisation, late weight-bearing mobilisation, and early weight-bearing mobilisation). The authors found that tendon elongation occurred for up to 26 weeks post-operative and that variable loading patterns (early versus late weight bearing) during the first 8 weeks after surgery did not significantly influence elongation. In addition, plantar-flexion strength, range of motion, gastrocnemius muscle size, Achilles Tendon Total Rupture Score (ATRS), or time to return to full duty at work were not affected by variable post-operative immobilisation and weight-bearing patterns [11]. Finally, Brorsson et al [12] evaluated long-term calf muscle performance after operative and non-operative management of Achilles tendon rupture. Seven years after injury, the injured limb had reduced calf muscle endurance and strength compared to the non-injured limb. No significant improvements in calf muscle strength and endurance occurred from 2 to 7 years post-injury, except for heel rise height. Additionally, no differences were found between patients treated operatively versus non-operatively [12].

Ankle instability

The operative treatment of lateral ligament instability of the ankle has recently included augmentation with suture tape to help increase stability (**Figure 12.2**). Porter et al [13] are the first to compare the ligament augmentation reconstruction system (LARS) to the traditional modified Brostrom–Gould (MBG) procedure in a level-I prospective RCT. Although patients improved after both procedures, the 22 patients randomised to the LARS procedure had significantly greater improvements in Foot and Ankle Outcome Score (FAOS) sport and quality of life sub-scores at 1, 2, and 5 years post-operative. Pain and activities of daily living were more significantly improved in the LARS group at 1 year, as well. All study participants were enrolled in an identical rehabilitation programme that allowed early range of motion (except inversion-supination) and weight bearing as tolerated in a functional brace after the first post-operative visit [13]. While this form of early rehabilitation is typical for the LARS, it may have been too aggressive for the MBG group, and thus influenced the results.

Osteochondral lesions of the talus

There has been much interest in the diagnosis and management of osteochondral lesions of the talus (OLT). It has recently been suggested that low vitamin D levels may

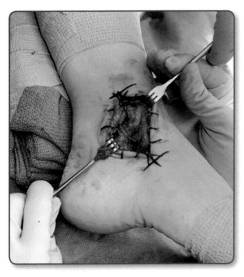

Figure 12.2 Suture tape augmentation for lateral ligament reconstruction.

be associated with the occurrence of OLT [14,15] Micro-fracture is a widely accepted treatment strategy and has demonstrated good to excellent results for small to medium sized OLT < 150 mm^2. Since the majority of studies are short-term with <2 years of follow-up, there is concern that any benefit from micro-fracture may deteriorate over time due to fibrocartilage being less durable than articular cartilage. Two recent studies reviewed mid-term outcomes after arthroscopic microfracture [16,17]. At an average follow-up of 47 months, visual analogue scale (VAS) and the American Orthopedic Foot and Ankle Society (AOFAS) scores were significantly improved, with incremental improvement for up to 2 years post-operative, but not after [16]. The largest series with 165 patients and long-term average follow-up of 6.7 years noted significant improvements in FAOS, AOFAS, SF-36, and VAS pain scores [17]. Therefore, even if the fibro-cartilage formed after micro-fracture is less durable than articular hyaline cartilage, this study demonstrated that it is sustained at intermediate follow-up of 6 years. Although 22 (13.3%) patients required repeat arthroscopy for recurrent pain. Of those that underwent repeat arthroscopy, four were considered treatment failures based on the repaired cartilage status being poor (grade 4), as per the Ferkel and Cheng staging system [17]. Another study by Shimozono et al [18] looked at mid-term clinical outcomes after micro-fracture for osteochondral lesions with specific attention to the influence of sub-chondral bone marrow oedema (BME). Mean FAOS score was significantly higher in patients without BME at 4 years post-operative. A moderate correlation was found between BME grade and FAOS scores at final follow-up. The authors suggest that while BME in the early post-operative period may be a physiologic healing response, its presence may be associated with poorer clinical outcomes at 4 years post-operative. For larger lesions >150 mm^2, osteochondral autograft transplantation (OAT) is commonly performed. Due to the potential risk of host graft site pain, allograft transplantation has more recently been utilised. Shimozono et al [19] found that OLT treated with allograft versus autograft transplantation demonstrated significant improvements in FAOS and SF-12 outcome scores from pre-operative to post-operative. However, sub-chondral cysts and cartilage degeneration were more prevalent and lower MOCART scores were identified in the allograft group [19]. A retrospective study by Nguyen et al [20] looked at OAT for large OLT in amateur and professional athletes. Of the 38 patients included, 11 professional and 22 amateur athletes returned to pre-injury level, four amateur returned to a lower level, and one amateur did not return to sport. The mean time that athletes returned to sport was 8 months, with professionals returning slightly earlier at 6 months. There is a paucity of literature comparing primary and secondary OAT for large osteochondral lesions. A study by Park et al [21] found no significant difference in VAS pain or FAOS outcome scores from pre-operative to final follow-up at a mean of 6 years. There was also no significant difference in revision surgeries performed. Lesion size > 225 mm^3 was found to be associated with clinical failure. Overall, this study found that patients who underwent a secondary OAT after failure of bone marrow stimulation had similar clinical outcomes to those who underwent primary OAT for large osteochondral lesions [21].

In 2017, an International Consensus Meeting on Cartilage Repair developed consensus statements on diagnosis, treatment options, rehabilitation and return to play, and follow-up [22–32]. A selection of the unanimous (100%) and strong (75–99%) consensus findings are included in **Table 12.2**. Grading of evidence was done based on **Table 12.3** [22–32].

Table 12.2 Selected consensus statements on cartilage repair. *Continues on pages 153–155*

Diagnosis	Statement	Consensus	Grade of evidence
Which radiographic/imaging studies can be utilised to evaluate a known or suspected cartilage lesion of the ankle?	Weight-bearing AP/lateral radiographs; standard CT and MRI. A CT scan with the ankle in full plantar flexion can be ordered to evaluate arthroscopic accessibility for pre-operative planning	Strong	A2
Conservative treatment			
In what cases can conservative management be considered for a cartilage lesion of the ankle?	(1) Asymptomatic lesions; (2) incidental findings; (3) non-displaced acute bone/cartilage injury; (4) older age with lower functional status; (5) signs of adjacent joint arthritis; and (6) a skeletally immature patient	Strong	E
What is the optimal protocol for conservative management (e.g. brace, cast, boot, PT, etc.) of an acute non-displaced cartilage lesion of the ankle?	Immobilisation for 4–6 weeks with touchdown weight bearing ± non-steroidal anti-inflammatory drugs (NSAIDs) in cases of significant pain and swelling. In cases with a significant bony component to an osteochondral injury, there is no use for a bone stimulator	Strong	B2
Debridement, curettage, bone marrow stimulation			
What are the ideal lesion size guidelines (diameter, depth, etc.) for the use of bone marrow stimulation in the primary surgical treatment of an osteochondral lesion of the talus?	Lesions <10 mm in diameter, <100 mm^2 in area, and <5 mm in depth. Bone marrow stimulation is less likely to succeed when used as a sole treatment in a lesion 15 mm in diameter or greater	Strong	Diameter, A1; Area, A1; Depth, B2
Can an awl or drill be utilised for bone marrow stimulation of the ankle, and what size should be used?	The use of an awl or a low-speed drill of 2 mm or less in size is recommended	Strong	C

	Table 12.2 *Continued*		
Diagnosis	**Statement**	**Consensus**	**Grade of evidence**
To what depth can the awl/drill holes be made in the ankle?	The awl/drill holes can be made to a depth that results in sub-chondral bone bleeding or presence of fat droplets	Strong	B1
What distance should be maintained between the awl/drill holes in the ankle?	The distance between the awl apertures should be 3–5 mm	Strong	B2
To what depth can a lesion be debrided before bone grafting is required in the ankle?	A lesion can be debrided to a depth of 5 mm before bone grafting is required	Strong	E
Fixation techniques			
In what cases/lesion types can fixation be considered for the surgical treatment of a cartilage lesion of the ankle?	Both acute and chronic lesions are indicated for fixation and can be considered in the following cases: (1) an intact osteochondral fragment > 10 mm in diameter and (2) a bony fragment of at least 3 mm in thickness. Fixation is contraindicated in cases of generalised osteoarthritis	Strong	C
Can fixation be performed in the case of a purely cartilaginous lesion?	It is possible but unlikely to be successful and therefore not recommended	Strong	C
Osteochondral autograft			
In what cases/lesion types can osteochondral autograft techniques be considered for the surgical treatment of cartilage pathology of the ankle?	Osteochondral autograft techniques can be considered in primary cystic lesions > 1 cm in diameter, as well as in revision scenarios after a failed primary procedure with a lesion size > 1 cm in diameter	Strong	B2
Is there a preferred osteochondral autograft donor site?	The lateral femoral condyle	Strong	C
Is donor site morbidity a concern after osteochondral autograft harvest? If so, can it be reduced?	The incidence of donor site morbidity after osteochondral graft harvest is generally <15% but warrants concern after graft harvest and should be discussed with patients, particularly in those with a higher BMI and larger lesion size. The following steps are recommended as potential means by which to reduce the incidence of donor site morbidity: (1) avoid iatrogenic damage to the articular cartilage, (2) avoid tight closure of the lateral capsule, (3) decrease soft-tissue manipulation, and (4) early rehabilitation and range of motion of the knee	Strong	C
Osteochondral allograft			
In what cases/lesion types can cylindrical osteochondral allograft plugs be considered in preference to autograft for the surgical treatment of cartilage pathology of the ankle?	Contained lesions > 1.5 cm in diameter, knee osteoarthritis, history of knee infection, and patients expressing concern with donor site morbidity of the knee	Strong	B1

Table 12.2 *Continued*			
What is the preferred type of allograft (storage, preservation, etc.) for use in the ankle?	Fresh and non-frozen allograft is preferred for use in the ankle	Strong	E (basic science)
Is there an optimal time for use of fresh osteochondral allograft? When is it too late to use secondary to loss of chondrocyte viability?	Fresh osteochondral allografts should not be used if older than 28 days. It is preferable to use grafts not older than 21 days	Strong	B2
What is the optimal method of fixation for a bulk osteochondral allograft in the ankle?	A conformed fit with headless compression screws	Strong	C
Scaffold-based therapies			
In what cases/lesion types can an autologous chondrocyte implantation (ACI) procedure be considered for a cartilage lesion of the ankle?	Large lesions > 1 cm^2, with or without cysts, including shoulder lesions	Strong	C
Rehabilitation			
Is there a benefit(s) to early versus delayed motion after cartilage repair of the ankle?	Early motion is beneficial and should be utilised after cartilage repair of the ankle. Early motion can begin within 1 week following surgery and should consist of free, active range of motion Manoeuvres such as forced passive movements that extend the patient beyond their available range of motion should be avoided	Strong	C
Post-treatment imaging			
For how long after cartilage repair of the ankle can clinicians and radiologists agree that there will be expected visualisation of post-operative sub-chondral oedema on imaging?	Even in asymptomatic patients, post-operative sub-chondral oedema may be seen on imaging for up to 2 years after treatment	Strong	C

Table 12.3 Grades of evidence for consensus statements on cartilage repair. With permission from the 2017 Consensus Meeting on Cartilage Repair [22–32]	
Grades of evidence	
A1	Multiple (two or more) Level-I RCTs with similar findings, or a meta-analysis
A2	A single Level-I RCT
B1	Prospective cohort study
B2	Any comparison group that is not Level-I (e.g. case-control)
C	Case series
D	Case report
E	Expert opinion/basic science
(RCTs, randomised controlled trials).	

Orthobiologics

Orthobiologics have become increasingly popular as patients and physicians seek viable alternatives or augmentation to surgery and accelerated return to activities and sports. Although the basic science theory behind their use is logical, few high quality clinical studies have been performed to support the use of orthobiologics in foot and ankle surgery. A double-blinded RCT evaluating injections for mid-substance Achilles tendinopathy favoured the use of PRP injection combined with eccentric training over eccentric training alone [33]. High-volume steroid injection was also evaluated in this study which showed better short-term outcomes than PRP injection. Another double-blinded RCT by Peerbooms et al [34] including 82 patients with chronic plantar fasciitis found that at 1 year, patients injected with PRP had significantly reduced pain and disability scores than those injected with corticosteroid. However, there were no differences in functional or quality of life scores between the two groups.

A retrospective study evaluated functional and radiographic outcomes after surgical treatment of talar osteochondral lesions [35]. Thirty patients had micro-fracture, while approximately half also received adjuvant bone marrow aspirate concentrate (BMAC), and 20 patients underwent treatment with juvenile allogenous articular cartilage with BMAC. Functional improvement was noted and healing of the lesions was confirmed on MRI with minimum 1 year follow-up. The repair tissue was primarily fibro-cartilage, with neither the addition of juvenile allogenous articular cartilage nor BMAC improving the quality of the repair tissue. There were also no differences in functional outcome relative to treatment group [35].

Synthetic bone graft has gained traction as an alternative to autograft at the time of arthrodesis to reduce post-operative morbidity. Based on a series of prospective RCTs, the use of recombinant human platelet-derived growth factor BB homodimer (rhPDGF-BB), better known by its brand name, "Augment Injectable Bone Graft" (Wright Medical Technologies, Franklin, TN), in combination with beta-tricalcium phosphate was found to be equivalent to autograft for ankle and hindfoot fusion, with less pain and morbidity than treatment with autograft [36].

MINIMALLY INVASIVE SURGERY AND ANALGESICS

Minimally invasive techniques have been implemented in many aspects of foot and ankle surgery in order to help to reduce wound complications and post-operative pain. Gutteck et al [37] compared open versus percutaneous calcaneal osteotomies in 122 consecutive patients. The open technique demonstrated wound complications in 9 (15.5%) patients, with 6 (10.3%) of them requiring operative irrigation and debridement. No patient in the percutaneous group had wound healing complications despite greater prevalence of diabetics and smokers. Adequate correction with improved pain and function was also reported by Veljkovic et al [38] in their retrospective case series of 41 patients after percutaneous endoscopically assisted calcaneal osteotomies. No post-operative wound complications or sural/lateral calcaneal nerve injuries were reported.

A RCT by Lee et al [39] compared the percutaneous chevron/Akin (PECA) and open scarf/Akin osteotomies for hallux valgus (HV) correction. Although follow-up was only 6 months, both groups demonstrated improvement in the HV and intermetatarsal (IM) angles, VAS pain, and patient reported outcome scores from pre-operative to final follow-up. The PECA group had less pain in the early post-operative period. These results were comparable to other studies comparing the PECA or minimally invasive chevron/Akin

(MICA) to the open scarf/Akin [40–42]. Post-operative wound complications were more common in the open procedure as compared to the PECA or MICA techniques [40,41]. Further, radiation time was increased and overall operative time decreased with the MICA or PECA technique [39–41]. However, hardware irritation and subsequent screw removal is more common after MICA and PECA compared to the open technique [39,40,42]. Further study is still needed to assess long-term outcomes after minimally invasive or percutaneous bunion correction.

Minimally invasive techniques are also utilised for hallux rigidus. A study by Stevens et al [43] compared MIS versus open cheilectomy of the first metatarsophalangeal joint (MTPJ). At a mean follow-up of 3 years, a higher proportion of MIS patients required a secondary procedure, most commonly being conversion to arthrodesis or secondary open cheilectomy. Overall there was no difference in wound complications between groups. All four of the MIS wound complications were due to residual bone particles, which is a known complication of the MIS technique [43]. This is similar to the results reported by Teoh et al [44] in which five out of the 12 re-operations were due to poor technique, including incomplete dorsal cheilectomy and residual bone slush left in the wound. The authors emphasise the learning curve that must be overcome in order to optimise results.

The opioid epidemic spurred many studies evaluating non-narcotic treatment of pain after foot and ankle surgery. Saini et al [45] identified that patients tended to receive nearly double the amount of pain pills that they required to manage post-operative pain. Patients that underwent regional anaesthesia tended to require less narcotic pain medication, and 30 narcotic tablets were recommended as an appropriate quantity to dispense in most cases [46]. Popliteal fossa nerve blocks were found by Schipper et al [47] to be more effective than peripheral ankle blocks in a RCT. Narcotic alternatives were also explored. Some providers elect to avoid non-steroidal anti-inflammatory drugs (NSAIDs) after fracture repair or arthrodesis operations because of the theory that it can cause delayed union or non-union. However, McDonald et al [48] evaluated ketorolac administration after ankle fracture open reduction and internal fixation (ORIF) in a RCT and there was no effect of ketorolac on radiographic time to union of the fractures. Acetaminophen may also be a good option for post-operative pain control and has been shown to have equivalent pain relieving effects with fewer side effects when compared to tramadol for treatment of pain associated with extremity fracture surgery [48].

ANKLE ARTHRITIS

Post-traumatic arthritis is the most common aetiology for a patient to require an ankle arthrodesis (AA) or TAA. A recent series of studies by Adams et al [49,50] demonstrated the changes in synovial fluid that occur after intra-articular ankle fractures. Pro-inflammatory cytokines rise steadily over the first 10 days, followed by matrix metalloproteinases, and cartilage degradation products. In addition, this pro-inflammatory environment may persist up to 6 months after the initial injury when the fracture is healed. Early evacuation of the joint with arthroscopic lavage may prove to be beneficial, and further study of these biologic markers as targets for therapeutic treatment is indicated.

Ankle arthritis can be a particularly challenging problem for younger patients. Although AA has traditionally been the gold standard, there is an increased interest in ankle motion preservation procedures. A 9-year follow-up study of 82 patients with a mean age of 44.3 years who underwent tibiotalar bipolar allograft osteochondral transplantation (OTA) found that survivorship of the OTA was 74.8% and 56% at 5 and

10 years, respectively, with a re-operation rate of 41% at a mean of 4.6 years due to OTA failure [51]. TAA is another motion preservation option that may lead to improved outcomes compared to AA. Hendy et al [52] reported that a higher range of motion after TAA correlated significantly with improved VAS pain, FAAM ADL and sports scores at varying intervals from 3 months to 2 years post-operative. A few studies have recently compared AA to TAA and found equivalent or improved outcomes in the TAA groups [53–55] Although when compared to arthroscopic arthrodesis, both open AA and TAA proved to result in improved outcomes [55]. Similarly, Brodsky et al [56] reported that those with significant pre-operative stiffness can make great gains in gait kinematics after TAA. In particular, they found that the change in pre-operative to post-operative motion was greatest in stiffer ankles.

With newer designs and broadening surgical indications, TAA continues to grow in popularity. In fact, two studies recently reported on the safety of performing TAA in the outpatient setting with adequate pain control and no difference in re-admission rates compared to those performed in the inpatient setting [57,58]. Additionally, patient-specific instrumentation (PSI) is now available and may help to improve the accuracy and reproducibility of implantation. The Prophecy technology (Wright Medical Technology, Memphis, TN) is the first foot and ankle navigation system to use pre-operative CT scan and computer-generated models to generate patient specific guides. A multi-centre, multi-surgeon retrospective study was performed by Daigre et al [59] to evaluate component alignment in 44 patients who underwent TAA with the INBONE II prosthesis using the Prophecy technology. A neutral alignment was reproduced in 93.2% of patients.

Significant deformity has traditionally been a contraindication to TAA, although acceptable parameters continue to evolve. Lee et al [60] evaluated outcomes after TAA utilising a Hintegra mobile-bearing prosthesis with either moderate coronal deformity of 5–15° versus severe deformity of 20–35°. Kaplan-Meier survival curve analysis demonstrated a survivorship of 92.3% in the severe group, and 90.7% in the moderate group. Overall, the authors reported similar functional outcomes and complications in both the moderate and severe coronal deformity groups. Further, Lee et al [61] evaluated 144 ankles with varying amounts of pre-operative coronal plane deformity including varus 0–20°, valgus 0–20°, and neutral <5°. At 7.3-years follow-up, the survivorship of the varus, valgus, and neutral groups were 97.7%, 81.1%, and 90.9%, respectively. The authors suggest that pre-operative deformity does not reduce clinical outcomes as long as a stable, neutral ankle is restored post-operatively [61].

Total ankle arthroplasty, although traditionally reserved for older patients, is now proving to be beneficial to those at younger ages, as well. Benich et al [53] found that younger and lighter patients had improved post-operative functional outcomes after TAA. Another study by Lee et al [62] compared TAA in patients younger and older than 55 years old. At a mean follow-up of 78 months, survivorship was not statistically different between the two groups, being 97.0% and 87.9% for the younger and older groups, respectively. Ankle range of motion and the tibiotalar angle improved more in the >55 years old age group, while complications were similar between both groups.

Lastly, the total talus is a more recent surgical option to treat the difficult problem of talus osteonecrosis. The study by Kanzaki et al [63] reported on 22 patients that underwent combined TAA with total talus. At mean follow-up of 34.9 months, range of motion and functional outcome scores all significantly improved from pre-operative measures. This study demonstrates promising results for a historically devastating problem, although more studies are needed.

Studies with more mid-term to long-term outcomes after TAA are now available. **Table 12.4** represents the most recent outcome studies based on implant type [64–72].

Table 12.4 Mid- and long-term outcome data after total ankle arthroplasty (TAA). Post-operative outcomes, complications, and survivorship are included for various fixed and mobile bearing implants. *Continues on pages 159–161*							
Citation	Implant	Population size (*n*)	Mean follow-up (months)	Significantly improved outcomes	Complications	Survivorship	Conclusions
Nunley et al [64] (2019); Level-I RCT	Integra Salto Talaris (FB) vs. Stryker STAR Ankle (MB)	84	54	*No difference:* range of motion, VAS pain, SF-36, FADI, SMFA, AOFAS	*STAR Ankle:* talar component lucency/cyst formation/ subsidence, HO, re-operations; *No difference:* tibial component lucency/ subsidence/ stress shielding, malalignment, tibiotalar angle, gutter impingement	N/A	There is no significant difference in improvement of clinical outcomes or range of motion based on radiographic evaluation between the mobile and fixed bearing TAA
Lefrancois et al [65] (2017); Level-II therapeutic	DePuy Agility* (FB), DePuy Mobility* (FB), Hintegra (FB), Stryker STAR Ankle (MB)	451	54	*Agility, Hintegra, STAR:* improved outcomes overall, AOS pain and disability, SF-36 mental and physical	*Agility and mobility:* higher metal component revision rates; *STAR:* polyethylene failure	STAR >hintegra >agility >mobility	TAA is a viable and reproducible procedure with subtle differences among the 4 prostheses types that a surgeon should be aware of when offering to their patients
Cody et al [66] (2018); Level-III retrospective	Wright IN BONE I and II (FB), Integra Salto Talaris (FB), Stryker STAR Ankle (MB)	538	36	N/A	Re-operation (25%), revision of metal components (6.4%). Most common reasons for revision: talar subsidence (41%), septic loosening (21%), excessive cyst formation (15%), excessive coronal deformity (12%)	5 years: 95.5%	Previous ankle fusion led to an eight-fold increased failure risk. Other risk factors for revision TAA included, use of the IN-BONE I prosthesis and an ipsilateral hindfoot fusion. Diabetes and severe valgus deformity were also associated with increased risk although not statistically significant

	Table 12.4 *Continued*						
Citation	Implant	Population size (n)	Mean follow-up (months)	Significantly improved outcomes	Complications	Survivor-ship	Conclusions
Koivu et al [67] (2017); Level-IV retrospective	Stryker STAR Ankle (MB)	34	159	Koefed ankle and pain (pre-operative to all follow-up intervals at 1, 5, 10, and 15 years)	Revision rate (including all re-operations): 44%; failure rate (exchange of metal components or conversion to arthrodesis only): 14.7%	5 years: 93.9%; 10 years: 86.7%; 15 years: 63.6%	The STAR implant demonstrates satisfactory long-term survival at over 13 years
Palanca et al [68] (2018); Level-IV case series	Stryker STAR Ankle (MB)	24	188	AOFAS Ankle/hindfoot; no limitations in walking distance (41%)	HO (61.9%), re-operation (52.4%), metal component failure (16.7%), progression of adjacent arthritis (14.3%), symptomatic/progressive bone cyst (14.3%), polyethylene fracture (14.3%)	5 years: 96%; 10 years: 90%; 15 years: 73%	The STAR component demonstrated a 73% metal component survivorship at 15 years follow-up with significant improvements in pain and minimal functional loss. Supplementary procedures are common
Loewy et al [69] (2018); Level-IV case series	Stryker STAR Ankle (MB)	138	106	AOFAS Ankle/hindfoot	Metal component failure rate: 15.2%; annual revision rate: 1.9%; re-operation (other than metal/poly failure) (12.3%), intra-operative fracture (9.4%), polyethylene fracture (6.5%), post-operative fracture (5.8%), deep infection (2.9%)	5 years: 90.4%; 10 years: 81.9%; 15 years: 76.7%	The STAR prosthesis demonstrated an overall survival of 84.8% at an average of 9–17 years, with improved patient reported outcomes, and low major complication rates
Stewart et al [70] (2017); Level-IV case series	Integra Salto Talaris (MB)	72	82	VAS pain, AOFAS Ankle/hindfoot, SF-36, SMFA dysfunction and bothersome index	Re-operation (19%)	95.8% (at mean follow-up of 82 months)	The Salto Talaris demonstrates improved pain and function at mid-term outcomes with excellent survivorship

Table 12.4 *Continued*							
Citation	Implant	Population size (n)	Mean follow-up (months)	Significantly improved outcomes	Complications	Survivor- ship	Conclusions
Usuelli et al [71] (2018); Level-IV case series	Zimmer-Biomet trabecular metal total ankle, trans-fibular (FB)	89	24	VAS pain, AOFAS, SF-12 mental and physical, range of motion, neutral alignment on post-operative radiographs	Re-operation (10%), delayed wound healing (2.2%), post-operative fracture (1.1%)	98.9% (at mean follow-up of 24 months)	At 2 years, the lateral transfibular approach to TAA is safe and provides pain relief and improved functional outcomes equivalent to the traditional anterior approach
Barg et al [72] (2018); Level-IV case series	Zimmer-Biomet trabecular metal total ankle, transfibular (FB)	55	27	PROMIS physical and pain, subjective "pain-free" (60%), range of motion	Tibia-prosthesis interface lucency (35%), tibia metal revision (5.5%), re-operation (18%), intra-operative fracture (3.6%), delayed wound healing (3.6%), superficial infection (3.6%)	1 year: 100%; 2 years: 93%	The transfibular TAA improves pain and motion, however, the increased tibia lucency is concerning and more long-term studies are needed

*no longer commercially available
(AOFAS, American Orthopedic Foot and Ankle Score; FADI, foot and ankle disability index; FB, fixed bearing; HO, heterotopic ossification; MB, mobile bearing; SF-36, 36-item short form survey; SMFA, short musculoskeletal function assessment; VAS, visual analogue scale).

Progression of adjacent joint hindfoot arthritis after TAA is another potential complication. Dekker et al [73] compared radiographic progression of adjacent joint hindfoot arthritis of three modern total ankle implants [Salto Talaris (Integra), IN-BONE (Wright), STAR (Stryker)]. The majority of patients had preexisting subtalar and talonavicular arthritis, yet did not show progression of arthritis at a minimum of 5 years postoperative. Those that did have progression of adjacent joint arthritis (27%) demonstrated an increase by only 1 Kellgren-Lawrence grade. Overall, a statistically significant progression of subtalar arthritis (11%) was seen compared to talonavicular arthritis (1%). When comparing types of implants, subtalar arthritis increased in 27%, 29%, and 22% with the IN-BONE, Salto Talaris, and STAR prostheses, respectively. Of those with progressive hindfoot arthritis, 7 IN-BONE, 5 Salto Talaris, and 4 STAR underwent secondary subtalar arthrodesis. However, all of the patients that went on to subsequent subtalar arthrodesis had pre-existent arthritis, whereas no patient without preexisting arthritis had post-operative subtalar pain or an arthrodesis. Although adjacent joint arthritis does occur after ankle

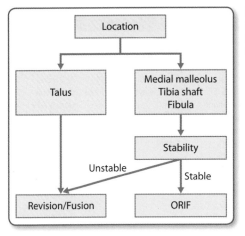

Figure 12.3 Treatment algorithm for the management of periprosthetic ankle fractures. ORIF, open reduction and internal fixation. With permission from Lazarides AL, et al (2019).

arthroplasty it does not appear to be clinically significant at 6.5 years follow-up, with an 11% and 1% risk of post-operative subtalar and talonavicular arthrodesis, respectively.

There is a paucity of literature on the management of periprosthetic fractures after TAA. A study by Lazarides et al [74] aimed to provide an algorithm for the treatment of fractures around a total ankle prosthesis (**Figure 12.3**). After review of all TAAs performed from 2000 to 2017, 32 post-operative fractures were identified, with a total incidence of 2%. The authors found that fractures most commonly occurred around the medial malleolus (59.4%) and 75% (24/32) of fractures were around a stable implant. Fractures were most commonly treated with ORIF or an IMN (75%), immobilisation (20.8%), and arthrodesis (4.2%). Interestingly, 80% of patients treated with immobilisation eventually went on to surgical fixation due to non-union, mal-union, or continued pain. 100% of fractures around the talus were unstable and required operative fixation.

Infection following TAA is a real challenge for both the patient and surgeon. In July 2018, an International Consensus Meeting took place and consensus statements were released on the topic of periprosthetic joint infections. The following are a selection of consensus statements pertaining to TAA [75–93].

CONSENSUS STATEMENTS FOR THE MANAGEMENT OF PERIPROSTHETIC JOINT INFECTIONS OF TOTAL ANKLE ARTHROPLASTY

Prevention

What are the important risk factors that predispose a patient to infection after TAA [75]?

- Inflammatory arthritis, prior ankle surgery, body mass index (BMI) < 19, and peripheral vascular disease
- There is conflicting evidence on obesity (BMI > 30), tobacco use, diabetes, duration of surgery, age <65 years, hypothyroidism, low pre-operative American Orthopaedic Foot and Ankle Society (AOFAS) hindfoot score, and chronic lung disease
- *Level of evidence*: Limited

- *Does intra-articular injection of the ankle with corticosteroids increase the risk of subsequent periprosthetic joint infection (PJI) following TAA [76]?*
  - The recommendation is to wait at least 3 months after corticosteroid injection and prior to performing TAA*
  - *Level of evidence*: Limited
- *What pre-operative optimisation should be implemented to reduce the risk of surgical site infection/periprosthetic joint infection (SSI/PJI) in patients undergoing TAA [77]?*
  - Skin cleansing, nutritional status enhancement, glycaemic control, BMI optimisation, smoking cessation, and management of immune-modulating co-morbidities
  - Preparation of the surgical site with an alcohol-containing agent, weight-based and timely administration of antibiotic prophylaxis, and reducing operating room traffic
  - *Level of evidence*: Moderate
- *What prophylactic antibiotic (type, dose and route of administration) should be administered peri-operatively for patients undergoing TAA [78]?*
  - Weight-based (of at least 2 g) cefazolin administered intravenously within 60 minutes before the procedure. It is unclear whether prophylaxis should be given as a single dose or as multiple doses
  - In patients with a β-lactam anaphylaxis, an appropriate alternative antibiotic effective against *Staphylococcus* can be used
  - *Level of evidence*: Strong
- *What is the optimal management of patients with prior septic arthritis of the ankle who are undergoing TAA [79]?*
  - Thorough history, physical examination, serologic tests, and possible aspiration; antibiotics should be added to the cement (if used), thoroughly cleanse the joint, obtain intra-operative cultures of bone and soft tissue
  - *Level of evidence*: Consensus

Diagnosis

- *What is the definition of acute and chronic periprosthetic joint infection (PJI) of TAA [80]?*
  - Any discussion of PJI after TAA is entirely reliant on the literature surrounding knee and hip arthroplasty*
  - *Level of evidence*: Consensus
- *What is the diagnostic "algorithm" for infected TAA [81]?*
  - Clinical signs/symptoms:
    - Likely: Pain, erythema, warmth, sinus tract, and abscess around the wound
    - Confirmative: Sinus tracts communicating with the ankle/subtalar joint
  - Elevated inflammatory markers [erythrocyte sedimentation rate (ESR) and C-reactive protein (CRP)] should prompt ankle joint aspiration for cell count, differential, and culture. The joint aspiration is to be repeated
    - *Confirmative*: If the same organism is identified in at least two cultures of synovial fluid
    - If the repeat aspiration is negative, further investigation is warranted
  - In patients not requiring operative intervention for other reasons, nuclear imaging should be considered for diagnosis

- If an operation is indicated, histologic examination (>5 neutrophils/high-power field) or synovial fluid analysis is conducted to confirm infection
- *Level of evidence*: Limited
- *What tests are useful to investigate a possible infection of TAA? What are their thresholds [82]?*
  - Joint aspiration or intra-operative tissue/synovial biopsies with micro-biological cultures are the most important*
  - *Level of evidence*: Strong
- *What are the indications for aspiration of a possibly infected TAA [83]?*
  - Whenever a PJI of a TAA is clinically possible or suspected. Especially with elevated ESR and CRP*
  - *Level of evidence*: Consensus

Treatment

- *What is the optimal protocol for performing debridement, antibiotics and implant retention (DAIR) in an infected total ankle arthroplasty (TAA) (type and volume of irrigation solution, and so on) [84]?*
  - Debridement, antibiotics, and implant retention (DAIR) in acute TAA infections may be an acceptable treatment option. If performed, DAIR should be done meticulously, ensuring that all necrotic or infected tissues are removed and modular parts of the prosthesis, if any, exchanged. The infected joint should also be irrigated with antiseptic solutions
  - *Level of evidence*: Consensus
- *What Determines the Type and Dose of Antibiotic that is Needed to be Added to the Cement Spacer in Patients with Infected TAA [85]?*
  - Antibiotics can be tailored to the infecting organism, if it has been identified, and added to cement spacers.* Vancomycin, gentamicin, and tobramycin are the most common antibiotics added to methylmethacrylate cement. Typical doses include, 2 or 4 g vancomycin, 2.4 g or 4.8 g tobramycin or 1 g daptomycin, 6 g clindamycin, 4 g ceftazidine, and 100–150 mg of amphotericin B added to a 40 g packet of cement to combat against gram positive [including methicillin-resistant *Staphylococcus aureus* (MRSA)], Gram negative (including P*seudomonas*), Gram negative and Gram positive (broad spectrum), Gram negative, and fungal organisms, respectively. The consensus recommends 2 g vancomycin and 2.4 g tobramycin to be added to every 40 g packet of cement as broad spectrum coverage for the treatment of periprosthetic infections in TAA
  - *Level of evidence*: Consensus
- *What are the predictors of treatment failure in patients who have undergone two-stage exchange for infected TAA [86]?*
  - Compromised soft tissues (e.g. sinus tract and exposed hardware), significant bone involvement/osteomyelitis, and insufficient timing of antibiotic course before re-implantation
  - *Level of evidence*: Moderate

Those recommendations marked with an asterisk (*) are derived from literature on PJI in hip and knee arthroplasty. Questions that require further study due to insufficient evidence are listed, below

"Insufficient Evidence"

- *Should routine mrsa, screening be in place prior to TAA [87]?*

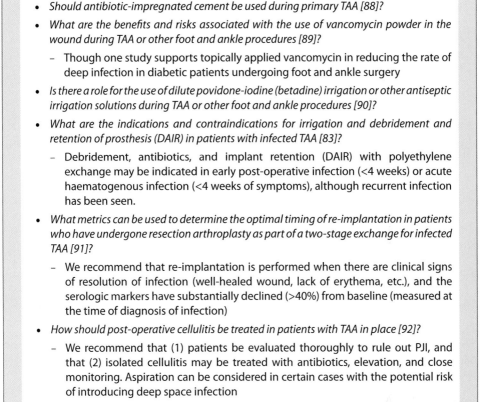

- *Should antibiotic-impregnated cement be used during primary TAA [88]?*
- *What are the benefits and risks associated with the use of vancomycin powder in the wound during TAA or other foot and ankle procedures [89]?*
  - Though one study supports topically applied vancomycin in reducing the rate of deep infection in diabetic patients undergoing foot and ankle surgery
- *Is there a role for the use of dilute povidone-iodine (betadine) irrigation or other antiseptic irrigation solutions during TAA or other foot and ankle procedures [90]?*
- *What are the indications and contraindications for irrigation and debridement and retention of prosthesis (DAIR) in patients with infected TAA [83]?*
  - Debridement, antibiotics, and implant retention (DAIR) with polyethylene exchange may be indicated in early post-operative infection (<4 weeks) or acute haematogenous infection (<4 weeks of symptoms), although recurrent infection has been seen.
- *What metrics can be used to determine the optimal timing of re-implantation in patients who have undergone resection arthroplasty as part of a two-stage exchange for infected TAA [91]?*
  - We recommend that re-implantation is performed when there are clinical signs of resolution of infection (well-healed wound, lack of erythema, etc.), and the serologic markers have substantially declined (>40%) from baseline (measured at the time of diagnosis of infection)
- *How should post-operative cellulitis be treated in patients with TAA in place [92]?*
  - We recommend that (1) patients be evaluated thoroughly to rule out PJI, and that (2) isolated cellulitis may be treated with antibiotics, elevation, and close monitoring. Aspiration can be considered in certain cases with the potential risk of introducing deep space infection

FOREFOOT

We continue to learn more about hallux valgus surgery, including patient factors that may affect outcomes, novel techniques, and the role of pronation correction. In particular, mental health is one area of increased interest. Shakked et al [93] found that VAS pain scores were higher pre-operatively and lower post-operatively in patients with depressive symptoms that underwent surgical bunionectomy. Interestingly, outcomes and satisfaction were more closely correlated to SF-12 mental (MCS) scores as opposed to history of depression. Since most patients are on medication to help control depression, practitioners should consider utilising a broader mental health questionnaire, such as the SF-12 MCS, to better evaluate a patient's current mental health status. A recent study by Conti et al [94] utilised a yaw-pitch-roll method to quantify pronation in three planes with yaw being the abduction-adduction axis, pitch being the dorsiflexion–plantar-flexion axis, and roll being the pronation axis. Overall, this study found that the modified Lapidus was an effective tool to change pronation of the first ray, with an average correction of 8.8°. Interestingly, the change in pronation was not associated with a change in sesamoid position. As such, the authors suggest that using sesamoid position and reduction alone to determine pronation correction may not actually be as useful as previously thought. Lastly, a study by McDonald

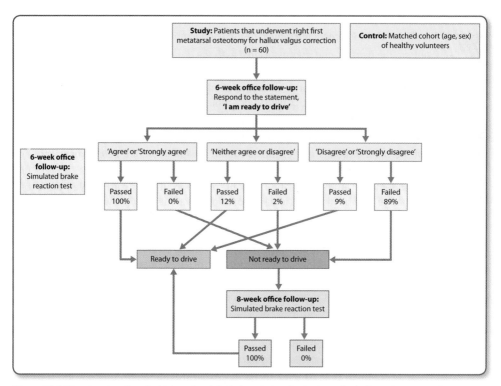

Figure 12.4 Time to return to safe driving after right first meta-tarsal osteotomy for hallux valgus correction. Sixty patients underwent a 6-week follow-up survey and simulated break reaction test (SBRT). 100% of those that responded 'agree' or 'strongly agree' also passed the SBRT, whereas 89% of those that responded 'disagree' or 'strongly disagree' failed the SBRT. By 8 weeks, all patients passed the SBRT

et al [95] evaluated time to return to safe driving after right first metatarsal osteotomy for hallux valgus correction. The results are summarised in **Figure 12.4**.

Surgical management of hallux rigidus entails much variability, seemingly due to the lack of correlation between grading systems and treatment success. For example, long-term success with significantly improved pain and high satisfaction was reported after dorsal cheilectomy for treatment of hallux rigidus Coughlin grades 1 through 3 [96]. Similarly, both a synthetic cartilage implant and arthrodesis may be appropriate choices in the treatment of moderate to severe hallux rigidus [97,98]. In particular, Coughlin grade was not found to correlate with treatment success after a synthetic implant or arthrodesis was performed [97]. Nonetheless, there seems to be no consensus on optimal treatment, with recent literature supporting polyvinyl alcohol (PVA) hydrogel hemi-arthroplasty (**Figure 12.5**), inter-positional arthroplasty, and arthrodesis for the treatment of hallux rigidus. Daniels et al [99] reported significantly improved patient reported outcomes, good to excellent patient satisfaction, and 96% survivorship at a mean of 5.4 years after PVA hydrogel hemi-arthroplasty. Similarly, Glazebrook et al [100] reported significant reductions in VAS pain and FAAM ADL/Sports scores, and maintenance of dorsiflexion from 2 years to 5 years post-operative. However, 9 (7.6%) of the 119 patients underwent

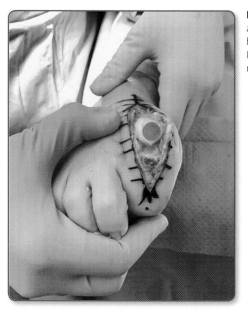

Figure 12.5 Polyvinyl alcohol (PVA) hydrogel hemi-arthroplasty. An intra-operative example of a PVA hydrogel hemi-arthroplasty [Cartiva (R) SCI, Wright Medical, Alpharetta, GA] used for the treatment of hallux rigidus.

implant removal and conversion to arthrodesis, with a reported survivorship of 84.9% at a mean age of 5.8 years. Other inter-positional arthroplasty techniques have also been reported with improvements in pain, functional outcomes, and patient satisfaction, including capsule and muscle interposition arthroplasty [101,102], or the use of a synthetic acellular dermal matrix [102]. The largest cohort of 133 patients with the longest follow-up to date of a mean of 62.2 months utilised a modified oblique Keller inter-positional arthroplasty with either a synthetic acellular dermal matrix or autograft using capsule and extensor hallucis brevis (EHB) tendon [102]. One hundred and one (76%) patients were able to return to fashionable or regular footwear afterwards. Both allograft and autograft inter-positional arthroplasty yielded excellent functional outcomes and satisfaction at final follow up. Finally, although arthrodesis tends to be reserved for more sedentary, heavier patients, Cunha et al [103] evaluated 2 years outcomes after first MTPJ fusion in healthy, active patients ages 18 through 55 years. Pre-operatively, 34.3% reported high impact activities, as opposed to 34.9% post-operatively. By final follow-up, patients were able to reach maximum participation in 88.6% of the physical activities at a median of 9–12 months. Further, patients reported participation in >10 hours of physical activity per week. This study demonstrates that first MTPJ arthrodesis is an option for athletic patients with moderate to severe hallux rigidus, with most being able to compensate post-operatively for the loss of motion.

Lastly, a retrospective series of 97 patients by Flint et al [104] reported on outcomes after plantar plate repair for lesser MTPJ instability (**Figure 12.6**). All plantar plate repairs were performed with suture and all but two also underwent a Weil osteotomy. Ninety percent of the 152 toes had concomitant procedures performed, most commonly for hallux valgus correction. In 80.4% of the feet, good to excellent satisfaction scores were reported, with higher satisfaction reported in those that had only a plantar plate repair and no additional procedures.

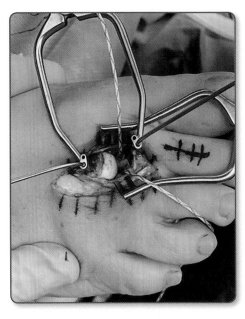

Figure 12.6 Plantar plate repair. An intra-operative example of a plantar plate repair for the treatment of lesser meta-tarsophalangeal joint (MTPJ) instability.

TRAUMA

Stabilisation techniques of the syndesmosis have been a focus of the recent literature involving lower extremity trauma. One study identified a malreduction rate of 27.8% based on post-operative CT scans and indicated that direction of malreduction related to version of the incisura [105]. An RCT concluded that suture button syndesmotic fixation was better than screw fixation with regard to functional outcome scores, pain levels, and long-term syndesmotic reduction [106]. The dynamic nature of suture button fixation may allow for a more anatomic reduction compared to rigid screw fixation. Suture button fixation was also shown to be better than screw fixation in a meta-analysis of 285 patients with regard to functional outcome scores and syndesmotic reduction with no difference in complication rates [107]. There continues to be controversy over whether to repair the deltoid ligament at the time of ankle fracture fixation. A retrospective cohort study showed decreased medial clear space and better functional outcome scores after deltoid repair compared to no deltoid repair in the setting of fibula fracture with associated syndesmotic instability and deltoid ligament tear [108]. Although sample sizes were small, there was a higher rate of medial ankle instability when the deltoid ligament was not fixed compared to those cases that underwent deltoid ligament repair in these cases. Of note, some patients were permitted to weight bear as early as 4 weeks post-operatively which may also have played a role in insufficient ligament healing. Furthermore, no differences were noted in the setting of a stable syndesmosis.

A large database study published by Bohl et al [109] identified independent risk factors for adverse events after ankle fracture fixation: greater age, female sex, chronic obstructive pulmonary disease (COPD), insulin-dependent diabetes, anaemia, and end-stage renal disease. Overall risk of adverse event after ankle fracture surgery was 6%. A risk stratification tool was also developed to help with pre-operative counselling and decision-making (**Tables 12.5** and **12.6**).

Table 12.5 Risk-stratification system from the nomogram analysis of the multivariate model (Development Cohort)*

Characteristic	Points in risk-stratification system
Age in years	
<40	+0
40–59	+1
60–79	+3
≥80	+5
Female sex	+1
COPD	+2
Insulin-dependent diabetes	+2
Anaemia†	+3
End-stage renal disease	+4

*Clinicians can use this table in conjunction with Table 12.6 to estimate risk for their own patients. COPD, chronic obstructive pulmonary disease.
†Defined as a pre-operative haematocrit value of <36% for females and <39% for males.
Source: Bohl DD, Idarraga AJ, Holmes GB, et al. Validated Risk-Stratification System for Prediction of Early Adverse Events Following Open Reduction and Internal Fixation of Closed Ankle Fractures. J Bone Joint Surg 2019; 101:1768–1774.

Table 12.6 Final estimation of the risk of occurrence of any adverse event (Combined Cohort)*

Total points	Risk	95% Confidence interval
0	1.9%	1.6–2.2%
1	2.5%	2.2–2.8%
2	3.2%	2.9–3.6%
3	4.2%	3.9–4.6%
4	5.5%	5.1–6.0%
5	7.2%	6.7–7.7%
6	9.2%	8.7–9.9%
7	11.9%	11.0–12.8% 9 19.1% 17.3–20.9%
8	15.2%	13.9–16.5%
9	19.1%	17.3–20.9%
10	23.8%	21.4–26.4%
11	29.2%	26.0–32.6%
12	35.3%	31.2–39.5%
13	41.9%	36.9–46.9%
14	48.8%	43.1–54.5%
15	55.7%	49.4–61.8%
16	62.4%	55.7–68.7%
17	68.7%	61.9–74.8%

*Clinicians can use this table in conjunction with Table III to estimate risk for their own patients.
Source: Bohl DD, Idarraga AJ, Holmes GB, et al. Validated Risk-Stratification System for Prediction of Early Adverse Events Following Open Reduction and Internal Fixation of Closed Ankle Fractures. J Bone Joint Surg 2019; 101:1768–1774.

There is growing evidence supporting the treatment of Lisfranc injuries with ORIF in the active population. In a retrospective review of 33 recreational athletes with Lisfranc injuries treated with ORIF (Lisfranc screw and bridge plate) Mora et al [110] found that 31 (94%) returned to some level of physical activity or sport post-operatively. Twenty two (67%) patients were able to participate at the same or higher level to pre-injury, while 11 (33%) participated less frequently. Cochran et al [111] compared outcomes of low energy Lisfranc injuries treated with primary arthrodesis (PA) versus ORIF in a young, active military population. Sixteen (89%) and 12 (86%) of patients in the ORIF and PA groups, respectively, were able to return to active duty at an average of 209 and 138 days, respectively. Those in the PA group were able to return to active duty 2 months sooner and had a post-injury run 29 seconds faster per mile than the ORIF group. Another study by Hawkinson et al [112] found that over two-thirds of their patient population of active military personnel were able to return to full duty, with there being no difference between PA or ORIF. They also found the timing of difference did not affect outcomes. In a large retrospective study of 217 patients, re-operation rates also seem to be comparable between PA and ORIF when planned re-operation with removal of hardware was excluded from the ORIF group [113].

DIABETES

Operative reconstructive techniques for Charcot neuroarthropathy-associated deformity continue to evolve with a trend towards robust internal fixation. Combined internal and external fixation has recently been shown to be a successful technique to achieve ankle arthrodesis in a recent retrospective study [114]. Twenty two patients (92%) went on to successful fusion and two developed stable non-unions after undergoing hybrid ring external fixation and TTC arthrodesis nail. TTC nailing was also shown to be an acceptable alternative to ORIF of certain diabetic ankle fractures [115]. In this series of high-risk patients with complicated diabetes, primary TTC nail fixation without joint preparation was performed which allowed for earlier weight bearing and acceptable outcomes. Limb salvage rate was 92.6% and weight bearing occurred around 6 weeks post-operative on average. The complication rate was relatively high at 18.5%, although the population is high risk and prior studies have shown complication rates after ORIF of ankle fractures in diabetics to range between 13% [116] and 42% [117]. Correction of Charcot deformity through the midfoot can be achieved using intra-medullary beaming as shown in a recent retrospective case series of 25 patients with 1 year follow-up [118]. Eighty four percent (21/25) achieved a successful result with a plantigrade foot and no ulcerations. Infections requiring re-operation occurred in six (24%) patients, all of whom had pre-operative ulceration. Intra-medullary beams may be a good alternative to ring fixation; however, it should be considered with caution in the setting of pre-operative ulceration. A large retrospective study published in 2017 by Pinzur et al [119] described a novel classification system for midfoot deformity that correlates with prognosis. Valgus midfoot deformity was associated with the highest success rate (87%) while varus midfoot deformity was associated with fewer successful outcomes (56%). Overall, nearly 80% of patients achieved acceptable results with the ability to ambulate independently in regular shoes [120].

CONCLUSION

The previous chapter is a summary of some of the most recent peer-reviewed studies in foot and ankle surgery published from 2017 to present. While the 2010 AAOS CPG highlight general recommendations for the treatment of acute Achilles tendon ruptures, there have been more recent studies to better define these previous recommendations. For example, Svedman et al reported that patients had improved pain and functional outcomes when repair was done within 48 hours from injury [7]. In addition, Trofa et al found that at 1 year post-Achilles tendon rupture and repair, professional athletes played significantly fewer games, had significantly reduced playing time, and performed worse. However, at 2 years post-operative, there was no difference, suggesting professional athletes may be able to return to play and compete at their pre-injury level by 2 years [2]. In regard to osteochondral lesions, there has been recent concern that the benefits of micro-fracture are deleterious over time due to the healing fibro-cartilage being less durable than hyaline articular cartilage. Most previous studies have only followed patients for up to 2 years post-operative. A study by Choi et al found that at a mean follow-up of 6.5 years, functional outcomes after micro-fracture were maintained without any clear sign of deterioration [17]. Further, in 2018 an International Consensus Meeting on Cartilage Repair was held and developed consensus statements on diagnosis, treatment options, rehabilitation and return to play, and follow-up [22–32]. Minimally invasive surgery has also been on the forefront recently for the theoretical benefit of reduced post-operative wound complications. However, MIS is not without consequence, especially with the inherent learning curve that exists with the introduction any new technique to one's practice. For example, re-operation and revision procedures are common, as well as hardware irritation often due to inadequate or poor technique [39,40,42,43]. A series of papers by Adams et al on the presence of pro-inflammatory cytokines after intra-articular ankle fracture leads one to believe that early evacuation of the joint with arthroscopic lavage may prove to be beneficial [49,50]. Further study of these biologic markers as targets for therapeutic treatment is indicated. Indications for TAA have also broadened. Lee et al found that pre-operative coronal deformity >20° is not a contraindication to TAA and that patients have reduced pain and improved function as long as there ankle joint is corrected to neutral [60]. In addition, patients both older and younger than 55 years old can have improved pain and function after TAA [61]. Mid- to long-term survivorship has also been reported for a number of TAA implants, including the STAR, Salto Talaris, Hintegra, and Agility [64–72]. An interesting study by Conti et al found that the modified Lapidus was an effective tool to change pronation of the first ray and that the change in pronation was not associated with a change in sesamoid position [94]. In addition, the syndesmotic suture button is growing in popularity with level-I evidence proving improved pain and function compared to the syndesmosis screw [100]. Finally, the opioid epidemic has been an important topic in the medical field. A few studies have reported on post-operative opioids after foot and ankle surgery. Saini et al identified that patients tended to receive nearly double the amount of pain pills that they required to manage post-operative pain [45]. In addition, patients that undergo regional anaesthesia tend to require less narcotic pain medication, and 30 narcotic tablets are recommended as an appropriate quantity to dispense in most cases [46].

REFERENCES

1. Wezenbeek E, Willems T, Mahieu N, et al. The Role of the Vascular and Structural Response to Activity in the Development of Achilles Tendinopathy: A Prospective Study. Am J Sports Med 2018; 46:947–954.
2. Trofa DP, Miller JC, Jang ES, et al. Professional Athletes' Return to Play and Performance After Operative Repair of an Achilles Tendon Rupture. Am J Sports Med 2017; 45:2864–2871.
3. Schipper ON, Anderson RB, Cohen BE. Outcomes After Primary Repair of Insertional Ruptures of the Achilles Tendon. Foot Ankle Int 2018; 39:664–668.
4. Chiodo CP, Glazebrook MM, Bluman EM, et al. Diagnosis and Treatment of Acute Achilles Tendon Rupture. Am Acad Ortho Surg 2010; 18:503–510.
5. Grassi A, Amendol A, Samuelsson K, et al. Minimally Invasive Versus Open Repair for Acute Achilles Tendon Rupture. J Bone Joint Surg 2018; 100:1969–1981.
6. Stavenuiter XJR, Lubberts B, Prince RM, et al. Postoperative Complications Following Repair of Acute Achilles Tendon Rupture. Foot Ankle Int 2019; 40:679–686.
7. Svedman S, Juthberg R, Edman G, Ackermann PW. Reduced Time to Surgery Improves Patient-Reported Outcome After Achilles Tendon Rupture. Am J Sports Med. 2018; 46:2929–2934.
8. Lim CS, Lees D, Gwynne-Jones DP. Functional Outcome of Acute Achilles Tendon Rupture With and Without Operative Treatment Using Identical Functional Bracing Protocol. Foot Ankle Int 2017; 38:1331–1336.
9. Heikkinen J, Lantto I, Flinkkila T, et al. Soleus Atrophy Is Common After the Nonsurgical Treatment of Acute Achilles Tendon Ruptures: A Randomized Clinical Trial Comparing Surgical and Nonsurgical Functional Treatments. Am J Sports Med 2017; 45:1395–1404.
10. Heikkinen J, Lantto I, Piilonen J, et al. Tendon Length, Calf Muscle Atrophy, and Strength Deficit After Acute Achilles Tendon Rupture. Journal Bone Joint Surg 2017; 99:1509–1515.
11. Eliasson P, Agergaard AS, Couppé C, et al. The Ruptured Achilles Tendon Elongates for 6 Months After Surgical Repair Regardless of Early or Late Weightbearing in Combination With Ankle Mobilization: A Randomized Clinical Trial. Am J Sports Med 2018; 46:2492–2502.
12. Brorsson A, Grävare Silbernagel K, Olsson N, Nilsson Helander K. Calf Muscle Performance Deficits Remain 7 Years After an Achilles Tendon Rupture. Am J Sports Med 2017; 46:470–477.
13. Porter M, Shadbolt B, Ye X, Stuart R. Ankle Lateral Ligament Augmentation Versus the Modified Broström-Gould Procedure: A 5-Year Randomized Controlled Trial. Am J Sports Med 2019; 99:1509–1515.
14. Telleria JJM, Ready LV, Bluman EM, Chiodo CP, Smith JT. Prevalence of Vitamin D Deficiency in Patients With Talar Osteochondral Lesions. Foot Ankle Int 2018; 39:471–478.
15. Fraissler L, Boelch SP, Schäfer T, et al. Vitamin D Deficiency in Patients With Idiopathic and Traumatic Osteochondritis Dissecans of the Talus. Foot Ankle Int 2019; 40:1309–1318.
16. Kim TY, Song SH, Baek JH, Hwang YG, Jeong BO. Analysis of the Changes in the Clinical Outcomes According to Time After Arthroscopic Microfracture of Osteochondral Lesions of the Talus. Foot Ankle Int 2018; 40:74–79.
17. Choi SW, Lee GW, Lee KB. Arthroscopic Microfracture for Osteochondral Lesions of the Talus: Functional Outcomes at a Mean of 6.7 Years in 165 Consecutive Ankles. Am J Sports Med 2019; 48:153–158.
18. Shimozono Y, Hurley ET, Yasui Y, Deyer TW, Kennedy JG. The Presence and Degree of Bone Marrow Edema Influence Midterm Clinical Outcomes After Microfracture for Osteochondral Lesions of the Talus. Am J Sports Med 2018; 46:2503–2508.
19. Shimozono Y, Hurley ET, Nguyen JT, Deyer TW, Kennedy JG. Allograft Compared with Autograft in Osteochondral Transplantation for the Treatment of Osteochondral Lesions of the Talus. J Bone Joint Surg 2018; 100:1838–1844.
20. Nguyen A, Ramasamy A, Walsh M, McMenemy L, Calder JDF. Autologous Osteochondral Transplantation for Large Osteochondral Lesions of the Talus Is a Viable Option in an Athletic Population. Am J Sports Med 2019; 47:3429–3435.
21. Park KH, Hwang Y, Han SH, et al. Primary Versus Secondary Osteochondral Autograft Transplantation for the Treatment of Large Osteochondral Lesions of the Talus. Am J Sports Med 2018; 46:1389–1396.
22. Van Bergen CJA, Baur OL, Murawski CD, et al. Diagnosis: History, Physical Examination, Imaging, and Arthroscopy: Proceedings of the International Consensus Meeting on Cartilage Repair of the Ankle. Foot Ankle Int 2018; 39:3S–8S.
23. Dombrowski ME, Yasui Y, Murawski CD, et al. Conservative Management and Biological Treatment Strategies: Proceedings of the International Consensus Meeting on Cartilage Repair of the Ankle. Foot Ankle Int 2018; 39:9S–15S.

24. Hannon CP, Bayer S, Murawski CD, et al. Debridement, Curettage, and Bone Marrow Stimulation: Proceedings of the International Consensus Meeting on Cartilage Repair of the Ankle. Foot Ankle Int 2018; 39:16S–22S.
25. Reilingh ML, Murawski CD, DiGiovanni CW, et al. Fixation Techniques: Proceedings of the International Consensus Meeting on Cartilage Repair of the Ankle. Foot Ankle Int 2018; 39:23S–27S.
26. Hurley ET, Murawski CD, Paul J, et al. Osteochondral Autograft: Proceedings of the International Consensus Meeting on Cartilage Repair of the Ankle. Foot Ankle Int 2018; 39:28S–34S.
27. Smyth NA, Murawski CD, Adams SB, et al. Osteochondral Allograft: Proceedings of the International Consensus Meeting on Cartilage Repair of the Ankle. Foot Ankle Int 2018; 39:35S–40S.
28. Rothrauff BB, Murawski CD, Angthong C, et al. Scaffold-Based Therapies: Proceedings of the International Consensus Meeting on Cartilage Repair of the Ankle. Foot Ankle Int 2018; 39:41S–47S.
29. Shimozono Y, Brown AJ, Batista JP, et al. Subchondral Pathology: Proceedings of the International Consensus Meeting on Cartilage Repair of the Ankle. Foot Ankle Int 2018; 39:48S–53S.
30. Mittwede PN, Murawski CD, Ackermann J, et al. Revision and Salvage Management: Proceedings of the International Consensus Meeting on Cartilage Repair of the Ankle. Foot Ankle Int 2018; 39:54S–60S.
31. D'Hooghe P, Murawski CD, Boakye LAT, et al. Rehabilitation and Return to Sports: Proceedings of the International Consensus Meeting on Cartilage Repair of the Ankle. Foot Ankle Int 2018; 39:61S–67S.
32. Van Dijk PAD, Murawski CD, Hunt KJ, et al. Post-treatment Follow-up, Imaging, and Outcome Scores: Proceedings of the International Consensus Meeting on Cartilage Repair of the Ankle. Foot Ankle Int 2018; 39:68S–73S.
33. Boesen AP, Hansen R, Boesen MI, Malliaras P, Langberg H. Effect of High-Volume Injection, Platelet-Rich Plasma, and Sham Treatment in Chronic Midportion Achilles Tendinopathy: A Randomized Double-Blinded Prospective Study. Am J Sports Med 2017; 45:2034–2043.
34. Peerbooms JC, Lodder P, den Oudsten BL, et al. Positive Effect of Platelet-Rich Plasma on Pain in Plantar Fasciitis: A Double-Blind Multicenter Randomized Controlled Trial. Am J Sports Med 2019; 7:3238–3246.
35. Karnovsky SC, DeSandis B, Haleem AM, et al. Comparison of Juvenile Allogenous Articular Cartilage and Bone Marrow Aspirate Concentrate Versus Microfracture With and Without Bone Marrow Aspirate Concentrate in Arthroscopic Treatment of Talar Osteochondral Lesions. Foot Ankle Int 2018; 39:393–405.
36. Daniels TR, Anderson J, Swords MP, et al. Recombinant Human Platelet–Derived Growth Factor BB in Combination With a Beta-Tricalcium Phosphate (rhPDGF-BB/β-TCP)-Collagen Matrix as an Alternative to Autograft. Foot Ankle Int 2019; 40:1068–1078.
37. Gutteck N, Zeh A, Wohlrab D, Delank KS. Comparative Results of Percutaneous Calcaneal Osteotomy in Correction of Hindfoot Deformities. Foot Ankle Int 2018; 40:276–281.
38. Veljkovic A, Symes M, Younger A, et al. Neurovascular and Clinical Outcomes of the Percutaneous Endoscopically Assisted Calcaneal Osteotomy (PECO) Technique to Correct Hindfoot Malalignment. Foot Ankle Int 2018; 40:178–184.
39. Lee M, Walsh J, Smith MM, et al. Hallux Valgus Correction Comparing Percutaneous Chevron/Akin (PECA) and Open Scarf/Akin Osteotomies. Foot Ankle Int 2017; 38:838–846.
40. Frigg A, Zaugg S, Maquieira G, Pellegrino A. Stiffness and Range of Motion After Minimally Invasive Chevron-Akin and Open Scarf-Akin Procedures. Foot Ankle Int 2019; 40:515–525.
41. Lai MC, Rikhraj IS, Woo YL, et al. Clinical and Radiological Outcomes Comparing Percutaneous Chevron-Akin Osteotomies vs Open Scarf-Akin Osteotomies for Hallux Valgus. Foot Ankle Int 2017; 39:311–317.
42. Holme TJ, Sivaloganathan SS, Patel B, Kunasingam K. Third-Generation Minimally Invasive Chevron Akin Osteotomy for Hallux Valgus. Foot Ankle Int 2019; 41:50–56.
43. Stevens R, Bursnall M, Chadwick C, et al. Comparison of Complication and Reoperation Rates for Minimally Invasive Versus Open Cheilectomy of the First Metatarsophalangeal Joint. Foot Ankle Int 2019; 41:31–36.
44. Teoh KH, Tan WT, Atiyah Z, et al. Clinical Outcomes Following Minimally Invasive Dorsal Cheilectomy for Hallux Rigidus. Foot Ankle Int 2018; 40:195–201.
45. Saini S, McDonald EL, Shakked R, et al. Prospective Evaluation of Utilization Patterns and Prescribing Guidelines of Opioid Consumption Following Orthopedic Foot and Ankle Surgery. Foot Ankle Int 2018; 39:1257–1265.
46. Gupta A, Kumar K, Roberts MM, et al. Pain Management After Outpatient Foot and Ankle Surgery. Foot Ankle Int 2017; 39:149–154.
47. Schipper ON, Hunt KJ, Anderson RB, et al. Ankle Block vs Single-Shot Popliteal Fossa Block as Primary Anesthesia for Forefoot Operative Procedures: Prospective, Randomized Comparison. Foot Ankle Int 2017; 38:1188–1191.

48. McDonald E, Winters B, Nicholson K, et al. Effect of Postoperative Ketorolac Administration on Bone Healing in Ankle Fracture Surgery. Foot Ankle Int 2018; 39:1135–1140.

49. Adams SB, Leimer EM, Setton LA, et al. Inflammatory Microenvironment Persists After Bone Healing in Intra-articular Ankle Fractures. Foot Ankle Int 2017; 38:479–484.

50. Adams SB, Reilly RM, Huebner JL, Kraus VB, Nettles DL. Time-Dependent Effects on Synovial Fluid Composition During the Acute Phase of Human Intra-articular Ankle Fracture. Foot Ankle Int 2017; 38:1055–1063.

51. French MH, McCauley JC, Pulido PA, Brage ME, Bugbee WD. Bipolar Fresh Osteochondral Allograft Transplantation of the Tibiotalar Joint. J Bone Joint Surg 2019; 101:821–825.

52. Hendy BA, McDonald EL, Nicholson K, et al. Improvement of Outcomes During the First Two Years Following Total Ankle Arthroplasty. J Bone Joint Surg 2018; 100:1473–1481.

53. Benich MR, Ledoux WR, Orendurff MS, et al. Comparison of Treatment Outcomes of Arthrodesis and Two Generations of Ankle Replacement Implants. J Bone Joint Surg 2017; 99:1792–1800.

54. Norvell DC, Ledoux WR, Shofer JB, et al. Effectiveness and Safety of Ankle Arthrodesis Versus Arthroplasty. J Bone Joint Surg 2019; 101:1485–1494.

55. Veljkovic AN, Daniels TR, Glazebrook MA, et al. Outcomes of Total Ankle Replacement, Arthroscopic Ankle Arthrodesis, and Open Ankle Arthrodesis for Isolated Non-Deformed End-Stage Ankle Arthritis. J Bone Joint Surg 2019; 101:1523–1529.

56. Brodsky JW, Kane JM, Taniguchi A, Coleman S, Daoud Y. Role of Total Ankle Arthroplasty in Stiff Ankles. Foot Ankle Int 2017; 38:1070–1077.

57. Borenstein TR, Anand K, Li Q, Charlton TP, Thordarson DB. A Review of Perioperative Complications of Outpatient Total Ankle Arthroplasty. Foot Ankle Int 2017; 39:143–148.

58. Mulligan RP, Parekh SG. Safety of Outpatient Total Ankle Arthroplasty vs Traditional Inpatient Admission or Overnight Observation. Foot Ankle Int 2017; 38: 825–831.

59. Daigre J, Berlet G, Van Dyke B, Peterson KS, Santrock R. Accuracy and Reproducibility Using Patient-Specific Instrumentation in Total Ankle Arthroplasty. Foot Ankle Int 2016; 38:412–418.

60. Lee GW, Lee KB. Outcomes of Total Ankle Arthroplasty in Ankles with >20° of Coronal Plane Deformity. J Bone Joint Surg 2019; 101:2203–2211.

61. Lee GW, Seon J, Kim NS, Lee KB. Comparison of Intermediate-Term Outcomes of Total Ankle Arthroplasty in Patients Younger and Older Than 55 Years. Foot Ankle Int 2019; 40:762–768.

62. Lee GW, Wang SH, Lee KB. Comparison of Intermediate to Long-Term Outcomes of Total Ankle Arthroplasty in Ankles with Preoperative Varus, Valgus, and Neutral Alignment. J Bone Joint Surg 2018; 100:835–842.

63. Kanzaki N, Chinzei N, Yamamoto T, et al. Clinical Outcomes of Total Ankle Arthroplasty With Total Talar Prosthesis. Foot Ankle Int 2019; 40:948–954.

64. Nunley JA, Adams SB, Easley ME, DeOrio JK. Prospective Randomized Trial Comparing Mobile-Bearing and Fixed-Bearing Total Ankle Replacement. Foot Ankle Int 2019; 40:1239–1248.

65. Lefrancois T, Younger A, Wing K, et al. A Prospective Study of Four Total Ankle Arthroplasty Implants by Non-Designer Investigators. J Bone Joint Surg 2017; 99:342–348.

66. Cody EA, Bejarano-Pineda L, Lachman JR, et al. Risk Factors for Failure of Total Ankle Arthroplasty with a Minimum Five Years of Follow-up. Foot Ankle Int 2018; 40:249–258.

67. Koivu H, Kohonen I, Mattila K, Loyttyniemi E, Tiusanen H. Long-term Results of Scandinavian Total Ankle Replacement. Foot Ankle Int 2017; 38:723–731.

68. Palanca A, Mann RA, Mann JA, Haskell A. Scandinavian Total Ankle Replacement: 15-Year Follow-up. Foot Ankle Int 2018; 39:135–142.

69. Loewy EM, Sanders TH, Walling AK. Intermediate-term Experience With the STAR Total Ankle in the United States. Foot Ankle Int 2018; 40:268–275.

70. Stewart MG, Green CL, Adams SB, et al. Midterm Results of the Salto Talaris Total Ankle Arthroplasty. Foot Ankle Int 2017; 38:1215–1221.

71. Usuelli FG, Maccario C, Granata F, et al. Clinical and Radiological Outcomes of Transfibular Total Ankle Arthroplasty. Foot Ankle Int 2018; 40:24–33.

72. Barg A, Bettin CC, Burstein AH, Saltzman CL, Gililland J. Early Clinical and Radiographic Outcomes of Trabecular Metal Total Ankle Replacement Using a Transfibular Approach. J Bone Joint Surg 2018; 100:505–515.

73. Dekker TJ, Walton D, Vinson EN, et al. Hindfoot Arthritis Progression and Arthrodesis Risk After Total Ankle Replacement. Foot Ankle Int 2017; 38:1183–1187.

74. Lazarides AL, Vovos TJ, Reddy GB, et al. Algorithm for Management of Periprosthetic Ankle Fractures. Foot Ankle Int 2019; 40:615–621.

75. Senneville E, Aiyer A, Smyth N. What Are the Important Risk Factors That Predispose a Patient to Infection After Total Ankle Arthroplasty (TAA)? Foot Ankle Int 2019; 40:2S–3S.

76. Uckay I, Hirose C, Assal M. Does Intra-articular Injection of the Ankle With Corticosteroids Increase the Risk of Subsequent Periprosthetic Joint Infection (PJI) Following Total Ankle Arthroplasty (TAA)? Foot Ankle Int 2019; 40:3S–4S.

77. Emara K, Hirose CB, Rogero R. What Preoperative Optimization Should Be Implemented to Reduce the Risk of Surgical Site Infection/Periprosthetic Joint Infection (SSI/PJI) in Patients Undergoing Total Ankle Arthroplasty (TAA)? Foot Ankle Int 2019; 40:6S–8S.

78. Sanchez M, Losada C. What Prophylactic Antibiotic (Type, Dose and Route of Administration) Should Be Administered Perioperatively for Patients Undergoing Total Ankle Arthroplasty (TAA)? Foot Ankle Int 2019; 40:8S–9S.

79. Winters B, Da Rin de Lorenzo F, O'Neil J. What Is the Optimal Management of Patients With Prior Septic Arthritis of the Ankle Who Are Undergoing Total Ankle Arthroplasty (TAA)? Foot Ankle Int 2019; 40:9S–10S.

80. Aynardi MC, Plöger MM, Walley KC, Arena CB. What Is the Definition of Acute and Chronic Periprosthetic Joint Infection (PJI) of Total Ankle Arthroplasty (TAA)? Foot Ankle Int 2019; 40:19S–21S.

81. Heidari N, Oh I, Malagelada F. What Is the Diagnostic "Algorithm" for Infected Total Ankle Arthroplasty (TAA)? Foot Ankle Int 2019; 40:21S–22S.

82. Uçkay I, Pedowitz D, Assal M, Stull JD. What Tests Are Useful to Investigate a Possible Infection of Total Ankle Arthroplasty (TAA)? What Are Their Thresholds? Foot Ankle Int 2019; 40:22S–23S.

83. Plöeger MM, Aiyer A. What Are the Indications for Aspiration of a Possibly Infected Total Ankle Arthroplasty (TAA)? Foot Ankle Int 2019; 40:24S–25S.

84. Embil JM, O'Neil JT. What Is the Optimal (Type, Dose and Route of Administration) Antibiotic Treatment for Patients With Infected Total Ankle Arthroplasty (TAA)? Foot Ankle Int 2019; 40:46S–47S.

85. Shakked R, Da Rin de Lorenzo F. What Determines the Type and Dose of Antibiotic That Is Needed to Be Added to the Cement Spacer in Patients With Infected Total Ankle Arthroplasty (TAA)? Foot Ankle Int 2019; 40:48S–52S.

86. McDonald E. What Are the Predictors of Treatment Failure in Patients Who Have Undergone Two-Stage Exchange for Infected Total Ankle Arthroplasty (TAA)? Foot Ankle Int 2019; 40:60S–61S.

87. Kaplan JRM, Slullitel G, Lopez V. Should Routine Methicillin-Resistant *Staphylococcus aureus (S. aureus)*, or MRSA, Screening Be in Place Prior to Total Ankle Arthroplasty (TAA)? Foot Ankle Int 2019; 40:4S–6S.

88. Richter J. Should Antibiotic-Impregnated Cement Be Used During Primary Total Ankle Arthroplasty (TAA)? Foot Ankle Int 2019; 40:12S.

89. Slullitel G, Tanaka Y, Rogero R, et al. What Are the Benefits and Risks Associated With the Use of Vancomycin Powder in the Wound During Total Ankle Arthroplasty (TAA) or Other Foot and Ankle Procedures? Foot Ankle Int 2019; 40:12S–14S.

90. Englund K, Heidari N. Is There a Role for the Use of Dilute Povidone-Iodine (Betadine) Irrigation or Other Antiseptic Irrigation Solutions During Total Ankle Arthroplasty (TAA) or Other Foot and Ankle Procedures? Foot Ankle Int 2019; 40:14S–15S.

91. Senneville E, Lopez V, Slullitel G. What Metrics Can Be Used to Determine the Optimal Timing of Reimplantation in Patients Who Have Undergone Resection Arthroplasty as Part of a Two-Stage Exchange for Infected Total Ankle Arthroplasty (TAA)? Foot Ankle Int 2019; 40:58S–60S.

92. Plöger MM, Murawski CD. How Should Postoperative Cellulitis Be Treated in Patients With Total Ankle Arthroplasty (TAA) in Place? Foot Ankle Int 2019; 40:61S–62S.

93. Shakked R, McDonald E, Sutton R, et al. Influence of Depressive Symptoms on Hallux Valgus Surgical Outcomes. Foot Ankle Int 2018; 39:795–800.

94. Conti M, Willett J, Garfinkel J, et al. Effect of the Modified Lapidus Procedure on Pronation of the First Ray in Hallux Valgus. Foot and Ankle International 2020; 41:125–132.

95. McDonald E, Shakked R, Daniel J, et al. Driving After Hallux Valgus Surgery. Foot Ankle Int 2017; 38:982–986.

96. Sidon E, Rogero R, Bell T, et al. Long-term Follow-up of Cheilectomy for Treatment of Hallux Rigidus. Foot Ankle Int 2019; 40:1114–1121.

97. Baumhauer JF, Singh D, Glazebrook M, et al. Correlation of Hallux Rigidus Grade With Motion, VAS Pain, Intraoperative Cartilage Loss, and Treatment Success for First MTP Joint Arthrodesis and Synthetic Cartilage Implant. Foot Ankle Int 2017; 38:1175–1182.

98. Goldberg A, Singh D, Glazebrook M, et al. Association Between Patient Factors and Outcome of Synthetic Cartilage Implant Hemiarthroplasty vs First Metatarsophalangeal Joint Arthrodesis in Advanced Hallux Rigidus. Foot Ankle Int 2017; 38:1199–1206.

99. Daniels TR, Younger ASE, Penner MJ, et al. Midterm Outcomes of Polyvinyl Alcohol Hydrogel Hemiarthroplasty of the First Metatarsophalangeal Joint in Advanced Hallux Rigidus. Foot Ankle Int 2016; 38:243–247.

100. Glazebrook M, Blundell CM, O'Dowd D, et al. Midterm Outcomes of a Synthetic Cartilage Implant for the First Metatarsophalangeal Joint in Advanced Hallux Rigidus. Foot Ankle Int 2018; 40:374–383.

101. Vulcano E, Chang AL, Solomon D, Myerson M. Long-Term Follow-up of Capsular Interposition Arthroplasty for Hallux Rigidus. Foot Ankle Int 2017; 39:1–5.

102. Aynardi MC, Atwater L, Dein EJ, et al. Outcomes After Interpositional Arthroplasty of the First Metatarsophalangeal Joint. Foot Ankle Int 2017; 38:514–518.

103. Da Cunha RJ, MacMahon A, Jones MT, et al. Return to Sports and Physical Activities After First Metatarsophalangeal Joint Arthrodesis in Young Patient. Foot Ankle Int 2019; 40:745–752.

104. Flint WW, Macias DM, Jastifer JR, et al. Plantar Plate Repair for Lesser Metatarsophalangeal Joint Instability. Foot Ankle Int 2016; 38:234–242.

105. Boszczyk A, Kwapisz S, Krümmel M, Grass R, Rammelt S. Correlation of Incisura Anatomy With Syndesmotic Malreduction. Foot Ankle Int 2017; 39:369–375.

106. Andersen MR, Frihagen F, Hellund JC, Madsen JE, Figved W. Randomized Trial Comparing Suture Button with Single Syndesmotic Screw for Syndesmosis Injury. J Bone Joint Surg 2018; 100:2–12.

107. Grassi A, Samuelsson K, D'Hooghe P, et al. Dynamic Stabilization of Syndesmosis Injuries Reduces Complications and Reoperations as Compared With Screw Fixation: A Meta-analysis of Randomized Controlled Trials. Am J Sports Med 2019; 48:1000–1013.

108. Woo SH, Bae SY, Chung HJ. Short-Term Results of a Ruptured Deltoid Ligament Repair During an Acute Ankle Fracture Fixation. Foot Ankle Int 2017; 39:35–45.

109. Bohl DD, Idarraga AJ, Holmes GB, et al. Validated Risk-Stratification System for Prediction of Early Adverse Events Following Open Reduction and Internal Fixation of Closed Ankle Fractures. J Bone Joint Surg 2019; 101:1768–1774.

110. Mora AD, Kao M, Alfred T, et al. Return to Sports and Physical Activities After Open Reduction and Internal Fixation of Lisfranc Injuries in Recreational Athletes. Foot Ankle Int 2018; 39:801–807.

111. Cochran G, Renninger C, Tompane T, Bellamy J, Kuhn K. Primary Arthrodesis versus Open Reduction and Internal Fixation for Low-Energy Lisfranc Injuries in a Young Athletic Population. Foot Ankle Int 2017; 38:957–963.

112. Hawkinson MP, Tennent DJ, Belisle J, Osborn P. Outcomes of Lisfranc Injuries in an Active Duty Military Population. Foot Ankle Int 2017; 38:1115–1119.

113. Buda M, Kink S, Stavenuiter R, et al. Reoperation Rate Differences Between Open Reduction Internal Fixation and Primary Arthrodesis of Lisfranc Injuries. Foot Ankle Int 2018; 39:1089–1096.

114. El-Mowafi H, Abulsaad M, Kandil Y, El-Hawary A, Ali S. Hybrid Fixation for Ankle Fusion in Diabetic Charcot Arthropathy. Foot Ankle Int 2017; 39:93–98.

115. Ebaugh MP, Umbel B, Goss D, Taylor BC. Outcomes of Primary Tibiotalocalcaneal Nailing for Complicated Diabetic Ankle Fractures. Foot Ankle Int 2019; 40:1382–1387.

116. Lovy AJ, Dowdell J, Keswani A, et al. Nonoperative Versus Operative Treatment of Displaced Ankle Fractures in Diabetics. Foot Ankle Int 2017; 38:255–260.

117. McCormack RG, Leith JM. Ankle fractures in diabetics. Complications of surgical management. J Bone Joint Surg Br 1998; 80:689–692.

118. Ford SE, Cohen BE, Davis WH, Jones CP. Clinical Outcomes and Complications of Midfoot Charcot Reconstruction With Intramedullary Beaming. Foot Ankle Int 2018; 40:18–23.

119. Pinzur MS, Schiff AP. Deformity and Clinical Outcomes Following Operative Correction of Charcot Foot: A New Classification With Implications for Treatment. Foot Ankle Int 2017; 39:265–270.

120. Daniels TR, Halai M, Matz J. What's New in Foot and Ankle Surgery. J Bone Joint Surg 2019; 101:859–867.

Chapter 13

What is new in orthopaedic oncology?

Joseph Ippolito, Valdis Lelkes, Francis Patterson

SARCOMA

Bone sarcoma

Osteosarcoma

Osteogenic sarcoma is the most common primary bone cancer in adults and in children, occurring most frequently during the second decade of life, with a second peak during the seventh and eighth decades. Since the advent of systemic chemotherapy in the 1960s, treatment of osteosarcoma continues to evolve. Complete en bloc resection of the tumour for local control of osteosarcoma is considered the standard of care, though there has been little agreement on how wide the margin of resection should be. Recent works suggest negative margins of <2 millimeters (mm) and <90% necrosis response to chemotherapy were the strongest predictors of local recurrence (LR) following osteosarcoma resection. These findings may highlight the utility of advanced functional imaging such as positron emission tomography/computed tomography (PET-CT) to evaluate chemotherapy response prior to surgical planning [1].

In patients with juxta-articular osteosarcoma at the knee, joint preserving allograft reconstruction following microwave ablation was associated with higher rates of knee function and lower rates of degenerative changes than with cryoablation, which was associated with a 100% of osteonecrosis. No difference in functional outcomes or complications was seen between patients without and with partial epiphyseal involvement, though nearly a third of patients had a residual limb length discrepancy of 1–3.5 cm [2].

Both local recurrence and metastasis of osteosarcoma influence overall survival. In prediction of metastasis, increasing evidence indicates that both tumour-associated elements as well as host-associated elements play important roles in the systemic cancer

Joseph Ippolito MD, Rutgers New Jersey Medical School, Orange Ave, Newark, US
Email: josephippolitoMD@gmail.com

Valdis Lelkes MD, Hackensack University Medical Center, Prospect Avenue, Hackensack, New Jersey, US
Email: valdislelkes@gmail.com

Francis Patterson MD, Hackensack University Medical Center, Prospect Avenue, Hackensack, New Jersey, US
Email: francis.patterson@hackensackmeridian.org

response. Circulating monocytes, derived from bone marrow, give rise to tissue-resident and inflammatory macrophages throughout the body, working to modulate the tumour micro-environment and promote tumour invasion and metastasis. Increasing neutrophils and/or decreasing counts of lymphocytes may suppress lymphocyte-activation, which may be detrimental to prognosis and survival. Higher tumour grade, circulating monocyte ratio > 1 and neutrophil to lymphocyte ratio > 1 has been found to be the most predictive of osteosarcoma metastasis [3].

Chrondrosarcoma

Chondrosarcomas are the third most common primary bone tumours and encompass a heterogeneous collective of neoplasms that produce cartilage matrix. Historically, challenges have persisted regarding classification of benign versus malignant cartilaginous lesions. Consequently, surgical decision-making can vary considerably dependent on pathologic diagnosis. In a retrospective review of patients with confirmed pelvic enchondroma or atypical cartilaginous lesions (ACT), endosteal scalloping, presence of calcifications, advanced age, and larger tumour size were shown to favour a diagnosis of ACT over enchondroma [4]. In a review of 89 patients with ACT or enchondroma of the long bones, no difference in local recurrence or overall survival was detected between curettage or wide resection, and authors concluded that curettage as index treatment yields sufficient local disease control and superior functional outcome [5]. In a large retrospective series, patients with conventional central chondrosarcoma of the pelvis were found to have a stepwise increase in risk of disease related death by increasing tumour grade (Grade 1: 3%; Grade 2: 33%, Grade 3: 54%) [6]. Although wide margins were more commonly obtained in hindquarter amputations compared with limb salvage procedures, this did not significantly influence outcomes. Authors urged consideration of obtainment of wide margins even in low grade chondrosarcoma, due to the frequency at which local recurrence of initially low-grade chondrosarcoma presented as intermediate or high grade [6].

Mesenchymal chondrosarcomas are historically associated with worse outcomes than classical chondrosarcoma variants. A recent study utilising the Surveillance, Epidemiology, and End Results (SEER) registry found appendicular and cranial tumours to be more strongly associated with long-term survival after treatment, with overall survival of 51% for the entire series. No difference was found in survival between skeletal and non-skeletal origin, though increase in tumour size, metastasis on presentation, and advanced age in presentation were associated with increased risk of death [7]. This study was limited by the lack of robust data regarding chemotherapy treatment, which may improve recurrence and survival rates in this sub-type.

Ewing's sarcoma

Ewing's sarcoma family of tumours (ESFT) is a family of small round cell sarcomas which occur most commonly in the first 2 decades of life and most frequently osseous in origin. Systemic chemotherapy combined with surgery and/or radiotherapy is typically performed for initial disease control. In a systemic review of children and adolescents with relapsed Ewing's sarcoma, treatment with high dose chemotherapy and autologous hematopoietic cell transplantation (as rescue for myelosuppression) found to confer greater survival advantage compared with conventional chemotherapy [8]. Following neo-adjuvant chemotherapy, post-treatment Magnetic resonance imaging (MRI) with use of non-enhanced T1 sequence may provide a more accurate assessment of tumour limits for planning surgical resection, as demonstrated in recent review of 20 patients comparing both pre- and post-treatment MRI [9]. Following neo-adjuvant chemotherapy and surgical treatment, decision-making for administration of adjuvant radiotherapy is multifactorial. Albergo and colleagues found that post-surgical radiotherapy in patients with intra-lesional or marginal resections decreased local recurrence, but did not influence LR or overall survival after wide resection, regardless of necrosis response to chemotherapy [10].

Soft-tissue sarcoma

Systemic therapy for soft-tissue sarcoma

The pursuit of more effective drug therapy for soft-tissue sarcomas continues. The Sarcoma Alliance through Research and Collaboration (SARC) group completed phase II study of Dasatinib in patients with alveolar soft part sarcoma, chondrosarcoma, chordoma, epithelioid sarcoma, and solitary fibrous tumour. In 109 patients treated with Dasatinib, there was failure of growth suppression in >50% of the patients for at least 6 months [11]. Prior studies have challenged whether synovial sarcoma patients benefit from chemotherapy. In a joint analysis of two prospective trials for children and adolescents with localised, small synovial sarcoma tumours which underwent complete resection, there was 90% event free survival at 3 years and overall survival of 100%. Authors concluded that paediatric patients with adequately excised ≤5 cm synovial sarcoma can avoid the use of adjuvant and neo-adjuvant radiation and chemotherapy without endangering their outcomes [12] Similarly, a review of 191 patients with synovial sarcoma found adjuvant chemotherapy to have no effect on disease-specific survival, local recurrence-free survivals, or metastasis-free survival. They identified grade 3 tumours ≥5 cm were associated with worse survival [13].

Considerable variability in use of chemotherapy and radiotherapy exists in treatment of soft-tissue sarcomas, with a multi-centre review of 3,752 patients finding use of radiation therapy among centres ranging from 48 to 82% and chemotherapy usage from 2 to 52%. Authors found radiation therapy decreased local recurrence, with greatest benefit in myxoid liposarcoma, vascular sarcoma, and myxofibrosarcoma. Chemotherapy provided a trend towards modest increase in overall survival that did not reach significance [14]. Similarly, in a meta-analysis of studies treating adult patients with resectable soft-tissue sarcoma, review of 10 studies with 3,157 patients found chemotherapy (neo-adjuvant or adjuvant) provided no benefit over surgical resection with or without radiation therapy in all-comers, or site-specific sub-groups [15].

Surgical treatment

Goals of limb sparing surgery include wide resection of all tumour tissue while preserving critical neurovascular structures, and many surgeons have chosen to include the biopsy tract during resection. A review of 180 biopsy tracts found increased risk of biopsy tract contamination in open versus needle biopsies, and in soft-tissue sarcoma versus bone sarcoma biopsies. Biopsy tract contamination appeared to correlate with an overall decreased local recurrence-free survival [16]. Wide resections often remove a large amount of tissue or skin, requiring soft-tissue coverage to achieve limb salvage, which can vary in size and invasiveness from skin graft all the way to free flap coverage. Similarly, an evaluation of patients treated with either local flap, free flap, or skin graft soft-tissue coverage following lower extremity soft-tissue sarcoma resection found no difference in wound complications or healing between coverage options, despite an overall 53% rate of wound healing problems and mean time to healing of 13 weeks [17]. There was no difference with regard to local recurrence of sarcoma or metastatic disease based off of the reconstructive technique [18].

Wide resection for curative treatment in non-metastatic soft-tissue sarcoma is widely accepted, but management of metastatic disease is not as well delineated. A review of 102 patients found metastatectomy of soft-tissue sarcoma to increase overall survival in eligible patients [19]. Successful surgical treatment of soft-tissue sarcoma is a complex undertaking requiring special skill and understanding of the disease process which may be better provided by high volume treatment centres. After controlling for patient, tumour, and treatment characteristics, a recent analysis of over 25,000 patients treated for soft-tissue sarcoma of the extremities found patients treated at higher volume centres to have overall lower risk of mortality and positive margins. Additionally, patients treated with radiation had higher likelihood of receiving it pre-operatively at higher volume centres [20].

Diagnostics

When evaluating patients for disease recurrence, advanced imaging is a cornerstone for sarcoma surveillance. New hybrid imaging modalities such as 18-F-FDG PET/MRI may help with diagnosis of recurrent soft-tissue sarcomas. This modality increased accuracy in diagnosis of recurrence versus MRI alone (96% vs. 81%) in a study of 41 patients [21]. Understanding which soft-tissue sarcomas are at risk of lymph node metastases can help to identify patients at risk of worse outcomes. In a new SEER database analysis of histologic sub-types of 15,525 patients with soft-tissue sarcomas, 5.5% of patients had nodal involvement. Most common sub-types to have nodal involvement were clear cell sarcoma, epithelioid sarcoma, rhabdomyosarcoma, and myxoid/round cell liposarcoma. Interestingly there was no increase in nodal involvement in patients with synovial sarcoma. Furthermore, lymph node metastases were associated with worse overall survival and patients that underwent lymphadenectomy in addition to limb salvage had better 5-year survival [22].

Oncologic outcomes

Interest has been generated in reviewing specific sub-groups of patients with soft-tissue sarcoma and identifying factors unique to these sub-groups related to their outcomes. Unplanned non-oncologic resection of a sarcoma is a complex problem that many orthopaedic oncologists will treat. In a retrospective comparison of patients treated with planned versus unplanned primary oncologic resection of the American Joint Committee on Cancer (AJCC) stage III extremity soft-tissue sarcomas, 19% of patients were found to have unplanned excision, with 83% of these patients having residual tumour upon resection of the previous tumour bed. There were no significant differences in local recurrence, metastasis-free survival, overall survival, or functional outcomes, though patients undergoing re-resection more frequently required wound coverage from plastic surgeons and had higher rates of amputation [23].

There exists discrepancy in the treatment of elderly compared with younger adult patients with soft-tissue sarcoma, with a recent study finding elderly patients less likely to undergo surgery, receive pre-operative radiation treatment, or receive adjuvant or neo-adjuvant chemotherapy. Elderly patients who did have surgery were less likely to have an R0 resection and had higher mortality rates after surgery compared to younger adults. Despite this, surgical treatment increased overall survival in the elderly population [24].

Patients with distal extremity soft-tissue sarcoma (DESTS) have involvement of the hand, fingers, foot, and toes. A recent review of the European sarcoma database found DESTS patients more likely to be younger, female, and have smaller tumours. Also, DESTS tumours were more likely to be grade 2 versus grades 1 or 3 at other sites, less likely to receive radiation, and more likely to receive chemotherapy as adjuvant, rather than neo-adjuvant, treatment. There were no statistical differences in recurrence, metastasis, or overall survival among patients with DESTS or with sarcoma at other locations [25].

There are concerns that patients with obesity who have a soft-tissue sarcoma may present with a larger tumour because the patient's body habits may mask the tumour. In a review of 85 patients with soft-tissue sarcoma, patients with BMI > 30 had 50% greater median tumour diameter on presentation, though no differences were demonstrated in local recurrence, metastasis, or overall survival. However, obese patients were more likely to have post-operative complications and more frequently required complex wound closures [26].

Follow-up and surveillance

Pre- and peri-operative nutritional status of patients with bone and soft-tissue tumours plays an important role in the recovery period following removal of disease and reconstructive efforts. Following surgical treatment for limb sarcomas, malnutrition as measured by hypoalbuminaemia may increase risk of post-operative complications [27]. Following treatment of sarcoma, patients had comparable rates of pain, sleep disturbance, anxiety, fatigue and lower rates of depression compared with the general US population, despite expected lower scores in physical function, as shown by a recent study utilising self-reported outcome scores [28]. Following tumour resection, some disparity exists among institutions with regard to frequency and intensity of surveillance imaging. Recent evidence from a randomised clinical trial of patients with limb sarcoma suggests that less intensive surveillance with chest X-ray (vs. CT) and follow-up intervals of 6 months (vs. 3 months) resulted in comparable rates of overall survival and detection of recurrence or metastasis [29].

BENIGN BONE TUMOURS

Chondroblastoma

Chondroblastoma is an uncommon, benign, locally aggressive tumour that occurs in the apophyses or epiphyses of long bones in young patients. Aggressive curettage is typically pursued for local control of disease, but may result in damage to the growth plate and articular cartilage over time. A series of 53 patients had 90% joint survival at 5 years, a 38% rate of arthritis development at a mean of 58 months, and a significantly increased risk of arthritis and requirement for arthroplasty in patients with disease at the proximal femur. Authors stated that degenerative changes at the joint may be higher than initially anticipated, and counsell patients on these risks at the proximal femur, including offering hip arthroplasty as an index treatment procedure [30].

Giant cell tumour

Representing 5% of all primary neoplasias of bone, giant cell tumour (GCT) of bone is a locally aggressive primary neoplasm which most commonly occurs in ages 20–45 years and at the knee. Deciding between curettage or resection of GCT includes consideration of tumour size, articular surface involvement, grade, and presentation with pathologic fracture which can increase difficulty of curettage. In surgical treatment at the knee, the use of structural sub-chondral allograft in addition to cement resulted in lower rates of peri-articular fracture and joint degeneration [31]. At the distal radius, treatment of GCT is associated with difficulty in local control due to its anatomic location. Extended intra-lesional curettage was found to be associated with higher functional outcomes although also higher rates of local recurrence compared with resection arthrodesis at the distal radius [32]. Despite recurrence rates, repeat curettage and joint preservation was feasible in most cases. These authors urged reservation of resection for Campanacci grade 3 tumours and recurrences.

While treatment of GCT with denosumab has become recently popularised, its use prior to curettage may increase risk for local recurrence [33]. Authors suggested the rim of new bone formed in denosumab treatment may contain tumour cells which may reactivate upon conclusion of systemic therapy. Although cryoablation remains an effective intra-operative adjuvant for tumour control, the use of liquid nitrogen poses potential risk of damage to adjacent tissues and peri-operative complications. A recent animal model evaluating the use of a nitrogen ethanol composite with less extreme freezing was found to have rates of ex vivo and in vivo tumour cryoablation comparable to liquid nitrogen, while theoretically mitigating some disadvantages of conventional cryotherapy [34].

Desmoid tumours

Management of desmoid tumours, a type of benign yet locally aggressive neoplasm, has included surgical treatment ranging from wide resection to excision, as well as medical management and radiation treatment. A meta-analysis reviewed outcomes in 16 studies encompassing 1,295 patients. Local recurrence rates were doubled in patients with residual positive margins following resection. Post-operative radiation decreased recurrence risk in these patients but did not impact outcomes in those with negative margins [35]. Over the last 2 decades changes in the approach to treating desmoid tumours have begun to include non-operative management as a mainstay in treatment. A series of 1,141 patients with extra-abdominal desmoid tumour found overall disease progression of 9% in patients treated non-operatively [36]. The percentage of patients treated non-surgically from 2009 to 2013 increased 12% compared to between years 1993 and 1998. Authors conclude that surveillance is a safe initial treatment option.

Chordoma

Following surgical resection of sacrococcygeal chordoma, the addition of radiotherapy to improve local control has been described. A series of 193 patients showed no improved recurrence, metastasis, or overall survival benefit in patients who received radiotherapy post-operatively, though higher rates of wound complication and sacral stress fractures were reported [37].

METASTATIC DISEASE

A focus of treating patients with osseous metastatic disease is centred around providing osseous stability and maintaining function. Understanding patient prognosis, risks of complications, and available interventions can aid the orthopaedic oncologist in providing the most appropriate care and provide the best functional results. A new prognostic model was developed using a patient's clinical profile, Karnofsky performance score, and presence of visceral, or brain metastases, which stratifies predicted patient survival [38] (**Figure 13.1**). Renal cell carcinoma long bone metastases can be treated with cryoablation for effective local oncologic control. In a review of 40 patients with metastatic appendicular renal cell carcinoma, treatment with cryoablation as associated with 82% local tumour control. Cryoablation can be a useful and effective alternative to metastatectomy [39].

Fixation of impending pathologic fractures can prevent the morbidity of a complete fracture. In a retrospective review from the US Veterans Administration database, 362 patients undergoing prophylactic fixation for an impending pathologic femur fracture had lower risk of death than 588 patients undergoing fixation for pathologic fracture. Authors report more study is needed to identify other associations that may lead to this improved survival [40]. In treatment of metastatic disease at the acetabular region, utilisation of acetabular cages with cemented dual mobility cups was associated with improvement in pain and function, comparing pre- and post-operative functional walking independence [41] (**Figure 13.2**).

RECONSTRUCTION

Computer-assisted surgery (navigation)

With advances in pre-operative and intra-operative imaging modalities, the incorporation of computer-assisted navigation has become increasingly popular, with an emphasis on pelvic tumour resection and acetabular reconstruction or preservation (**Figure 13.3**) [42]. Navigation-

1. Clinical profile	Favourable				Moderate				Unfavourable			
2. Karnofsky	80–100		≤70		80–100		≤70		80–100		≤70	
3. Visceral/ brain metastases	No	Yes	No	Yes	No	Yes	No	Yes	No	Yes	No	Yes
Survival (95% CI; months)	27 – 34	12 – 23	10 – 16	6 – 9	9 – 14	5 – 14	4 – 6	2 – 4	3 – 8	4 – 5	2 – 3	2 – 3
Category	A	A	A	B	B	B	C	C	C	C	D	D

Figure 13.1 Tabular data for stratification of patients with long-bone metastatic disease. With permission from Willeumier JJ, van der Linden YM, van der Wal CWPG, et al. An easy-to-use prognostic model for survival estimation for patients with symptomatic long bone metastases. J Bone Joint Surg Am 2018; 100:196–204.

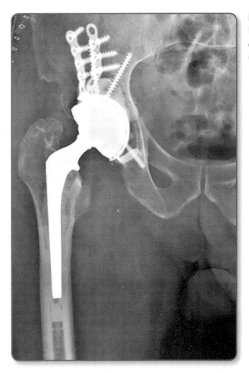

Figure 13.2 Post-operative X-ray. Modular dual mobility liner (Stryker) cemented into restoration GAP II acetabular cage (Stryker). With permission from Plummer D, et al. (2019).

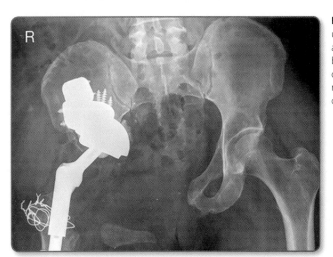

Figure 13.3 Reconstruction with use of a highly porous tantalum acetabular component, numerous buttresses, and off-label use of a dual-mobility construct following resection of a large periacetabular chondrosarcoma in a 61-year-old.

guided resection of sarcoma or chordoma of the pelvis and sacrum was recently associated with a 100% rate of negative bony margins and low navigation-related complication rate [43]. In a historically controlled study, higher rates of adequate bony margins were obtained using navigation (81% vs. 50%) [44]. In both studies, navigation does not appear to have a defined advantage in obtaining soft-tissue margins [43,44]. In addition to lower rates of local recurrence, use of navigation was found to have lower blood loss and shorter operating time [45].

In cases of locally aggressive tumour at metaphyseal or epiphyseal appendicular locations where the articular surface can be preserved, early results suggest use of navigation may improve rates of obtainment of negative margins, though no benefit was demonstrated in function or local recurrence rate after treatment [46].

Patient-specific cutting guides

Utilising CT and MRI, performance of wide resection of bone tumours with custom cutting guides was associated with 100% rate of negative margins and a maximum of 3-mm cutting error, and all cuts were performed without requirement of intra-operative fluoroscopy [47]. Authors reported these guides may be particularly beneficial prior to utilisation of three-dimensional (3D) printed custom implants to ensure ideal fit (**Figure 13.4**). In a comparison of computer-assisted surgery (CAS), patient-specific instrumentation (PSI), and freehand technique in pelvic resection, both CAS and PSI were found to increase accuracy of resection [48]. However, authors found that PSI yielded the best surgical accuracy while being the fastest method of resection.

Endoprosthetic reconstruction

Following peri-acetabular malignant tumour resection, the incorporation of porous tantalum components (cups, augments, and buttresses) recently popularised in revision

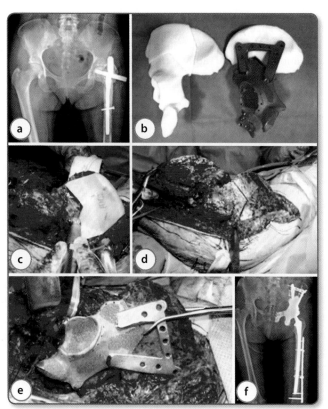

Figures 13.4 Bone tumour resection guide using three-dimensional printing for limb salvage surgery (a to d). With permission from Park JW, et al. (2018).

total joint arthroplasty has been associated with promising short-term outcomes, including return to ambulation in all living patients at latest follow-up [49]. The use of a stemmed acetabular pedestal cup or 'ice-cream cone' prosthesis, which relies upon residual ilium bone stock, was associated with a mean 71% MSTS score and 6% rate of aseptic loosening [50]. Due to residual bone and soft-tissue defects, these methods of reconstruction have been associated with high rates of dislocation, frequently addressed with the use of constrained liners [49,50]. Following resection of tumour at the distal femur or proximal tibia, long-term outcomes with endoprosthetic reconstruction at the knee included 79.3% implant survival at 10 years and 90% limb salvage at latest follow-up [51]. Hydroxyapatite coating of stems was found to diminish risk for aseptic loosening and requirement for revision. Following tumour resection at the proximal humerus, reverse shoulder endoprostheses have demonstrated excellent medium-term survivorship and pain relief, with mean abduction and forward flexion of 62° and 71° degrees, respectively [52]. Following peri-acetabular resection, the spectrum of local micro-organisms may be affected by the proximity of the abdominal cavity and peri-anal region. Patients with deep infection of endoprosthetic reconstruction at the pelvis may be at increased risk for gram-negative and polymicrobial colonisation suggesting consideration of specific pre- and peri-operative infection prevention measures in this patient population (**Figure 13.5**) [53].

Allograft and autograft reconstruction

Following tumour resection at the proximal tibia, recent evidence suggests comparable 5- and 10-year survival between endoprosthetic (5-year: 88%, 10-year: 56%) and massive osteoarticular allograft (5-year: 73%, 10-year: 68%) reconstruction. Authors highlighted that reconstructive decisions are multi-factorial, urging consideration of retaining bone stock and extensor mechanism function with allograft in young patients, immediate restoration of weight-bearing in older patients, and chemo- and radiotherapy requirement in both

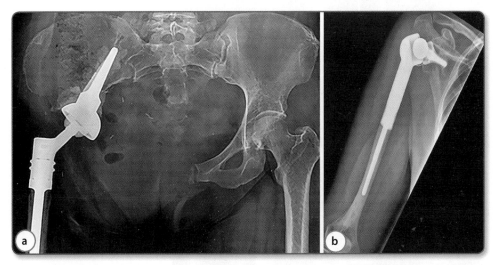

Figures 13.5 Advances in implant design have supported restoration of function following large tumor resections at the axial and appendicular skeleton, shown by (a) Stemmed pedestal cup reconstruction after periacetabular and ischial resection. (b) Segmental reverse total shoulder arthroplasty after proximal humerus resection.

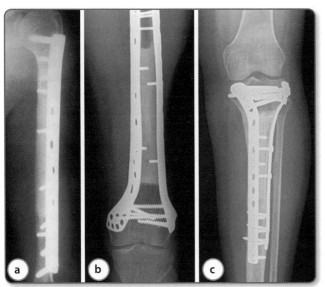

Figure 13.6 Intercalary allograft augmented with IM cement (a to c). With permission from Gupta S, et al. (2017).

patient groups [54]. Following massive allograft at the knee, 10-year graft retention was 60%, with higher complication rates following reconstruction at the proximal tibia than the distal femur. Most commonly, allograft failure at the proximal tibia was due to infection and due to fracture at the distal femur [55]. Following resection of diaphyseal tumour, augmentation with intra-medullary cement prior to plate fixation may decrease complications of non-union and fracture previously seen with intercalary allograft reconstruction (**Figure 13.6**) [56].

FUNCTIONAL OUTCOMES

Patient functional outcomes are an important measure following treatment for sarcoma. Authors have continued to evaluate the use of surgeon-reported outcome scores such as the Musculoskeletal Tumour Society (MSTS) score and Toronto Extremity Salvage Score (TESS) as self-reported outcomes scores such as the Patient Reported Outcomes Measurement Information System (PROMIS). A recent series of 150 patients undergoing longitudinal evaluation of MSTS and TESS scores highlights the potential value of obtaining these scores in more than one point in time. Authors found MSTS and TESS significantly improved post-operatively and identified 24 months as a cut-off value for when scores become stable. Both scores were related to patient age, with patients older than 47 years generally having poorer functional outcome [57].

CONCLUSION

Recent collaborative works have contributed to numerous advances in the field of musculoskeletal oncology, including use of diagnostic imaging, surgical treatment planning, and implementation of computer assisted navigation and patient specific instrumentation. New evidence suggests there may be considerable benefit in utilisation of advanced functional imaging such as PET-CT to evaluate chemotherapy response prior to surgical planning in osteosarcoma treatment. In a review of patients treated with curettage of atypical cartilaginous lesions or enchondroma of the long bones, curettage as index treatment was shown to yield sufficient local disease control and superior functional outcome. In patients with metastatic soft tissue sarcoma, metastatectomy may increase overall survival in eligible patients. In a comparison of computer assisted surgery and patient specific instrumentation in pelvic tumor resection, patient specific instrumentation yielded the best surgical accuracy while leading to the fasted method of reconstruction. Following tumor resection, authors have long used MSTS and TESS scores to evaluate patient functional outcomes. A recent study suggests the value of completion of these outcome scores at multiple timepoints, with 24 months identified as a cutoff timepoint for when scores become stable.

REFERENCES

1.   Byun BH, Kong CB, Lim I, et al. Combination of 18F-FDG PET/CT and diffusion-weighted MR imaging as a predictor of histologic response to neoadjuvant chemotherapy: preliminary results in osteosarcoma. J Nucl Med 2013; 54:1053–1059.
2.   Li J, Wang Z, Ji C, et al. What are the Oncologic and Functional Outcomes After Joint Salvage Resections for Juxtaarticular Osteosarcoma About the Knee? Clin Orthop Relat Res 2017; 475:2095–2104.
3.   Wang S, Zheng S, Hu K, et al. A predictive model to estimate the pretest probability of metastasis in patients with osteosarcoma. Medicine (Baltimore). 2017; 96:e5909.
4.   Alfaro PA, Ciani G, Herrera CA, et al. Differential diagnosis and treatment of enchondromas and atypical cartilaginous tumours of the pelvis: analysis of 21 patients. Eur J Orthop Surg Traumatol 2020; 30:25–30.
5.   Errani C, Tsukamoto S, Ciani G, et al. Risk factors for local recurrence from atypical cartilaginous tumour and enchondroma of the long bones. Eur J Orthop Surg Traumatol 2017; 27:805–811.
6.   Bus MPA, Campanacci DA, Albergo JI, et al. Conventional Primary Central Chondrosarcoma of the Pelvis: Prognostic Factors and Outcome of Surgical Treatment in 162 Patients. J Bone Joint Surg Am 2018; 100:316–325.
7.   Schneiderman BA, Kliethermes SA, Nystrom LM. Survival in Mesenchymal Chondrosarcoma Varies Based on Age and Tumor Location: A Survival Analysis of the SEER Database. Clin Orthop Relat Res 2017; 475:799–805.
8.   Tenneti P, Zahid U, Iftikhar A, et al. Role of High-Dose Chemotherapy and Autologous Hematopoietic Cell Transplantation for Children and Young Adults with Relapsed Ewing's Sarcoma: A Systematic Review. Sarcoma 2018; 2018:2640674.
9.   Thévenin-Lemoine C, Destombes L, Vial J, et al. Planning for Bone Excision in Ewing Sarcoma: Post-Chemotherapy MRI More Accurate Than Pre-Chemotherapy MRI Assessment. J Bone Joint Surg Am 2018; 100:13–20.
10.   Albergo JI, Gaston CLL, Parry MC, et al. Risk analysis factors for local recurrence in Ewing's sarcoma: when should adjuvant radiotherapy be administered? Bone Joint J 2018; 100-B:247–255.
11.   Schuetze SM, Bolejack V, Choy E, et al. Phase 2 study of dasatinib in patients with alveolar soft part sarcoma, chondrosarcoma, chordoma, epithelioid sarcoma, or solitary fibrous tumor. Cancer 2017; 123:90–97.
12.   Ferrari A, Chi YY, De Salvo GL, et al. Surgery alone is sufficient therapy for children and adolescents with low-risk synovial sarcoma: A joint analysis from the European paediatric soft tissue sarcoma Study Group and the Children's Oncology Group. Eur J Cancer 2017; 78:1–6.
13.   Outani H, Nakamura T, Murata H, et al. Localized synovial sarcoma: A single institutional study of 191 patients with a minimum follow-up of 5 years for survivors. J Surg Oncol 2019; 119:850–855.
14.   Callegaro D, Miceli R, Bonvalot S, et al. Impact of perioperative chemotherapy and radiotherapy in patients with primary extremity soft tissue sarcoma: retrospective analysis across major histological subtypes and major reference centres. Eur J Cancer 2018; 105:19–27.
15.   Istl AC, Ruck JM, Morris CD, et al. Call for improved design and reporting in soft tissue sarcoma studies: A systematic review and meta-analysis of chemotherapy and survival outcomes in resectable STS. J Surg Oncol 2019; 119:824–835.

16. Barrientos-Ruiz I, Ortiz-Cruz EJ, Serrano-Montilla J, et al. Are Biopsy Tracts a Concern for Seeding and Local Recurrence in Sarcomas? Clin Orthop Relat Res 2017; 475:511–518.

17. Kapoor T, Banuelos J, Adabi K, et al. Analysis of clinical outcomes of upper and lower extremity reconstructions in patients with soft-tissue sarcoma. J Surg Oncol 2018; 118:614–620.

18. Bridgham KM, El Abiad JM, Lu ZA, et al. Reconstructive limb-salvage surgery after lower extremity soft tissue sarcoma resection: A 20-year experience. J Surg Oncol 2019; 119:708–716.

19. Wigge S, Heißner K, Steger V, et al. Impact of surgery in patients with metastatic soft tissue sarcoma: A monocentric retrospective analysis. J Surg Oncol 2018; 118:167–176.

20. Lazarides AL, Kerr DL, Nussbaum DP, et al. Soft Tissue Sarcoma of the Extremities: What Is the Value of Treating at High-volume Centers? Clin Orthop Relat Res 2019; 477:718–727.

21. Erfanian Y, Grueneisen J, Kirchner J, et al. Integrated 18F-FDG PET/MRI compared to MRI alone for identification of local recurrences of soft tissue sarcomas: a comparison trial. Eur J Nucl Med Mol Imaging 2017; 44:1823–1831.

22. Jacobs AJ, Morris CD, Levin AS. Synovial Sarcoma Is Not Associated With a Higher Risk of Lymph Node Metastasis Compared With Other Soft Tissue Sarcomas. Clin Orthop Relat Res 2018; 476:589–598.

23. Traub F, Griffin AM, Wunder JS, et al. Influence of unplanned excisions on the outcomes of patients with stage III extremity soft-tissue sarcoma. Cancer 2018; 124:3868–3875.

24. Gingrich AA, Bateni SB, Monjazeb AM, et al. Extremity soft tissue sarcoma in the elderly: Are we overtreating or undertreating this potentially vulnerable patient population? J Surg Oncol 2019; 119:1087–1098.

25. Mattei JC, Brouste V, Terrier P, et al. Distal extremities soft tissue sarcomas: Are they so different from other limb localizations? J Surg Oncol 2019; 119:479–488.

26. Montgomery C, Harris J, Siegel E, et al. Obesity is associated with larger soft-tissue sarcomas, more surgical complications, and more complex wound closures (obesity leads to larger soft-tissue sarcomas). J Surg Oncol 2018; 118:184–191.

27. Park A, Lans J, Raskin K, et al. Is malnutrition associated with postoperative complications in patients with primary bone sarcomas? J Surg Oncol 2019; 119:324–328.

28. Wilke B, Cooper A, Scarborough M, et al. An Evaluation of PROMIS Health Domains in Sarcoma Patients Compared to the United States Population. Sarcoma 2019; 2019:9725976.

29. Puri A, Ranganathan P, Gulia A, et al. Does a less intensive surveillance protocol affect the survival of patients after treatment of a sarcoma of the limb? updated results of the randomized TOSS study. Bone Joint J 2018; 100-B:262–268.

30. Farfalli GL, Slullitel PA, Muscolo DL, et al. What Happens to the Articular Surface After Curettage for Epiphyseal Chondroblastoma? A Report on Functional Results, Arthritis, and Arthroplasty. Clin Orthop Relat Res 2017; 475:760–766.

31. Benevenia J, Rivero SM, Moore J, et al. Supplemental Bone Grafting in Giant Cell Tumor of the Extremity Reduces Nononcologic Complications. Clin Orthop Relat Res 2017; 475:776–783.

32. Abuhejleh H, Wunder JS, Ferguson PC, et al. Extended intralesional curettage preferred over resection-arthrodesis for giant cell tumour of the distal radius. Eur J Orthop Surg Traumatol 2020; 30:11–17.

33. Errani C, Tsukamoto S, Leone G, et al. Denosumab May Increase the Risk of Local Recurrence in Patients with Giant-Cell Tumor of Bone Treated with Curettage. J Bone Joint Surg Am 2018; 100:496–504.

34. Wu PK, Chen CF, Wang JY, et al. Freezing Nitrogen Ethanol Composite May be a Viable Approach for Cryotherapy of Human Giant Cell Tumor of Bone. Clin Orthop Relat Res 2017; 475:1650–1663.

35. Janssen ML, van Broekhoven DL, Cates JM, et al. Meta-analysis of the influence of surgical margin and adjuvant radiotherapy on local recurrence after resection of sporadic desmoid-type fibromatosis. Br J Surg 2017; 104:347–357.

36. van Broekhoven DLM, Verschoor AJ, van Dalen T, et al. Outcome of Nonsurgical Management of Extra-Abdominal, Trunk, and Abdominal Wall Desmoid-Type Fibromatosis: A Population-Based Study in the Netherlands. Sarcoma 2018; 2018:5982575.

37. Houdek MT, Rose PS, Hevesi M, et al. Low dose radiotherapy is associated with local complications but not disease control in sacral chordoma. J Surg Oncol 2019; 119:856–863.

38. Willeumier JJ, van der Linden YM, van der Wal CWPG, et al. An Easy-to-Use Prognostic Model for Survival Estimation for Patients with Symptomatic Long Bone Metastases. J Bone Joint Surg Am 2018; 100:196–204.

39. Gardner CS, Ensor JE, Ahrar K, et al. Cryoablation of Bone Metastases from Renal Cell Carcinoma for Local Tumor Control. J Bone Joint Surg Am 2017; 99:1916–1926.

40. Philipp TC, Mikula JD, Doung YC, Gundle KR. Is There an Association Between Prophylactic Femur Stabilization and Survival in Patients with Metastatic Bone Disease? Clin Orthop Relat Res 2020; 478:540–546.

41. Plummer D, Passen E, Alexander J, et al. Rapid return to function and stability with dual mobility components cemented into an acetabular reconstructive cage for large osseous defects in the setting of periacetabular metastatic disease. J Surg Oncol 2019; 119:1155–1160.

42. Sternheim A, Kashigar A, Daly M, et al. Cone-Beam Computed Tomography-Guided Navigation in Complex Osteotomies Improves Accuracy at All Competence Levels: A Study Assessing Accuracy and Reproducibility of Joint-Sparing Bone Cuts. J Bone Joint Surg Am 2018; 100:e67.

43. Abraham JA, Kenneally B, Amer K, et al. Can Navigation-assisted Surgery Help Achieve Negative Margins in Resection of Pelvic and Sacral Tumors? Clin Orthop Relat Res 2018; 476:499–508.

44. Bosma SE, Cleven AHG, Dijkstra PDS. Can Navigation Improve the Ability to Achieve Tumor-free Margins in Pelvic and Sacral Primary Bone Sarcoma Resections? A Historically Controlled Study. Clin Orthop Relat Res 2019; 477:1548–1559.

45. Laitinen MK, Parry MC, Albergo JI, et al. Is computer navigation when used in the surgery of iliosacral pelvic bone tumours safer for the patient? Bone Joint J 2017; 99-B:261–266.

46. Farfalli GL, Albergo JI, Piuzzi NS, et al. Is Navigation-guided En Bloc Resection Advantageous Compared With Intralesional Curettage for Locally Aggressive Bone Tumors? Clin Orthop Relat Res 2018; 476:511–517.

47. Park JW, Kang HG, Lim KM, et al. Bone tumor resection guide using three-dimensional printing for limb salvage surgery. J Surg Oncol 2018; 118:898–905.

48. Bosma SE, Wong KC, Paul L, et al. A Cadaveric Comparative Study on the Surgical Accuracy of Freehand, Computer Navigation, and Patient-Specific Instruments in Joint-Preserving Bone Tumor Resections. Sarcoma 2018; 2018:4065846.

49. Abdel MP, von Roth P, Perry KI, et al. Early Results of Acetabular Reconstruction After Wide Periacetabular Oncologic Resection. J Bone Joint Surg Am 2017; 99:e9.

50. Hipfl C, Stihsen C, Puchner SE, et al. Pelvic reconstruction following resection of malignant bone tumours using a stemmed acetabular pedestal cup. Bone Joint J 2017; 99-B:841–848.

51. Bus MP, van de Sande MA, Fiocco M, et al. What Are the Long-term Results of MUTARS. Clin Orthop Relat Res 2017; 475:708–718.

52. Maclean S, Malik SS, Evans S, et al. Reverse shoulder endoprosthesis for pathologic lesions of the proximal humerus: a minimum 3-year follow-up. J Shoulder Elbow Surg 2017; 26:1990–1994.

53. Sanders PTJ, Bus MPA, Scheper H, et al. Multiflora and Gram-Negative Microorganisms Predominate in Infections Affecting Pelvic Endoprostheses Following Tumor Resection. J Bone Joint Surg Am 2019; 101:797–803.

54. Albergo JI, Gaston CL, Aponte-Tinao LA, et al. Proximal Tibia Reconstruction After Bone Tumor Resection: Are Survivorship and Outcomes of Endoprosthetic Replacement and Osteoarticular Allograft Similar? Clin Orthop Relat Res 2017; 475:676–682.

55. Aponte-Tinao LA, Ayerza MA, Albergo JI, et al. Do Massive Allograft Reconstructions for Tumors of the Femur and Tibia Survive 10 or More Years after Implantation? Clin Orthop Relat Res 2020; 478:517–524.

56. Gupta S, Kafchinski LA, Gundle KR, et al. Intercalary allograft augmented with intramedullary cement and plate fixation is a reliable solution after resection of a diaphyseal tumour. Bone Joint J 2017; 99-B:973–978.

57. Oh E, Seo SW, Han KJ. A Longitudinal Study of Functional Outcomes in Patients with Limb Salvage Surgery for Soft Tissue Sarcoma. Sarcoma 2018; 2018:6846275.

Chapter 14

What is new in robotic knee arthroplasty?

Gregg R Klein, Harlan B Levine

INTRODUCTION

Total knee arthroplasty (TKA) is an excellent surgical procedure for the treatment of end-stage knee arthritis. However, not all patients are satisfied with their surgical results. Studies have shown that up to 20% of patients are not satisfied with their knee replacements [1–3]. New surgical techniques and protocols are constantly evolving with the goals to improve the results of TKA. This chapter will review the current literature on robotic knee arthroplasty published in the last 4 years.

Over the past few years, robotic TKA has gained increasing popularity [4–6]. In a recent study, 3,21,522 patients in Medicare Severity Diagnosis Related Groups 469 and 470 who underwent primary total hip arthroplasty (THA) ($n = 1,33,472$) or primary TKA or unicompartmental knee arthroplasty (UKA) ($n = 1,88,050$) between 2008 and 2015 in the New York Statewide Planning and Research Cooperative System (SPARCS) were evaluated. The proportion of cases using technology assistance increased every year from 2.8% (knee 4.3% and hip 0.5%) in 2008 to 8.6% (knee 11.6% and hip 5.2%) in 2015. The proportion of hospitals and surgeons using robotic assistance also increased during the study period, increasing from 16.2% of hospitals and 6.2% of surgeons in 2008 to 29.2% of hospitals and 17.1% of surgeons in 2015. This study also found that technology assistance was more common for knee (7.3%) than hip (1.9%) arthroplasty and was more likely to be used for patients with private insurance (5.9%) compared with Medicare or Medicaid and for patients at high-volume or very high-volume facilities [5].

Similarly, Antonios identified 6,060,901 patients who underwent TKA from 2005 to 2014. The use of technology-assisted TKAs steadily increased over the study period, from 1.2% in 2005 to 7.0% in 2014. The authors found that computer navigation was more likely to be used in the Western United States, whereas robot-assisted TKAs were more commonly performed in the Northeast [4]. Naziri compared robotic TKAs and non-robotic TKAs for

Gregg R Klein MD, Vice-Chairman, Department of Orthopedic Surgery, Hackensack University Medical Center, Associate Professor, Department of Orthopedic Surgery, Hackensack Meridian School of Medicine, Rothman Orthopedic Institute, Paramus NJ
Email: gregg.klein@rothmanortho.com

Harlan B Levine MD, Hackensack University Medical Center, Assistant Professor, Department of Orthopedic Surgery, Hackensack Meridian School of Medicine, Rothman Orthopedic Institute, Paramus, NJ
Email: harlan.levine@rothmanortho.com

utilisation and institutional trends using the NYS SPARCS database. Robotic assistance increased by 500% from the time period of 2009–2013. In this study, 80% of robotic TKAs were performed in teaching hospitals [6].

The hopeful goals of this evolving technology include – improved implant position and limb alignment, improved survivorship, and improved patient outcomes while maintaining patient safety and controlling costs. There is still controversy in the literature – both supporting the benefits and results of robotic surgery and while some manuscripts showing no benefit [7].

ALIGNMENT AND COMPONENT POSITIONS

Alignment in TKA has been studied and documented for many years. Proponents of the mechanical alignment philosophy advocate restoration of the mechanical axis to decrease wear and improve survivorship [8,9]. As navigated TKA has gained popularity, there are an increasing number of manuscripts demonstrating its benefit in regard to improving alignment and decreasing the number of outliers [10].

Ren performed a systematic review and meta-analysis of seven studies with a total of 517 knees undergoing TKA. Compared with conventional surgery, active robotic TKA showed better more precise mechanical alignment and implant position, with a lower number of outliers [11]. In an another systematic review of 22 studies, Agarawal found robotic-assisted TKA results in more accurate postoperative alignment of implants [12].

Marchand has reported on a single surgeon's experience with correcting severe coronal deformities using the robotic-assisted TKA. There were a total of 261 varus knees, 46 valgus knees, and 23 cases had neutral alignment. The authors focussed on severe deformity of 7° or greater. 129 of these patients had an initial severe varus deformity and seven patients with an initial severe valgus deformity of 7° or greater. All 132 knees with initial varus deformity of <7° were corrected to neutral. 64% with 7°or greater varus deformity were corrected to neutral. Of the patients not corrected to neutral, 30% of patients with severe deformity were still corrected within a couple of degrees of neutral. There were seven knees with 7° or greater valgus deformity, and all were corrected to neutral. In this study, all knees were corrected in the appropriate direction within a few degrees of neutral, and no knees were overcorrected [13].

Casper assessed the accuracy of a novel imageless semiautonomous handheld robotic sculpting system in performing bone resection and preparation in TKA by comparing the planned and final implant placement in 18 cadavers. A quantitative analysis was performed to determine the translational, angular, and rotational differences between the planned and achieved positions of the implants. The mean femoral flexion, varus/valgus, and rotational error were −2.0°, −0.1°, and −0.5°, respectively. The mean tibial posterior slope, and varus/valgus error was −0.2°, and −0.2°, respectively [14].

Cho reported on 351 patients (390 knees), 155 patients undergoing robotic TKA, and 196 patients treated with conventional TKA with a mean follow-up of 11.0 years. The conventional TKA group showed a significantly higher number of outliers compared with the robotic TKA group. However, overall survival was not different at this time period [15]. Similarly, Bollars has reported on 77 TKAs a novel image-free handheld robotic sculpting system and compared to a control group of mechanical alignment. The authors found significantly less outliers compared to the conventional technique [16].

In a review of 173 knee performed with robotic navigation, Figuerora evaluated implant position and alignment using computed tomography (CT). The authors evaluated – femoral coronal alignment (FCA), femoral sagittal alignment (FSA), femoral rotational alignment (FRA), tibial coronal alignment (TCA), tibial sagittal alignment (TSA), and hip-knee-ankle (HKA) angle. The mean differences between the navigated reported and the CT positions were not significant for FCA, FRA, and TCA. However, statistically significant results showed that the FSA was more flexed 1.5 ± 0.3, TCA was in 0.7 ± 1.1° more varus, and the TSA showed −1.3 ± 1.5 more negative slope [17].

In a cadaveric study, Hampp compared bone cut and final-component positioning errors relative to preoperative plans. When compared with manual instrumentation, Robotic arm-assisted TKA demonstrated more accurate and precise bone cuts and implant positioning to plan [17].

Parratte performed a cadaveric study of 30 knees in 15 specimens. Eight trained, board-certified orthopaedic surgeons performed robotically assisted TKA implantation using the same robotic protocol with three different implant designs. The target angles obtained from the intraoperative planning were then compared to the angles of the bone cuts performed using the robotic system and measured with the computer-assisted system considered to be the gold standard. All angle mean differences were below 1° and standard deviations below 1°. For all six angles, the mean differences between the target angle and the measured values were not significantly different from 0 except for the femoral flexion angle which had a mean difference of 0.95°. All resection mean differences were below 0.7 mm and standard deviations below 1.1 mm [18].

Sultan evaluated a series of 43 consecutive robotic-arm assisted and 39 manual total knee arthroplasties performed by seven fellowship-trained joint reconstructive surgeons in regards to restoration of posterior femoral offset and the Insall–Salvati index (ISI). The mean postoperative posterior offset was statistically larger in manual TKA when compared to the robotic-assisted cohort. In addition, the number of patients who had postoperative ISI outside of the normal range (0.8–0.12) was higher in the manual cohort (12 vs. 4). In addition, these patients were less likely to have values outside of normal ISI, which means they are less likely to develop patella baja [19].

Many different surgical techniques and alignment methods can be used when performing robotic-assisted TKA. Yeo randomly assigned to patients undergo robotic-assisted TKA using either mechanical (30 patients) or kinematic (30 patients) alignment method. Clinical outcomes between the two groups showed no significant difference in HSS, WOMAC, ROM, KS pain, or function score at the last follow-up. No significant difference in varus and valgus laxity assessment, mechanical alignment of the lower limb, or perioperative complications was shown between the two groups. In gait analysis, no significant difference in kinematic or kinetic parameters was found except for varus angle and mediolateral ground reaction force. Results of this study show that mechanical and kinematic knee alignment methods provide comparable clinical and radiological outcomes after robotic TKA with an average follow-up of 8 years. There was no functional difference during walking between the two alignment methods either [20].

More complex procedures can benefit from robotic assistance. Sodhi has presented a case series of three patients with extra-articular deformity. The robotic software was able to plan for the extra-articular deformity in the preoperative and real-time updated intraoperative plans. The surgeon was able to achieve balanced and aligned TKA [21].

Seidenstein has reported on a cadaveric study using a new robotic-assisted system for TKA comparing 14 robotically assisted to 20 conventional TKAs. The robotic group showed more accurate results and fewer outliers. 100% of the robotic cases were within 3° and 93% were within 2° when evaluating final limb alignment. The accuracy of bone resection angles was below 0.6° and bone resection levels were below 0.7 mm [22].

OUTCOMES

Patient satisfaction can be measured in many different forms. Obtaining well aligned and positioned components is important but patient satisfaction and high outcome scores are the true measure of a successful arthroplasty. Over the past few years, many manuscripts have been published evaluating these patient's outcomes.

In a randomised study evaluating 31 robotic assisted and 29, Liow found that both robotic-assisted and conventional TKA displayed significant improvements in majority of the functional outcome scores at 2 years. The robotic-assisted group displayed a trend towards higher scores in SF-36 quality of life (QoL) measures, with significant differences in SF-36 vitality, role emotional and a larger proportion of patients achieving SF-36 vitality minimally clinically important differences [23].

Kayani prospectively evaluated 40 consecutive patients undergoing conventional jig-based TKA followed by 40 consecutive patients receiving robotic-arm-assisted TKA. All surgical procedures were done by the same surgeon with the same surgical exposure and same implant design with standardised postoperative inpatient rehabilitation protocols. There were no significant differences in baseline characteristics between the conventional jig-based TKA and robotic-arm-assisted TKA treatment groups. Robotic-arm-assisted TKA was associated with reduced postoperative pain, decreased analgesia requirements, decreased reduction in postoperative haemoglobin levels, shorter time to straight leg raise, decreased number of physiotherapy sessions, and improved maximum knee flexion at discharge compared with conventional jig-based TKA. Discharge from the hospital was also faster in the robotic cohort [24].

Marchand compared 53 consecutive robotic-arm-assisted TKAs to 53 consecutive manual TKAs using a modified Western Ontario and McMaster Universities Osteoarthritis Index satisfaction survey preoperatively and at 1-year postoperatively. The robotic group had significantly improved mean total and physical function scores when compared with the manual group. The mean pain score for the robotic group was also lower than that for the manual cohort. Using backward linear regression analyses, robotic surgery was found to be significantly associated with more improved total, function, and pain scores. The robotic group was found to have the strongest association with improved scores when compared with age, gender, and body mass index (BMI). This study suggests that robotic assisted TKA patients patients may have short-term improvements at minimum 1 year postoperatively [25].

In a meta-analysis of 517 robotic-assisted TKA, Ren found better functional score (Western Ontario and McMaster University, Knee Society Score functional score) and less drainage in patients undergoing robotic-assisted TKA as compared to conventional methods. No significant differences were observed when comparing the operation time, range of motion, and complication rates [11]. Similarly, in a meta-analysis, Agarwal has found that robotic-assisted TKA results in greater improvements in postoperative

Hospital for Special Surgery score and Western Ontario and McMaster Universities scores compared to conventional TKA indicating improved postoperative outcomes [12].

LONG-TERM RESULTS

Yang compared clinical and radiological results between 71 robotic TKA and 42 conventional TKA with a cruciate-retaining implant at 10-year follow-up. The clinical outcomes and long-term survival rates were similar between the two groups. However, the robotic TKA group had significantly fewer postoperative leg alignment outliers and fewer radiolucent lines than the conventional TKA group. The authors concluded that both robotic and conventional TKAs resulted in good clinical outcomes and postoperative leg alignments [26].

Cho evaluated 351 patients (390 knees), 155 patients undergoing robotic TKA, and 196 patients treated with conventional TKA with a mean follow-up of 11 years. Clinical results were similar in the two groups. Radiographically, the conventional TKA group showed a significantly higher number of outliers compared with the robotic TKA group. The cumulative survival was not significantly different [15].

In a prospective randomised trial of robotic-assisted TKA, Kim followed 750 knees receiving robotic-assisted TKA and 766 knees receiving conventional TKA at an average follow-up of 13 years and found no differences between robotic-assisted TKA and conventional TKA in terms of functional outcome scores, aseptic loosening, overall survivorship, and complications [27].

GAP BALANCING

Robotic surgery now has the potential to help the surgeon more accurately and quantitatively balance soft tissue gaps. Theoretically, a more balanced articulation may improve outcomes and longevity [28]. Gap balancing has theoretical advantages of not relying on traditional femoral landmarks that have been shown to be quite variable. Using a robotic system for gap balancing now allows the surgeon to quantitate and balance the gaps in real time. Historically, one of the disadvantages of gap balancing has been reliance on the tibial cut. If the tibial cut is not accurate, balance will be difficult. Robot systems have been shown to have improved accuracy and diminished outliers in executing these cuts [11,12,14,15].

Shalhoub evaluated robotic-assisted, gap-balancing TKA in 14 cadaveric specimens. The native tibiofemoral gaps were measured using a robotic tensioner that dynamically tensioned the soft-tissue envelope throughout the arc of flexion. The femoral implant was then aligned to balance the gaps at 0° and 90° of flexion. The postoperative gaps were then measured using the system and found the native gaps increased by 3.4 mm medially and 3.7 mm laterally from full extension to 20° of flexion and then remained consistent through the remaining arc of flexion. The authors found that gap balancing after TKA produced equal gaps at 0° and 90° of flexion, but the gap laxity in mid-flexion was 2–4 mm greater than at 0° and 90°. They concluded that balancing the knee with equal gaps at 0° and 90° of flexion produced equal gaps in extension and flexion with larger gaps in mid-flexion [29].

Shalhoub more recently has used robotic-assisted gap balancing in 121 consecutive knees. About 90% of knees were found to have mediolateral balance within 2 mm across the flexion range. Gaps at 0° flexion were 2 mm smaller than the gaps at 90°. This difference decreased to <1 mm when comparing the tibiofemoral gaps at 10°, 45°, and 90°. This technique allowed the authors to predict postoperative gaps before femoral resections and virtually plan femoral implant alignment and optimise gap balance throughout the range of motion [30].

Nodzo has reported on 233 patients undergoing robotic arm-assisted TKA in regards to femoral component rotation. The authors concluded that intraoperative measured flexion space balance through femoral component positioning did not correlate with the implants relationship to the native thoracic epidural analgesia (TEA) or principal component analysis (PCA). Furthermore, when looking specifically at varus knees, the preoperative mechanical axis alignment correlated with an increase in femoral component external rotation to the TEA and PCA. For valgus knees, the severity of preoperative lateral distal femoral angle correlated with the rotational relationship of the femoral component to the PCA only [31].

LEARNING CURVE

Sodhi has evaluated the effect on the learning curve and operative time by evaluating two surgeons' operative times in a series of 240 robotic-assisted TKAs. For each surgeon, mean operative times for their first 20 and last 20 robotic-assisted cases were compared with 20 randomly selected manual cases performed by that surgeon as controls prior to the initiation of the robotic-assisted cases. For both surgeons, the mean operative time was significantly higher in the first 20 cases as compared to mechanical instrumentation and the last 20 cases were not different than their standard instrumented cases. The authors concluded that within a few months, a board-certified orthopaedic joint arthroplasty surgeon should be able to adequately perform robotic TKA without adding any operative times [32].

Kayani prospectively evaluated 60 consecutive conventional jig-based TKAs followed by 60 consecutive robotic-arm-assisted TKAs performed by a single surgeon. Robotic-arm-assisted TKA was associated with a learning curve of seven cases for operative times and surgical team anxiety levels. The use of a robotic-arm-assisted TKA led to increased operative times and heightened levels of anxiety among the surgical team for the initial seven cases but there was no learning curve for achieving the planned implant positioning. The authors also found that robotic-arm-assisted TKA improved accuracy of implant positioning and limb alignment compared to conventional jig-based TKA [33].

Similarly, vermue performed a systematic review of 11 previously published studies and reported that the operating time of robotic TKA and UKA is associated with a learning curve of between 6–20 cases and 6–36 cases, respectively. The stress level of the surgical team showed a learning curve of seven cases in TKA and six cases for UKA. Experience with the robotic systems did not influence implant positioning, preoperative planning, and postoperative complications [34].

SOFT TISSUE PROTECTION

Khlopas evaluated the effects of robotic-arm-assisted TKA in regards to ligament protection. Six robotic-assisted TKAs with a stereotactic boundary were compared to seven standard TKAs with mechanical instrumentation. An experienced surgeon performed a visual evaluation and palpation of the posterior cruciate ligament (PCL), medial collateral ligament (MCL), lateral collateral ligament (LCL), and the patellar ligament after the procedures. There were no ligament injuries in the robotic group and found two knees with slight disruption of the PCL that did not compromise its function integrity [35].

UNICOMPARTMENTAL ARTHROPLASTY

Alignment and component positions

Gaudiani reviewed the clinical and radiographic information of 94 robotic-assisted UKA surgeries for balancing of sagittal and coronal knee anatomy using radiographic parameters, such as posterior condylar offset ratio, posterior tibial slope (PTS), femoral-tibial angle, and joint line, and found that PTS was significantly lower after UKA compared to the native knee (4.91° vs. 2.28°). In the coronal plane, pre- and post-operative mechanical axes were significantly different (5.43° of varus vs. 2.76° of varus). The authors concluded that robotic surgery was helpful as they were able to accurately modify modifying PTS, while maintaining the posterior condylar offset [36].

In a prospective study evaluating implant position, Kayani found robotic-arm-assisted UKA improved accuracy of femoral and tibial implant positioning with no additional risk of postoperative complications compared to conventional jig-based UKA [37].

Maintaining the joint line

Maintaining the joint line is extremely important in unicondylar arthroplasty to ensure proper mechanics and range of motion. Herry retrospectively compared 80 patients receiving a resurfacing UKA either a robotic-assisted or conventional. The authors found restitution of joint line height was significantly improved in the robotic-assisted group compared than the control group [38].

Outcomes

In a randomised clinical trial comparing robotic arm-assisted unicompartmental UKA for medial compartment osteoarthritis (OA) of the knee with manual UKA performed using traditional surgical jigs, Blyth randomised 139 knees and found that from the 1st post-operative day through to week 8 post-operatively, the median pain scores for the robotic arm-assisted group were 55.4% lower than those observed in the manual surgery group. At 3 months post-operatively, the robotic arm-assisted group had better American knee society scores (KSS). But at 1 year, there was no difference. This study concluded that robotic arm-assisted surgery results in improved early pain scores and early function scores in some patient-reported outcomes measures, but no difference was observed at 1 year post-operatively [39].

There has been debate about the effects of obesity on longevity and outcomes after UKA. Plate specifically looked at the influence of obesity on the outcomes of UKA with a robotic-assisted system at a minimum follow-up of 24 months. Almost 746 medial robotic-assisted UKAs were reviewed and the authors found that BMI did not influence the rate of revision surgery to TKA (5.8%), type of prosthesis used, mean postoperative Oxford knee score, or readmission rate. There was a significant correlation with higher opioid medication requirements and a higher number of physical therapy session needed to reach discharge goals [40].

In a prospective cohort study, Kayani has reported on 146 patients (73 consecutive patients undergoing conventional jig-based mobile-bearing UKA followed by 73 consecutive patients receiving robotic-arm-assisted fixed bearing UKA). Robotic-arm-assisted UKA was associated with decreased postoperative pain, reduced opiate analgesia requirements, improved early functional rehabilitation, and shorter time to hospital discharge compared with conventional jig-based UKA. There was no difference in postoperative complications between the two groups within 90 days' follow-up [41].

In a cohort study, Clement reported 30 patients undergoing robotic UKA who were propensity score matched to 90 patients undergoing manual TKA for isolated medial compartment arthritis. Patients with isolated medial compartment arthritis had a greater knee-specific functional outcome and generic health with a shorter length of hospital stay after robotic UKA when compared to manual TKA [42].

Chin has performed a systematic review and meta-analysis comparing radiological and functional outcomes of TKA and UKA using either robotic assistance or conventional methods. Robot-assisted TKA and UKA were associated with significantly better component angle alignment accuracy at the cost of significantly greater operation time. The manuscript concluded that robot-assisted TKA and UKA lead to better radiological outcomes without differences in mid- and long-term functional outcomes compared with conventional methods for the former [43].

In contrast, Gaudiani performed a systematic review and meta-analysis of robotic-assisted UKA and found that the robotic and manual UKAs offer comparable improvements in pain, functional outcome scores, and revision rates [44].

Not all studies have shown significantly improved outcomes. Some manuscripts have demonstrated no significance differences between standard and robotic surgery. However, worse outcomes have not been shown. Gilmour reviewed the clinical outcomes of a single-centre, prospective, randomised controlled trial, comparing robotic-arm-assisted UKA with conventional surgery. At 2 years, there were no significant differences for any of the outcome measures. Survivorship was 100% in robotic-arm-assisted group and 96.3% in the manual group. The authors concluded that participants achieved an outcome equivalent to the most widely implanted UKA in the United Kingdom [45]. Wong retrospectively reviewed 176 consecutive fixed-bearing medial UKAs (118 conventional and 58 robotic procedures and found at 2 years, there was no significant difference between the robotic and conventional groups). The robotic cohort had a significantly longer operative time and a higher early revision [46].

Return to activities

In a small retrospective study, Canetti compared the return to sports after 11 lateral UKA performed with robotic-assisted technique and 17 with conventional technique. Robotic-assisted surgical technique provided significantly quicker return to sports than conventional technique. Patients returned to similar sports as those done pre-operatively. These activities were mainly low- and mid-impact sports (hiking, cycling, swimming, and skiing) [47].

Jinnah prospectively followed 30 consecutive robotic UKA in regards to returning to work. The mean time to return to work was 6.4 weeks and concluded that most patients can return to work 6 weeks following robotic-assisted UKA [48].

Survivorship

In a prospective multicentre study review of 1,135 robotic-assisted medial UKA, Pearle showed a survivorship of 98.8% at 2.5 years. Of all patients without revision, 92% were either very satisfied or satisfied with their knee function [49].

Kleeblad has reported on a prospective, multicentre study of 528 knee that underwent robotic-arm-assisted medial UKA at a mean follow-up of 5.7 years and have reported a 97% survivorship. The mean time to revision was 2.27 years. The most common failure mode was aseptic loosening and was seen in 7 of the 13 failures. Of the unrevised patients, 91% were either very satisfied or satisfied with their knee function [50].

Cool evaluated hospital admissions for revision surgeries associated with robotic arm-assisted UKA (rUKA) versus manually instrumented UKA (mUKA) and found that at 24 months after the primary UKA procedure, patients who underwent rUKA had fewer revision procedures, and a shorter mean length of stay [51].

Battenberg has reported on a handheld robotic system used for UKA for 128 patients at a mean follow-up period of 2.3 years. The overall survivorship of the knee implant was 99.2% [52].

Burger has reported the mid-term results of robotic-assisted unicompartmental arthroplasty. The 5-year survivorship of medial UKA ($n = 802$) and lateral UKA ($n = 171$) was 97.8% and 97.7%, respectively. Component loosening and progression of OA were the most common reasons for revision [53].

Mergenthaler has reported the results of 200 robotic-assisted UKA and 191 conventional UKA. At the most recent follow-up, revision rates were 4% for robotic-assisted UKA and 11% for conventional UKA. Complication rates for stiffness and infection were comparable in both groups. The KSS function scores were higher following robotic-assisted UKA. Satisfaction rates and contralateral OA were comparable in the two groups [54].

Zambianchi has reported on a multicentre, retrospective, observational study of a large cohort of robotic-arm-assisted medial and lateral UKAs at short-term follow-up and concluded that robotic-assisted medial and lateral UKAs demonstrated satisfactory clinical outcomes and excellent survivorship at 3-year follow-up [55].

Learning curve

Kayani prospectively followed 60 consecutive conventional jig-based UKAs compared with 60 consecutive robotic-arm-assisted UKAs for medial compartment knee OA and found that robotic-arm-assisted UKA was associated with a learning curve of six cases for operating time and surgical team confidence levels [37].

Cost-effectiveness

Nherera performed a cost-effectiveness study comparing non-CT robotic UKA to traditional unicompartmental knee arthroplasty (tUKA) using a 5-year four-state Markov model to evaluate the expected costs and outcomes of the two strategies in patients aged 65 years. For a high-volume orthopaedic centre that performs 100 UKA operations per year, non-CT rUKA was more costly than tUKA but offered better clinical outcomes. The manuscript concluded that non-CT robotic UKA is cost-effective compared with tUKA over a 5-year period. However, the results were dependent on case volumes and follow-up period and were better in younger (age < 55) age groups [56].

SOFT-TISSUE PROTECTION

Complications

Lonner has reported on the report on a series of 1,064 consecutive UKAs performed by one surgeon with either one of two commercially available semiautonomous robotic systems. There was no soft tissue, bone injuries, or other complications related to the use of the robotic bone preparation method. There were six complications related to the use of navigation pins occurred (0.6%) – one pseudoaneurysm of a branch of the tibialis anterior artery, one tibial metaphyseal stress fracture, and four areas of pin site irritation/superficial infection that resolved with a short course of oral antibiotics [57].

CONFLICT OF INTEREST

Cavinatto reviewed the literature in regard to publications related to robotic UKA and found that manuscripts, in which UKA was performed with the assistance of a robot, were more likely to be industry funded or be written by authors with financial conflicts of interest and published in less prestigious journals. There were no differences in scientific quality or influence between the two groups [58].

REFERENCES

1. Anderson JG, Wixson RL, Tsai D, et al. Functional outcome and patient satisfaction in total knee patients over the age of 75. J Arthroplasty 1996; 11:831–840.
2. Noble PC, Conditt MA, Cook KF, et al. The John Insall Award: Patient expectations affect satisfaction with total knee arthroplasty. Clin Orthop Relat Res 2006; 452:35–43.
3. Bourne RB, Chesworth BM, Davis AM, et al. Patient satisfaction after total knee arthroplasty: who is satisfied and who is not? Clin Orthop Relat Res 2010; 468:57–63.
4. Antonios JK, Korber S, Sivasundaram L, et al. Trends in computer navigation and robotic assistance for total knee arthroplasty in the United States: an analysis of patient and hospital factors. Arthroplast Today 2019; 5:88–95.
5. Boylan M, Suchman K, Vigdorchik J, et al. Technology-Assisted Hip and Knee Arthroplasties: An Analysis of Utilization Trends. J Arthroplasty 2018; 33:1019–1023.
6. Naziri Q, Burekhovich SA, Mixa PJ, et al. The trends in robotic-assisted knee arthroplasty: A statewide database study. J Orthop 2019; 16:298–301.
7. Kim YH, Park JW, Kim JS. 2017 Chitranjan S. Ranawat Award: Does Computer Navigation in Knee Arthroplasty Improve Functional Outcomes in Young Patients? A Randomized Study. Clin Orthop Relat Res 2018; 476:6–15.
8. Collier MB, Engh CA Jr, McAuley JP, et al. Factors associated with the loss of thickness of polyethylene tibial bearings after knee arthroplasty. J Bone Joint Surg Am 2007; 89:1306–1314.
9. Hsu RW, Himeno S, Coventry MB, et al. Normal axial alignment of the lower extremity and load-bearing distribution at the knee. Clin Orthop Relat Res 1990:215–227.
10. Hetaimish BM, Khan MM, Simunovic N, et al. Meta-analysis of navigation vs conventional total knee arthroplasty. J Arthroplasty 2012; 27:1177–1182.
11. Ren Y, Cao S, Wu J, et al. Efficacy and reliability of active robotic-assisted total knee arthroplasty compared with conventional total knee arthroplasty: a systematic review and meta-analysis. Postgrad Med J 2019; 95:125–133.
12. Agarwal N, To K, McDonnell S, et al. Clinical and Radiological Outcomes in Robotic-Assisted Total Knee Arthroplasty: A Systematic Review and Meta-Analysis. J Arthroplasty 2020; 35:3393–3409.e2.
13. Marchand RC, Sodhi N, Khlopas A, et al. Coronal Correction for Severe Deformity Using Robotic-Assisted Total Knee Arthroplasty. J Knee Surg 2018; 31:2–5.
14. Casper M, Mitra R, Khare R, et al. Accuracy assessment of a novel image-free handheld robot for Total Knee Arthroplasty in a cadaveric study. Comput Assist Surg (Abingdon) 2018; 23:14–20.

15. Cho KJ, Seon JK, Jang WY, et al. Robotic versus conventional primary total knee arthroplasty: clinical and radiological long-term results with a minimum follow-up of ten years. Int Orthop 2019; 43:1345–1354.
16. Bollars P, Boeckxstaens A, Mievis J, et al. Preliminary experience with an image-free handheld robot for total knee arthroplasty: 77 cases compared with a matched control group. Eur J Orthop Surg Traumatol 2020; 30:723–729.
17. Hampp EL, Chughtai M, Scholl LY, et al. Robotic-Arm Assisted Total Knee Arthroplasty Demonstrated Greater Accuracy and Precision to Plan Compared with Manual Techniques. J Knee Surg 2019; 32:239–250.
18. Parratte S, Price AJ, Jeys LM, et al. Accuracy of a New Robotically Assisted Technique for Total Knee Arthroplasty: A Cadaveric Study. J Arthroplasty 2019; 34:2799–2803.
19. Sultan AA, Samuel LT, Khlopas A, et al. Robotic-Arm Assisted Total Knee Arthroplasty More Accurately Restored the Posterior Condylar Offset Ratio and the Insall-Salvati Index Compared to the Manual Technique; A Cohort-Matched Study. Surg Technol Int 2019; 34:409–413.
20. Yeo JH, Seon JK, Lee DH, et al. No difference in outcomes and gait analysis between mechanical and kinematic knee alignment methods using robotic total knee arthroplasty. Knee Surg Sports Traumatol Arthrosc 2019; 27:1142–1147.
21. Sodhi N, Khlopas A, Ehiorobo JO, et al. Robotic-Assisted Total Knee Arthroplasty in the Presence of Extra-Articular Deformity. Surg Technol Int 2019; 34:497–502.
22. Seidenstein A, Birmingham M, Foran J, et al. Better accuracy and reproducibility of a new robotically-assisted system for total knee arthroplasty compared to conventional instrumentation: a cadaveric study. Knee Surg Sports Traumatol Arthrosc 2020; 29:859–866.
23. Liow MHL, Goh GS, Wong MK, et al. Robotic-assisted total knee arthroplasty may lead to improvement in quality-of-life measures: a 2-year follow-up of a prospective randomized trial. Knee Surg Sports Traumatol Arthrosc 2017; 25:2942–2951.
24. Kayani B, Konan S, Tahmassebi J, et al. Robotic-arm assisted total knee arthroplasty is associated with improved early functional recovery and reduced time to hospital discharge compared with conventional jig-based total knee arthroplasty: a prospective cohort study. Bone Joint J 2018; 100-B:930–937.
25. Marchand RC, Sodhi N, Anis HK, et al. One-Year Patient Outcomes for Robotic-Arm-Assisted versus Manual Total Knee Arthroplasty. J Knee Surg 2019; 32:1063–1068.
26. Yang HY, Seon JK, Shin YJ, et al. Robotic Total Knee Arthroplasty with a Cruciate-Retaining Implant: A 10-Year Follow-up Study. Clin Orthop Surg 2017;9:169–176.
27. Kim YH, Yoon SH, Park JW. Does Robotic-assisted TKA Result in Better Outcome Scores or Long-Term Survivorship Than Conventional TKA? A Randomized, Controlled Trial. Clin Orthop Relat Res 2020; 478:266–275.
28. Fang DM, Ritter MA, Davis KE. Coronal alignment in total knee arthroplasty: just how important is it? J Arthroplasty 2009; 24:39–43.
29. Shalhoub S, Moschetti WE, Dabuzhsky L, et al. Laxity Profiles in the Native and Replaced Knee-Application to Robotic-Assisted Gap-Balancing Total Knee Arthroplasty. J Arthroplasty 2018; 33:3043–3048.
30. Shalhoub S, Lawrence JM, Keggi JM, et al. Imageless, robotic-assisted total knee arthroplasty combined with a robotic tensioning system can help predict and achieve accurate postoperative ligament balance. Arthroplast Today 2019; 5:334–340.
31. Nodzo SR, Staub TM, Jancuska JM, et al. Flexion Space Balancing Through Component Positioning and Its Relationship to Traditional Anatomic Rotational Landmarks in Robotic Total Knee Arthroplasty. J Arthroplasty 2020; 35:1569–1575.
32. Bautista M, Manrique J, Hozack WJ. Robotics in Total Knee Arthroplasty. J Knee Surg 2019; 32:600–606.
33. Kayani B, Konan S, Huq SS, et al. Robotic-arm assisted total knee arthroplasty has a learning curve of seven cases for integration into the surgical workflow but no learning curve effect for accuracy of implant positioning. Knee Surg Sports Traumatol Arthrosc 2019; 27:1132–1141.
34. Vermue H, Lambrechts J, Tampere T, et al. How should we evaluate robotics in the operating theatre? Bone Joint J 2020; 102-B:407–413.
35. Khlopas A, Chughtai M, Hampp EL, et al. Robotic-Arm Assisted Total Knee Arthroplasty Demonstrated Soft Tissue Protection. Surg Technol Int 2017; 30:441–446.
36. Gaudiani MA, Nwachukwu BU, Baviskar JV, et al. Optimization of sagittal and coronal planes with robotic-assisted unicompartmental knee arthroplasty. Knee 2017; 24:837–843.
37. Kayani B, Konan S, Pietrzak JRT, et al. The learning curve associated with robotic-arm assisted unicompartmental knee arthroplasty: a prospective cohort study. Bone Joint J 2018; 100-B:1033–1042.
38. Herry Y, Batailler C, Lording T, et al. Improved joint-line restitution in unicompartmental knee arthroplasty using a robotic-assisted surgical technique. Int Orthop 2017; 41:2265–2271.

39. Blyth MJG, Anthony I, Rowe P, et al. Robotic arm-assisted versus conventional unicompartmental knee arthroplasty: Exploratory secondary analysis of a randomised controlled trial. Bone Joint Res 2017; 6:631–639.

40. Plate JF, Augart MA, Seyler TM, et al. Obesity has no effect on outcomes following unicompartmental knee arthroplasty. Knee Surg Sports Traumatol Arthrosc 2017; 25:645–651.

41. Kayani B, Konan S, Tahmassebi J, et al. An assessment of early functional rehabilitation and hospital discharge in conventional versus robotic-arm assisted unicompartmental knee arthroplasty: a prospective cohort study. Bone Joint J 2019; 101-B:24–33.

42. Clement ND, Bell A, Simpson P, et al. Robotic-assisted unicompartmental knee arthroplasty has a greater early functional outcome when compared to manual total knee arthroplasty for isolated medial compartment arthritis. Bone Joint Res 2020; 9:15–22.

43. Chin BZ, Tan SSH, Chua KCX, et al. Robot-Assisted versus Conventional Total and Unicompartmental Knee Arthroplasty: A Meta-analysis of Radiological and Functional Outcomes. J Knee Surg 2020; 34:1064–1075.

44. Gaudiani MA, Samuel LT, Kamath AF, et al. Robotic-Assisted versus Manual Unicompartmental Knee Arthroplasty: Contemporary Systematic Review and Meta-analysis of Early Functional Outcomes. J Knee Surg 2020; 34:1048–1056.

45. Gilmour A, MacLean AD, Rowe PJ, et al. Robotic-Arm-Assisted vs Conventional Unicompartmental Knee Arthroplasty. The 2-Year Clinical Outcomes of a Randomized Controlled Trial. J Arthroplasty 2018; 33:S109–S115.

46. Wong J, Murtaugh T, Lakra A, et al. Robotic-assisted unicompartmental knee replacement offers no early advantage over conventional unicompartmental knee replacement. Knee Surg Sports Traumatol Arthrosc 2019; 27:2303–2308.

47. Canetti R, Batailler C, Bankhead C, et al. Faster return to sport after robotic-assisted lateral unicompartmental knee arthroplasty: a comparative study. Arch Orthop Trauma Surg 2018; 138:1765–1771.

48. Jinnah AH, Augart MA, Lara DL, et al. Decreased Time to Return to Work Using Robotic-Assisted Unicompartmental Knee Arthroplasty Compared to Conventional Techniques. Surg Technol Int 2018; 32:279–283.

49. Pearle AD, van der List JP, Lee L, et al. Survivorship and patient satisfaction of robotic-assisted medial unicompartmental knee arthroplasty at a minimum two-year follow-up. Knee 2017; 24:419–428.

50. Kleeblad LJ, Borus TA, Coon TM, et al. Midterm Survivorship and Patient Satisfaction of Robotic-Arm-Assisted Medial Unicompartmental Knee Arthroplasty: A Multicenter Study. J Arthroplasty 2018; 33:1719–1726.

51. Cool CL, Needham KA, Khlopas A, et al. Revision Analysis of Robotic Arm-Assisted and Manual Unicompartmental Knee Arthroplasty. J Arthroplasty 2019; 34:926–931.

52. Battenberg AK, Netravali NA, Lonner JH. A novel handheld robotic-assisted system for unicompartmental knee arthroplasty: surgical technique and early survivorship. J Robot Surg 2020; 14:55–60.

53. Burger JA, Kleeblad LJ, Laas N, et al. Mid-term survivorship and patient-reported outcomes of robotic-arm assisted partial knee arthroplasty. Bone Joint J 2020; 102-B:108–116.

54. Mergenthaler G, Batailler C, Lording T, et al. Is robotic-assisted unicompartmental knee arthroplasty a safe procedure? A case control study. Knee Surg Sports Traumatol Arthrosc 2020; 29:931–938.

55. Zambianchi F, Franceschi G, Rivi E, et al. Clinical results and short-term survivorship of robotic-arm-assisted medial and lateral unicompartmental knee arthroplasty. Knee Surg Sports Traumatol Arthrosc 2020; 28:1551–1559.

56. Nherera LM, Verma S, Trueman P, et al. Early Economic Evaluation Demonstrates That Noncomputerized Tomography Robotic-Assisted Surgery Is Cost-Effective in Patients Undergoing Unicompartmental Knee Arthroplasty at High-Volume Orthopaedic Centres. Adv Orthop 2020; 2020:3460675.

57. Lonner JH, Kerr GJ. Low rate of iatrogenic complications during unicompartmental knee arthroplasty with two semiautonomous robotic systems. Knee 2019; 26:745–749.

58. Cavinatto L, Bronson MJ, Chen DD, et al. Robotic-assisted versus standard unicompartmental knee arthroplasty-evaluation of manuscript conflict of interests, funding, scientific quality and bibliometrics. Int Orthop 2019; 43:1865–1871.

Chapter 15

Coronavirus disease 2019: An orthopaedic perspective

Paul M Sousa, Chad A Krueger

INTRODUCTION

The novel severe acute respiratory syndrome-related coronavirus 2 (SARS-CoV-2) virus has wreaked havoc on society since early in 2020. It has been attributed to millions of deaths worldwide and caused healthcare systems to undergo drastic changes or, in many instances, become overwhelmed by the large number of patients effected by the virus. These changes have had a large trickle-down effect on the practice of orthopaedic surgery. In this chapter, we will review some of the challenges our profession has faced in light of coronavirus disease 2019 (COVID-19).

IMPACT TO PATIENTS

In the Spring of 2020, there was a unified movement by state and national governments to prepare for the already spreading viral pandemic. While preparedness was the key focus on all fronts, many other aspects of healthcare fell by the wayside. Elective surgery was postponed across the country for variable periods of time, which was supported by key healthcare societies. Along with guidance from the White House, American College of Surgeons issued recommendations for the management of elective surgical procedures [1], and the American Academy of Orthopaedic Surgeons issued, at that time, an indefinite ban on elective surgery [2]. In Europe, a survey of 272 member of either European Hip or Knee Association showed that nearly 70% of surgeons cancelled all elective surgeries for a period of time, and 93% of responders cancelled all primary total hip and total knee arthroplasty (TKA) [3]. Furthermore, a survey performed by the American Academy of Hip and Knee Surgeons showed over 90% of hospitals across the United States followed suit and ceased elective medical procedures, at least initially [4].

The initial response delayed access to care for many elective procedures. Total hip and TKA was significantly impacted. Moreover, there remains skepticism to seek medical care

Paul M Sousa MD, Rothman Orthopaedic Institute, Thomas Jefferson University Hospital, Philadelphia, PA
Email: Paul.Sousa@thecoreistitute.com

Chad A Krueger MD, Rothman Orthopaedic Institute, Assistant Professor, Orthopaedic Surgery, Sidney Kimmel Medical College
Philadelphia, PA
Email: Chad.krueger@rothmanortho.com

during the ongoing crisis. One recent study attempted to quantify the unmet need during this time period. National Inpatient Sample data was used to approximate the population-level volume of hospital-based total hip and TKA in the United States. Using modeled predictions for total knee and total hip volume in 2020 prior to the ban on elective surgery, the study estimated 1,55,293 total hip and TKA cases were delayed for the 6 weeks following March 15th, and 3,72,706 cases through June of 2020. Furthermore, time needed to meet the pent up demand for these procedures was approximated to be 9–36 months, albeit with numerous assumptions [5].

Delay in the treatment of end-stage osteoarthritis of the hip and knee has been shown to have numerous deleterious effects on physical function [6] and psychological health [7]. In addition, pain and disability significantly increase while waiting for a TKA [8]. When patients are surveyed about their current health while awaiting total joint arthroplasty, 19% of future total hip patients and 12% of total knee patients describe their health state as "worse than death" [9]. However, patients seem to understand that the pandemic is truly unprecedented, and delays in elective surgery were unavoidable. A recent study attempted to characterise certain sentiment of patient sentiment during the COVID pandemic whose surgery was delayed by the ban on elective surgery. Over 90% of respondents felt that the delay was in their best interest, and 45% said they would not want surgery immediately following the resumption of elective arthroplasty. However, 67% reported emotional distress about their surgical delay. Further, 46% wanted their surgery immediately, despite the pandemic [10]. There are multiple modalities for non-operative care during such circumstances, but their effectiveness is modest, and can be costly. Nearly one quarter of patients who had a TKA or total hip arthroplasty (THA) delayed due to COVID-19 demonstrated increased analgesic intake [10]. While increased opioid usage has yet to be demonstrated for these patients, there is an obvious potential risk for patients and providers alike to use opioid analgesia while awaiting surgery, which has been associated with complications and worse outcomes [11,12].

IMPACT TO PROVIDERS

The novel coronavirus had impacted every industry and profession, orthopaedic surgeons are no exception. While these providers have been somewhat shielded from the intensive care required for some COVID-19 patients, providers have been impacted in other ways. Specifically, some providers have been repurposed to assume care in the crisis setting, and while others have seen drastic changes to their practice, with numerous financial considerations.

In a recent practice review article from three prominent private practice, academic affiliated orthopaedic groups, each group provided insight into the drastic and wide sweeping measures required to maintain solvency amid the pandemic. All three groups, Midwest Orthopaedics at Rush, OrthoCarolina, and the Rothman Institute all made substantial decreases to all employees, including physicians, and mid-level providers. Practitioners and employees alike saw more than a 30% reduction in compensation for most of the second fiscal quarter of 2020, if they were not furloughed, which were considered for all three of the practices. As mentioned above, the financial impact to orthopaedic physicians and practices seemed to be consistent throughout the country. At least initially, 74% of arthroplasty surgeons were effectively not working due to institutional or self-imposed deferral of elective surgeries, as reported in an April survey of the American Association of Hip and Knee Surgeons (AAHKS) members [4]. For year 2020 overall, most members of the American Association of Hip and Knee Surgeons described a reduction in surgical volume of at least 20% for 2020. Moreover, the disruption to practices was sweeping, requiring adoption of novel practices. Physician had to quickly adopt telemedicine practices in order to continue providing care.

Historical data on musculoskeletal care shows that elective musculoskeletal care represents significant revenue and net income to hospitals and health systems. The National Inpatient Sample (NIS) for 2017 showed that elective musculoskeletal care represents 39% of reimbursement for elective surgery and 35% of net income for hospitals and 23% of net income overall for hospital-based encounters [13]. While the focus of this article is the impact to orthopaedic practices, hospital and healthcare systems are integrally connected to their providers. As such, the financial impact to hospitals in general warrants mention. The largest financial impact to healthcare systems was the ban on elective surgery. In general, over 30% of hospital revenue is generated from elective surgical procedures [14]. While an increase in demand for COVID-related care was noted across the country, the increased revenue for care of these patients does not compare to the lost revenue from elective surgery [15]. The situation in rural hospitals is more precarious. As of 2019, one in five rural hospitals is at risk of closure due financial difficulties [16].

SAFE PRACTICES AND RECOMMENDATIONS FOR ORTHOPAEDIC SURGERY

Patient selection and provider screening, use of personal protective equipment (PPE), social distancing, and practice ergonomics can be implemented to reduce potential exposure.

Early on in the spring of 2020 elective surgery was restrictive not only in the United States, but throughout much of the world to preserve resources and prepare for the demands of global pandemic. While these restrictions were critical to assess and bolstered resources, they also offered providers an opportunity to critically evaluate a safe methods to provide care. Healthcare providers, and even more so, their patients are vulnerable populations. Given the average age of total hip and TKA patients, and large proportion of musculoskeletal care in the United States, the risk of COVID-19 complications and death are higher in this group compared to the general population [17]. Furthermore, providers have the capacity to shed viral particles to high risk populations very rapidly based on the large number of patients that they interact with on a daily basis. With such high stakes, resuming care for musculoskeletal disease should be comprehensive. With this in mind, multiple societies have provided thoughtful recommendations for patients and providers alike to balance the demands of pandemic while providing care to the general public. The European Society for Sports, Traumatology, Knee Surgery, and Arthroscopy released guidelines in March 2020 and further guidelines have been provided from specialty societies, such as the European Hip and Knee Societies, as well as the International consensus committee and the American Association of Hip and Knee Surgeons. Careful consideration should be given to regulatory authorities, current demands to provide care for COVID patients, as well as hospital and health system preparedness. Furthermore, providers should apply a comprehensive approach to limit the spread of COVID-19 within their own practice.

CRITERIA FOR RESUMING ELECTIVE SURGERY

Governing bodies should be consulted and collaborated with in the decision making process. State and local authorities centralised resources for information and guidance. Their role is important for allocating resources such as a PPE, ventilators, as well as hospital-based resources, such as available beds in each intensive care unit. The European Hip and Knee Societies, the International Consensus Group (ICM) and AAHKS research committee, and the European Society of Sports Traumatology, Knee Surgery and Arthroscopy (ESSKA) all recommend close co-ordination with state and local regulatory bodies [18–20]. With this co-ordinated effort, providers and health systems can modulate their capacity with regard to the demands of the pandemic. The Centers for Disease Control and Prevention (CDC) has provided recommendations for reopening healthcare facilities to elective practices when there is a downward trajectory in positive cases, as well as the percentage of positive cases [21]. These recommendations are universally supported by both AAHKS and the European Hip and Knee Societies [18,20]. Lastly, hospitals and health systems need to be prepared. Preparedness is multi-faceted, including a robust-testing programme, adequate reserve of PPE, available ICU and non-ICU beds, an adequate workforce to delivery comprehensive care, and in general, the ability to provide care to COVID patients without "Crisis" [18,20]. Crisis is loosely defined, but relates to hospitals overwhelmed by patient demand. Providers would have to resort to rationing care, which would provide care that is below the general standard of care.

Beyond the general guidelines for resuming elective surgery, healthcare providers and systems had specific tools to limit viral spread, while providing high quality and efficient care for their patients. Consideration should be given to intercept and control interactions that can transmit the virus from person to person. Specific recommendations have been provided for triaging patient care, patient and provider screening, personal protective measures, and limiting unnecessary patient and provider exposure.

PATIENT TRIAGE

Although somewhat arbitrary, the degree of emergency can be assigned to each surgical case; Emergent, Urgent, Urgent/Somewhat Elective, or Elective.

Patient selection should stratify patients by known risk factors for adverse outcomes associated with COVID-19 infection. Age and comorbidities have been consistently associated with increased morbidity and mortality. The initial reports from the epicenter in China showed 81% of all mortalities occurred in patients over the age of 60 years [22]. Beyond age, there are other risk factors that require attention. Hypertension, cardiovascular disease, lung disease, diabetes, cancer, liver and kidney disease have all been correlated with worse outcomes following COVID exposure [23]. There is evidence that obesity is another significant risk factor for severe forms of COVID-19 [22]. In addition, socio-economic factors may impact patient triage as well. Discharge to long-term care or skilled-nursing facilities poses risk to not only the patient themselves, but also risk to other residents. Other factors to consider are urgency of the surgical intervention, the patient's COVID exposure status. Obviously, there are emergent and urgent conditions that should not be delayed due to the pandemic such as life-or-limb-threatening infections, hip and femur fractures, compartment syndrome, etc. However, a major component of orthopaedic procedures are considered elective. COVID exposure status should prioritise patients who have not been exposed, as well as patients who have been exposed and fully recovered. There is speculation on how long immunity lasts following recovery, and there are anecdotal reports of patients having been reinfected some time following an initial infection [24]. Moreover, the European Hip Society and the European Knee Society described priority indications for elective hip and knee arthroplasty [20]. Examples of such indications include acute fracture, periprosthetic joint infection, amputation for failed arthroplasty, osteonecrosis with femoral collapse, functional impairment compromising patient autonomy or independent ambulation. Regardless, priority for elective surgery remains patients without active infection.

SCREENING AND TESTING AVAILABLE FOR PATIENTS AND PRACTICES

Screening and contact tracing remain the critical tools to prevent spread of the COVID-19 virus. Transmission from asymptomatic carriers remains a substantial source of ongoing infection, representing 25–50% new cases [25]. Although there are multiple techniques to screen patients, none are 100% sensitive and specific. Therefore, a multi-layer approach offers the best opportunity to deliver care and lower the risk of viral transmission.

Patient and provider check-in are the first layer screening. Questions about potential exposure and current symptoms are easy to perform, and are low cost. A recent consensus statement from ICM and the Research Committee of AAHKS provided recommendations [18]. Prior to elective surgery patients should be asked about travel to regions with high COVID prevalence, occupations placing them at high risk for contact with COVID-19, contact with people with a known COVID-19 infection, or close proximity with people with known COVID-19 infection. In addition, patients should be screened for active symptoms of COVID-19, which include, but are not limited to, fever, cough, shortness of breath, loss of smell or taste, diarrhoea, headache, and sore throat. Objective screening, such as temperature testing and pulse oximetry are helpful adjuncts for the check-in process. There was over 98% consensus for using both screening questions, and objective tools for patients undergoing elective surgery [18].

There are multiple testing options now available to rapidly screen for active COVID-19 infection [26]. Moreover, testing capacity has greatly increased in the United States since the start of the pandemic [27]. Screening tests include real-time polymerase chain reaction (RT-PCR) and molecular testing. RT-PCR has demonstrated excellent specificity, but sensitivity has been variable [28]. Both nasopharyngeal and oropharyngeal swabs have been used, and early forms demonstrated lower sensitivity of oropharyngeal form. There was 100% consensus on the use of RT-PCR as a screening tool for patients undergoing elective orthopaedic surgery [18]. Tests should be performed within a reasonable window prior to surgery, 48–72 hours. This window allows ample time to report results of the RT-PCR, and limits the amount of time for potential exposure between testing and surgery. Antigen testing can be performed and reported at the site of care, and some are able to produce results within 15 minutes. However, early commercial forms were unregulated and marketed direct-to-consumer. Although antibody testing for COVID-19 has been readily available from early on in the pandemic, its utility remains questionable for preoperative screening. The major disadvantages are variable sensitivity, and it remains unknown whether the presence of antibodies confers immunity to the virus. There is building evidence about waning titres of antibodies over time [29]. Moreover, there is evidence to suggest genetic variability with different strains of COVID-19 [18].

Lastly, there are imaging modalities available for further screening. For patients with conflicting results, such as a negative RT-PCR test and unexplained symptoms consistent with COVID-19, a chest radiograph or chest CT scan may be beneficial. There are specific features of moderate to severe COVID-19 infection in the lungs, which may be helpful in such situations. These tests are not without costs, and when used in isolation show variable sensitivity [18].

Anaesthesia

Intubation generates large and small aerosolised particles, which place healthcare providers at increased risk [30]. As such, regional anaesthesia remains a preferred method if at all possible. Prior to the pandemic, spinal anaesthetic has become the preferred approach to primary hip and knee arthroplasty [31]. Furthermore, spinal anaesthesia has been reported safe for patients with active COVID-19 infection [32].

Personal protective equipment

Personal protective equipment has become a household word throughout much of the world. These low cost barriers are a simple way to reduce potential contact with the virus. For routine interactions, a surgical mask is recommended for patients and providers, and providers should also have protective eyewear [33]. Single-use face masks and surgical masks offer limited protection from airborne transmission, and typically are only capable of filtering larger droplets, >3 μm in size. Furthermore, emergent or urgent surgeries required for active COVID patients, or patients with an unknown COVID status require further precaution. The gold standard in such cases is the use of an N95, FFP2, or P3 masks, which have the capacity to filter airborne particle >0.3 μm in size [34]. Gloves and eye protection may be warranted in certain situations. Personnel in close proximity to the operative field, or the airway during intubation should use eye protection, gloves, and an advanced level of airway protection, N95 or equivalent.

EARLY DISCHARGE AND OUTPATIENT PROCEDURES

Whenever possible outpatient or early discharge to home should be considered. Elective hip and knee arthroplasty has shown a trend towards more outpatient surgery. Enhanced recovery protocols have been shown to be safe and effective at reducing overall hospital length of stay [35–37]. Recently, Centers for Medicare and Medicaid Services has recently removed total hip and TKA from the inpatient only list [38]. Recent consensus (100% agreement) from ICM and the AAHKS research committee recommended to minimise hospital length of stay, encourage discharge to home whenever possible, self-directed home physical therapy, and using telehealth to minimise postoperative contact, unless a face-to-face encounter is warranted [18]. These recommendations are supported by the European Hip and Knee Societies as well [20].

ROLE OF TELEHEALTH DURING THE PANDEMIC AND POTENTIALLY THEREAFTER

Prior to the current pandemic, telehealth services had seen a slow and limited adoption for healthcare delivery. A recent report showed only 6.6 telehealth visits per year were performed for every 1,000 medical practitioners in the United States [39]. Since the rapid spread of the COVID-19 virus across the globe, much has changed, and there is a new spotlight on "Telehealth".

Telehealth offers specific advantages, especially during the COVID-19 pandemic. Telehealth is a structured way to follow social distancing by using physical barriers to protect patients and providers alike. Furthermore, virtual encounters through telecommunications reduce the utilisation of PPE, and healthcare resources. While the waves of infections have varied by state and nation, virtual clinics are being used across the country and abroad [40,41].

Previously, telehealth had been used to follow patients post-operatively, including routine monitoring, to schedule follow-up, and to address post-operative concerns that may not warrant a face-to-face interaction. One example is wound-related questions, and studies have shown telehealth to be an effective modality in this area. Moreover, telehealth has repeatedly shown high levels of patient satisfaction in addition to substantial cost savings. A recent randomised control trial demonstrated no difference in patient satisfaction between telehealth and face-to-face encounters in a cohort of orthopaedic trauma patients. The US Department of Health and Human Resources has expanded the use of telehealth to a broader range of patient encounters, including remote wound evaluation, pre-operative visits when imaging is adequate and surgery has already been indicated [41,42].

However, wide spread use of telemedicine presents some challenges. The most prevalent concerns remain technical issues, patient and provider education, and the limitations of a virtual encounter. Technical issues arise in multiple ways. Providers must have access to new resources; two-way video and audio communications, bandwidth capacity for telecommunications, and methods to ensure patient confidentiality. Furthermore, there are limits to the virtual orthopaedic evaluation, most commonly when a direct treatment or physical examination is required. Tanaka et al have developed standardised methods to improve the accuracy and efficiency of a virtual physical examination, but challenges persist [41]. One orthopaedic department, formalised a triage to determine patients eligible for a virtual visit. In their experience, the patients that were ineligible for a telehealth visit require suture or staple removal, cast application or change, or the need for a hands-on evaluation by a provider [42].

CONCLUSION

The effects of COVID-19 on the orthopaedic surgery profession are likely to be felt for some time. While some of the changes ushered in by the virus (such as telemedicine) may lead to a long-term improvement in patient care, many others (such as the financial ramifications of the pandemic) are likely to have a negative impact for some time. It remains to be seen how quickly society will be able to get relative control of the disease and, until that happens, many of the changes brought on by the SARS-CoV-2 viruses are likely to remain in place.

REFERENCES

1.   American College of Surgeons. Clinical Issues and Guidance. Chicago, IL: The American College of Surgeons, 2020. https:// www.facs.org/COVID-19/clinical-guidance/elective-surgery [Last accessed 28 April 2022].

2.   American Academy of Orthopedic Surgeons. COVID-19: Information for our members / AAOS guidelines for elective surgery. United States: American Academy of Orthopedic Surgeons, 2022. https://www.aaos.org/about/covid-19-information-for-our-members/aaos-guidelines-for-elective-surgery/ [Last accessed 28 April 2022].

3.   Thaler M, Khosravi I, Hirschmann MT, et al. Disruption of joint arthroplasty services in Europe during the COVID-19 pandemic: an online survey within the European Hip Society (EHS) and the European Knee Associates (EKA). Knee Surg Sports Traumatol Arthrosc 2020; 28:1712–1719.

4.   2020;Pageshttp://www.aahks.org/aahks-surveys-members-on-COVID-19-impact/. Visited on May 24 2022. Survey completed on Apr 16 2020. American Association of Hip and Knee Surgeons.

5.   Wilson JM, Schwartz AM, Farley KX, et al. Quantifying the Backlog of Total Hip and Knee Arthroplasty Cases: Predicting the Impact of COVID-19. HSS J 2020; 1–7.

6.   Kapstad H, Rustoen T, Hanestad BR, et al. Changes in pain, stiffness and physical function in patients with osteoarthritis waiting for hip or knee joint replacement surgery. Osteoarthritis Cartilage 2007; 15:837–843.

7.   Ackerman IN, Bennell KL, Osborne RH. Decline in Health-Related Quality of Life reported by more than half of those waiting for joint replacement surgery: a prospective cohort study. BMC Musculoskelet Disord 2011; 12:108.

8.   Ho KW, Pong G, Poon WC, et al. Progression of health-related quality of life of patients waiting for total knee arthroplasty. J Eval Clin Pract 2020.

9.   Sloan M, Premkumar A, Sheth NP. Projected Volume of Primary Total Joint Arthroplasty in the U.S., 2014 to 2030. J Bone Joint Surg Am 2018; 100:1455–1460.

10. Wilson JM, Schwartz AM, Grissom HE, et al. Patient Perceptions of COVID-19-Related Surgical Delay: An Analysis of Patients Awaiting Total Hip and Knee Arthroplasty. HSS J 2020; 1–7.

11. Kim K, Chen K, Anoushiravani AA, et al. Preoperative Chronic Opioid Use and Its Effects on Total Knee Arthroplasty Outcomes. J Knee Surg 2020; 33:306–313.

12. Sodhi N, Anis HK, Acuna AJ, et al. Opioid Use Disorder Is Associated with an Increased Risk of Infection after Total Joint Arthroplasty: A Large Database Study. Clin Orthop Relat Res 2020; 478:1752–1759.

13. Best MJ, Aziz KT, McFarland EG, Anderson GF, Srikumaran U. Economic implications of decreased elective orthopaedic and musculoskeletal surgery volume during the coronavirus disease 2019 pandemic. Int Orthop 2020; 44:2221–2228.

14. Weiss A, Elixhauser A, Andrews R. Characteristics of operating room procedures in US hospitals, 2011. 2011.

15. Khullar D, Bond AM, Schpero WL. COVID-19 and the Financial Health of US Hospitals. JAMA 2020; 323:2127–2128.

16. Mosley D, DeBehnke D. Rural Hospital Sustainability: New Analysis Shows Worsening Situation for Rural Hospitals, Residents, Navigant — February 2019. https://guidehouse.com/-/media/www/site/insights/healthcare/2019/navigant-rural-hospital-analysis-22019.pdf [Last accessed on 28 April 2022].

17. Katzenschlager S, Zimmer AJ, Gottschalk C, et al. Can we predict the severe course of COVID-19 - a systematic review and meta-analysis of indicators of clinical outcome? medRxiv 2020.

18. Parvizi J, Gehrke T, Krueger CA, et al. Resuming Elective Orthopaedic Surgery During the COVID-19 Pandemic: Guidelines Developed by the International Consensus Group (ICM). J Bone Joint Surg Am 2020; 102:1205–1212.

19. Mouton C, Hirschmann MT, Ollivier M, Seil R, Menetrey J. COVID-19 - ESSKA guidelines and recommendations for resuming elective surgery. J Exp Orthop 2020; 7:28.

20. Kort NP, Barrena EG, Bedard M, et al. Resuming elective hip and knee arthroplasty after the first phase of the SARS-CoV-2 pandemic: the European Hip Society and European Knee Associates recommendations. Knee Surg Sports Traumatol Arthrosc 2020; 28:2730–2746.

21. Centers for Medicare and Medicaid Services. Opening Up America Again: Centers for Medicare & Medicaid Services (CMS) Recommendations--Re-opening Facilities to Provide Non-emergent Non-COVID-19 Healthcare: Phase I, 2020. https://www.cms.gov/files/document/COVID-flexibility-reopen-essential-non-COVID-services.pdf [Last accessed 28 April 2022].

22. Garg S, Kim L, Whitaker M, et al. Hospitalization Rates and Characteristics of Patients Hospitalized with Laboratory-Confirmed Coronavirus Disease 2019 - COVID-NET, 14 States, March 1-30, 2020. MMWR Morb Mortal Wkly Rep 2020; 69:458–464.
23. Karimi M, Haghpanah S, Zarei T, et al. Prevalence and severity of Coronavirus disease 2019 (COVID-19) in Transfusion Dependent and Non-Transfusion Dependent beta-thalassemia patients and effects of associated comorbidities: an Iranian nationwide study. Acta Biomed 2020; 91:e2020007.
24. Gousseff M, Penot P, Gallay L, et al. Clinical recurrences of COVID-19 symptoms after recovery: Viral relapse, reinfection or inflammatory rebound? J Infect 2020; 81:816–846.
25. Bai Y, Yao L, Wei T, et al. Presumed Asymptomatic Carrier Transmission of COVID-19. JAMA 2020; 323:1406–1407.
26. Wiersinga WJ, Rhodes A, Cheng AC, Peacock SJ, Prescott HC. Pathophysiology, Transmission, Diagnosis, and Treatment of Coronavirus Disease 2019 (COVID-19): A Review. JAMA 2020; 324:782–793.
27. Pulia MS, O'Brien TP, Hou PC, Schuman A, Sambursky R. Multi-tiered screening and diagnosis strategy for COVID-19: a model for sustainable testing capacity in response to pandemic. Ann Med 2020; 52:207–214.
28. Lin C, Xiang J, Yan M, et al. Comparison of throat swabs and sputum specimens for viral nucleic acid detection in 52 cases of novel coronavirus (SARS-Cov-2)-infected pneumonia (COVID-19). Clin Chem Lab Med 2020; 58:1089–1094.
29. Kissler SM, Tedijanto C, Goldstein E, Grad YH, Lipsitch M. Projecting the transmission dynamics of SARS-CoV-2 through the postpandemic period. Science 2020; 368:860–868.
30. Lie SA, Wong SW, Wong LT, Wong TGL, Chong SY. Practical considerations for performing regional anesthesia: lessons learned from the COVID-19 pandemic. Can J Anaesth 2020; 67:885–892.
31. Zhong HY, Zhang WP. Effect of intravenous magnesium sulfate on bupivacaine spinal anesthesia in preeclamptic patients. Biomed Pharmacother 2018; 108:1289–1293.
32. Zhong Q, Liu YY, Luo Q, et al. Spinal anaesthesia for patients with coronavirus disease 2019 and possible transmission rates in anaesthetists: retrospective, single-centre, observational cohort study. Br J Anaesth 2020; 124:670–675.
33. Massey PA, McClary K, Zhang AS, Savoie FH, Barton RS. Orthopaedic Surgical Selection and Inpatient Paradigms During the Coronavirus (COVID-19) Pandemic. J Am Acad Orthop Surg 2020; 28:436–450.
34. Coimbra R, Edwards S, Kurihara H, et al. European Society of Trauma and Emergency Surgery (ESTES) recommendations for trauma and emergency surgery preparation during times of COVID-19 infection. Eur J Trauma Emerg Surg 2020; 46:505–510.
35. Soffin EM, YaDeau JT. Enhanced recovery after surgery for primary hip and knee arthroplasty: a review of the evidence. Br J Anaesth 2016; 117:iii62–iii72.
36. Wainwright TW, Gill M, McDonald DA, et al. Consensus statement for perioperative care in total hip replacement and total knee replacement surgery: Enhanced Recovery After Surgery (ERAS((R))) Society recommendations. Acta Orthop 2020; 91:3–19.
37. Zhu S, Qian W, Jiang C, Ye C, Chen X. Enhanced recovery after surgery for hip and knee arthroplasty: a systematic review and meta-analysis. Postgrad Med J 2017; 93(1106): 736–742.
38. Courtney PM, Froimson MI, Meneghini RM, Lee GC, Della Valle CJ. Can Total Knee Arthroplasty Be Performed Safely as an Outpatient in the Medicare Population? J Arthroplasty 2018; 33:S28–S31.
39. Barnett ML, Ray KN, Souza J, Mehrotra A. Trends in Telemedicine Use in a Large Commercially Insured Population, 2005-2017. JAMA 2018; 320:2147–2149.
40. Buvik A, Bugge E, Knutsen G, Smabrekke A, Wilsgaard T. Patient reported outcomes with remote orthopaedic consultations by telemedicine: A randomised controlled trial. J Telemed Telecare 2019; 25:451–459.
41. Tanaka MJ, Oh LS, Martin SD, Berkson EM. Telemedicine in the Era of COVID-19: The Virtual Orthopaedic Examination. J Bone Joint Surg Am 2020; 102:e57.
42. Loeb AE, Rao SS, Ficke JR, et al. Departmental Experience and Lessons Learned With Accelerated Introduction of Telemedicine During the COVID-19 Crisis. J Am Acad Orthop Surg 2020; 28:e469–e476.